Primary Care
Oncology

Primary Care Oncology

Kathryn L. Boyer, MS, PA-C
Leukemia Department
The University of Texas
M.D. Anderson Cancer Center
Houston, Texas

Melissa Belle Ford, MSN, RN, CS, FNP
Pre-doctoral Fellow, Department of Epidemiology
The University of Texas
M.D. Anderson Cancer Center
Houston, Texas

Alice F. Judkins, MS, RN
Coordinator, Breast Evaluation Clinic/Surgical Breast Services
The University of Texas
M.D. Anderson Cancer Center
Houston, Texas

Bernard Levin, MD
Vice President for Cancer Prevention
Professor of Medicine
Division of Cancer Prevention
The University of Texas
M.D. Anderson Cancer Center
Houston, Texas

W.B. SAUNDERS COMPANY
A Division of Harcourt Brace & Company
Philadelphia   London   Toronto   Montreal   Sydney   Tokyo

W.B. SAUNDERS COMPANY
A Division of Harcourt Brace & Company

The Curtis Center
Independence Square West
Philadelphia, Pennsylvania 19106

Library of Congress Cataloging-in-Publication Data

Primary care oncology/[edited by] Kathryn L. Boyer . . . [et al.].

    p.   cm.

    ISBN 0–7216–7316–3

  1. Cancer.   2. Primary care (Medicine).   I. Boyer, Kathryn L. [DNLM:
    1. Neoplasms.   2. Primary Health Care.   QZ 200 P9517 1999]

  RC261.P725   1999   616.99′4—dc21
  DNLM/DLC   98-5822

PRIMARY CARE ONCOLOGY   ISBN 0–7216–7316–3

Printed in the United States of America.

Last digit is the print number: 9   8   7   6   5   4   3   2   1

Contributors

Robert J. Amato, DO
Associate Professor, and Deputy Chairman, Genitourinary Oncology Department, The University of Texas M.D. Anderson Cancer Center, Houston, Texas
Testicular Cancer

Kathryn L. Boyer, MS, PA-C
Physician Assistant, Leukemia Department, The University of Texas M.D. Anderson Cancer Center, Houston, Texas
Acute and Chronic Leukemias—A Concise Review

Thomas Burke, MD
Associate Professor of Gynecologic Oncology, Department of Gynecologic Oncology, The University of Texas M.D. Anderson Cancer Center, Houston, Texas
Invasive Gynecologic Cancers

David L. Callender, MD, MBA
Associate Professor of Surgery, Department of Head and Neck Surgery, The University of Texas M.D. Anderson Cancer Center, Houston, Texas
Head and Neck Cancer

Gwendolyn Killiam Corrigan, MSN, RN, FNP
Formerly Department of Gynecologic Oncology, The University of Texas M.D. Anderson Cancer Center, Houston, Texas
Preinvasive Disease of the Female Genital Tract

Yvette DeJesus, MSN, RN
Clinical Faculty and Clinical Coordinator of the Practice Outcomes Program, The University of Texas M.D. Anderson Cancer Center, Houston, Texas
Invasive Gynecologic Cancers

Paula DeMasi, MSN, RN, CNS
Department of Neurosurgery, The University of Texas M.D. Anderson Cancer Center, Houston, Texas
Tumors of the Central Nervous System

Franco DeMonte, MD, FRCS(C), FACS
Assistant Professor of Neurosurgery, Department of Neurosurgery, The University of Texas M.D. Anderson Cancer Center, Houston, Texas
Tumors of the Central Nervous System

Carmen P. Escalante, MD
Associate Professor of Medicine; Chief, Section of General Internal
Medicine; and Medical Director, Ambulatory Treatment Center, The
University of Texas M.D. Anderson Cancer Center, Houston, Texas
Complications of Cancer Treatment

Douglas B. Evans, MD
Associate Professor and Chief of Pancreas and Endocrinology,
Department of Surgical Oncology, The University of Texas M.D.
Anderson Cancer Center, Houston, Texas
Endocrine Cancer: The Thyroid, Parathyroid, Adrenal Glands, and Pancreas;
Pancreatic Cancer

Patricia Ewert-Flannagan, MSN, RN, BA, OCN, CNS
Adjunct Faculty, University of Texas School of Nursing; Clinical Nurse
Specialist and Nurse Endoscopist, The University of Texas M.D.
Anderson Cancer Center, Houston, Texas
Colorectal Cancer

Melissa Belle Ford, MSN, RN, CS, FNP
Pre-doctoral Fellow, Department of Epidemiology, The University of
Texas M.D. Anderson Cancer Center, Houston, Texas
Cancer Epidemiology

Debra Schoenberg Foreman, BS, PA-C
Coordinator, Physician Assistant Education Program, and Physician
Assistant, The University of Texas M.D. Anderson Cancer Center,
Houston, Texas
Head and Neck Cancer

Frank Fossella, MD
Associate Professor and Medical Director, Thoracic Oncology Care
Center, The University of Texas M.D. Anderson Cancer Center,
Houston, Texas
Lung Cancer

Sandra C. Henke, MSN, RN, CS, ANP
Thoracic Oncology Care Center, The University of Texas M.D.
Anderson Cancer Center, Houston, Texas
Lung Cancer

Elizabeth Hossan, MS, RN, C-FNP
Clinical Nurse Specialist, Genitourinary Oncology Department, The
University of Texas M.D. Anderson Cancer Center, Houston, Texas
Testicular Cancer

Mary K. Hughes, BS, MS
Clinical Faculty, The University of Texas–Houston Health Science
Center; Clinical Nurse Specialist, The University of Texas M.D.
Anderson Cancer Center, Houston, Texas
Medical Decision Making at the End of Life: Hospice Care and Care of the
Terminally Ill

Lawrence Hutchinson, MSN, RN, GNP
Clinical Nurse Specialist, Breast Medical Oncology, The University of
Texas M.D. Anderson Cancer Center, Houston, Texas
Testicular Cancer

Alice F. Judkins, MS, RN
Coordinator, Breast Evaluation Clinic/Surgical Breast Services, The
University of Texas M.D. Anderson Cancer Center, Houston, Texas
Cancer of the Breast

Hagop Kantarjian, MD
Professor of Medicine and Chairman, Leukemia Department, The
University of Texas M.D. Anderson Cancer Center, Houston, Texas
Acute and Chronic Leukemias—A Concise Review

Carol Lacey, PA-C
Physician Assistant, Department of Surgical Oncology, The University
of Texas M.D. Anderson Cancer Center, Houston, Texas
Melanoma

Bernard Levin, MD
Vice President for Cancer Prevention and Professor of Medicine,
Division of Cancer Prevention, The University of Texas M.D.
Anderson Cancer Center, Houston, Texas
Cancers of the Upper Gastrointestinal Tract; Colorectal Cancer

Jeanette Adams McNeill, DrPH, MSN
Associate Professor and Department Chair, Nursing for Target
Populations; Track Director, Oncology, The University of
Texas–Houston Health Science Center, School of Nursing; Clinical
Assistant Professor, The University of Texas M.D. Anderson Cancer
Center, Houston, Texas
Health Promotion for Cancer Survivors

Paul Mansfield, MD
Assistant Professor of Surgery, Department of Surgical Oncology, The
University of Texas M.D. Anderson Cancer Center, Houston, Texas
Melanoma

Michele Follen Mitchell, MD, MS
Associate Professor, Department of Gynecologic Oncology; Division
Director, Department of Obstetrics, Gynecology, and Reproductive
Science; and Director of Colposcopy, The University of Texas M.D.
Anderson Cancer Center and The University of Texas–Houston Health
Science Center, Houston, Texas
Cancer Epidemiology; Preinvasive Disease of the Female Genital Tract

Laura A. Murphy-Fertak, BS, PA-C
Formerly Physician Assistant, Orthopedic Oncology Section,
Department of Surgical Oncology, The University of Texas M.D.
Anderson Cancer Center, Houston, Texas
Bone Tumors

Richard Payne, MD
Formerly Department of Neuro-Oncology, The University of Texas
M.D. Anderson Cancer Center, Houston, Texas
Pain and Symptom Management

Janet Pinner, MSN, RN
Formerly Department of Neurosurgery, The University of Texas M.D.
Anderson Cancer Center, Houston, Texas
Tumors of the Central Nervous System

Louis L. Pisters, MD
Assistant Professor of Urology, Department of Urology, The University
of Texas M.D. Anderson Cancer Center, Houston, Texas
Genitourinary Cancers

Peter W.T. Pisters, MD
Assistant Professor, Department of Surgical Oncology, The University
of Texas M.D. Anderson Cancer Center, Houston, Texas
Soft Tissue Sarcoma

Alejandro Preti, MD
Formerly Lymphoma Section, Department of Hematology, The
University of Texas M.D. Anderson Cancer Center, Houston, Texas
Hodgkin's Disease; Non-Hodgkin's Lymphoma

Paula Respondek, MS, PA-C
Physician Assistant, Sarcoma Center, Department of Surgical
Oncology, The University of Texas M.D. Anderson Cancer Center,
Houston, Texas
Soft Tissue Sarcoma

Paula Trahan Rieger, MSN
Cancer Detection Specialist, Department of Clinical Cancer
Prevention, The University of Texas M.D. Anderson Cancer Center,
Houston, Texas
Complications of Cancer Treatment

Amelia Ritty, PA-C
Formerly Physician Assistant, Department of Breast Oncology, The
University of Texas M.D. Anderson Cancer Center, Houston, Texas
Non-Hodgkin's Lymphoma

Alma C. Sbach, MSN, RN, CS, FNP
Clinical Cancer Detection Specialist/Nurse Colposcopist, The
University of Texas M.D. Anderson Cancer Center, Houston, Texas
Preinvasive Disease of the Female Genital Tract

Shellie M. Scott, PA-C
Physician Assistant, Department of Urology, The University of Texas
M.D. Anderson Cancer Center, Houston, Texas
Genitourinary Cancers

Deborah E. Seigler, PA-C
Physician Assistant, Department of Gastrointestinal Oncology, The
University of Texas M.D. Anderson Cancer Center, Houston, Texas
Hodgkin's Disease

S. Eva Singletary, MD
Professor of Surgery and Chief, Surgical Breast Service, The
University of Texas M.D. Anderson Cancer Center, Houston, Texas
Cancer of the Breast

Patricia Spencer-Cisek, MS, RN, CS, ANP, OCN
Division of Cancer Prevention, The University of Texas M.D.
Anderson Cancer Center, Houston, Texas
Cancers of the Upper Gastrointestinal Tract

Pamela A. Stanford, MN, RN, OCN
Clinical Nurse Specialist, Department of Surgery, The University of
Texas M.D. Anderson Cancer Center, Houston, Texas
*Endocrine Cancer: The Thyroid, Parathyroid, Adrenal Glands, and Pancreas;
Pancreatic Cancer*

Deborah M. Thorpe, PhD, RN, CS
Department of Pain and Syndrome Management, The University of
Texas M.D. Anderson Cancer Center, Houston, Texas
Pain and Symptom Management

Elisabeth S. Waxman, RN, MSN, OCB, CNS
Lymphoma Section, Department of Hematology, The University of
Texas M.D. Anderson Cancer Center, Houston, Texas
Multiple Myeloma and Other Plasma Cell Dyscrasias

Donna M. Weber, MD
Assistant Professor, Department of Lymphoma and Myeloma, The
University of Texas M.D. Anderson Cancer Center, Houston, Texas
Multiple Myeloma and Other Plasma Cell Dyscrasias

Sharon Weinstein, MD
Assistant Professor of Medicine (Neurology), and Assistant Professor,
Management and Policy Sciences, The University of Texas Health
Science Center School of Public Health; Assistant Neurologist,
Department of Neuro-Oncology, Section of Pain and Symptom
Management, The University of Texas M.D. Anderson Cancer Center,
Houston, Texas
*Medical Decision Making at the End of Life: Hospice Care and Care of the
Terminally Ill*

Alan W. Yasko, MD
Associate Professor, Chief of Orthopedic Oncology Section,
Department of Surgical Oncology, The University of Texas M.D.
Anderson Cancer Center, Houston, Texas
Bone Tumors

Foreword

For the past 12 years I have worked as a Physician Assistant in the Department of Urology at The University of Texas M.D. Anderson Cancer Center. During that time I had the privilege and advantage of being able to call on my colleagues, physician assistants, nurse practitioners, and clinical nurse specialists to readily answer any questions and update me on the latest information about cancers in their subspecialties. This text now offers advanced care providers everywhere the same clear, concise, and practical information. Some of the topics covered in this book include prevention, early detection, epidemiology, risk factors, clinical presentation, physical findings, histology, pathology, staging, differential diagnosis, treatment modalities, and referral criteria for all the major cancers. The authors are advanced care providers who work independently or collaboratively with physicians to assess and treat oncology patients.

In today's health care environment, practitioners are fulfilling an ever-expanding role in patient care, extending from the most complex tertiary levels of cancer management to the front lines of primary care. Now your colleagues have created a comprehensive yet practical guide to primary care oncology, using the latest information available to them, and placed it at your fingetips.

Robert B. Evans, BS, PA-C

Charter Member of Physician
Assistants in Oncology,
Department of Urology,
The University of Texas
M.D. Anderson Cancer Center,
Houston, Texas

Preface

The practice of medicine continues to undergo major changes. Whereas the initial emphasis of managed care was targeted primarily at cost reduction, more recently we have begun to observe a welcome concern about quality of care and cost-effectiveness. As more individuals survive cancer, there is also a shift occurring from inpatient to outpatient management. For these and other reasons, we believe that advanced practitioners (PAs, NPs, CNSs) are well suited to play a vital role in the long-term management of the patient with cancer.

This volume provides a comprehensive guide for the outpatient management of the individual with cancer, including diagnostic procedures, treatment outlines, posttreatment follow-up, and surveillance plans. We have also incorporated prevention approaches and early detection methods as well as guidelines for appropriate subspecialty referrals. As is becoming very familiar, we have included comprehensive management guidelines for specific disease sites.

We have attempted to facilitate the work of advanced practitioners and the care of their patients in all primary care settings from rural areas to highly specialized tertiary care centers. We have also taken into account the needs of the advanced practitioner working independently or in close collaboration with a physician.

It is our ultimate objective to greatly enhance the quality of care of the patient with cancer. We are very grateful to our many contributors and consultants who have given generously of their time and expertise.

Kathryn L. Boyer, MS, PA-C
Melissa Belle Ford, MSN, RN, CS, FNP
Alice F. Judkins, MS, RN
Bernard Levin, MD

Acknowledgments

The editors and contributors of *Primary Care Oncology* would like to gratefully acknowledge the Department of Scientific Publications at The University of Texas M.D. Anderson Cancer Center, under the direction of Walter Pagel, for their expertise and guidance in the development of this landmark text in oncology for the advanced care practitioner.

Contents

Chapter 1

Cancer Epidemiology

*Melissa Belle Ford, MSN, RN, CS, FNP, and
Michele Follen Mitchell, MD, MS*

OVERVIEW

The Problem

It is estimated that more than 7.4 million Americans alive today have a history of cancer. Approximately one in three persons now living in the United States will develop cancer, and one in four will die of it. Cancer is actually a group of diseases characterized by the uncontrolled development and proliferation of abnormal cells. If growth of these cells is not checked, a precancerous or cancerous growth will develop. Cancers can become invasive and metastasize, leading to death if untreated. External (environmental) and internal (host) factors may act together or in sequence to promote carcinogenesis.[1]

The Impact

Cancer and its sequelae often cause substantial mortality and morbidity, resulting in tremendous emotional and financial burdens for the individual and for society as a whole. At the current fiscal rate, the National Cancer Institute (NCI) estimates overall costs for cancer at $104 billion per year; this includes direct medical costs, costs associated with morbidity or lost productivity, and mortality costs. Of the direct medical costs, more than half derive from the treatment of breast, lung, and prostate cancers. Another $3 to $4 billion is spent annually on cancer screening, including mammography, Papanicolaou (Pap) smears, and colorectal examinations. Although the expenditure for screening activities is significant, cost recovery can be realized in terms of reduced suffering and number of lives saved if cancer is detected at an early, treatable stage.[1]

The Challenge

Although most cancers can be treated by surgery, radiation, chemotherapy, hormone therapy, immunotherapy, or a combination thereof, the best method of cancer control is prevention. Researchers estimate that if everything known about cancer prevention were applied, up to two thirds of cancers would not occur. Regular screening and self-examinations can detect cancers of the breast, head and neck, colorectal area, cervix, prostate, testes, and skin early, when treatment is most likely to be successful. These cancers alone represent more than half of all new cases. Currently, about two thirds of patients with these cancers survive 5 years or longer, but the American Cancer Society (ACS) estimates that with early detection about 95% would survive. Moreover, it is estimated that up to 80% of cancers in the United States may be caused in part by factors that relate to lifestyle and the environment and are thus potentially preventable. This estimate does not preclude coexisting genetic factors, but it does suggest that avoidance of these external factors could be sufficient to prevent or delay many cancers.[1]

Colditz and Gortmaker[2] suggest that the scientific basis for cancer prevention rests on two fundamental components: (1) a knowledge of biologic processes and epidemiology as a basis for understanding the causes of cancer, and (2) a knowledge of the effectiveness of interventions to prevent cancer by changing modifiable risks.[2]

Familiarity with cancer epidemiology is fundamental to understanding the origin of disease, causal relationships, risk, prevention and early detection, treatment, and care of those with cancer. Table 1–1 provides a glossary of basic terms related to the study of epidemiology.[3] Once the course of carcinogenesis and patterns of disease progression are identified, individual and public health interventions can be implemented to eliminate or lessen the risk of cancer.[4] One way to reduce the human suffering, early deaths, and economic loss from cancer is to avoid exposure to known carcinogens. Screening and early detection and diagnosis of cancer can improve the prospects for cure with the use of available treatment modalities.[5]

NATURAL HISTORY OF CANCER

At the cellular level, development of cancer is quite rare; 10 or more years may pass between exposure or mutation of a cell and the presence of clinically detectable cancer. Of the billions of cells in any organ site, a single cell may undergo malignant transformation and through a multistep process may eventually produce clinical disease. Indeed, many epidemiologic, pathologic, and molecular biologic studies indicate that a cell must undergo a series of changes before it can become malignant.[4] Therefore, although the probability that cancer will develop during a person's lifetime is appreciable, the chance of a single cell's becoming cancerous is exceedingly small.[4]

Normal cells reproduce in an orderly, controlled fashion at a steady rate, with the overall number of cells remaining almost constant. Regulating the growth of normal cells are feedback mechanisms that stimulate or inhibit cell division. However, the body's normal regulatory mechanisms are usually unable to control the proliferation of cancerous cells once malignant transformation has taken place. Unlike normal cells, which undergo physical and structural changes as they develop to form different tissues of the body, cancer cells become less differentiated.[5]

The extent to which cancer cells lose the ability to differentiate varies among tumors. The process by which a normal cell undergoes malignant transformation, known as *carcinogenesis*, involves progressive changes, usually after genetic damage or alteration of cellular DNA.[5] Carcinogenesis may involve both initiating and promoting factors: an "initiator" transforms a normal cell into a malignant cell, and a "promoter" gives the transformed cell advantages that favor its growth and development.[4]

Agents capable of triggering the events of cellular transformation into cancer are called carcinogens. Factors strongly implicated as carcinogens include environmental, genetic, and viral factors.[5] Environmental factors are usually referred to as exogenous or nonhost factors, and genetic and viral factors are considered endogenous or host factors. The early stage of carcinogenesis, known as *initiation*, involves an irreversible alteration of the genetic makeup of a cell as a result of induction by a particular agent or factor. Initiation alone does not cause malignant transformation of cells, but the resulting alteration in cellular structure can be passed on to the next generation of cells as a clone, which does have the potential to become cancerous. However, initiation of carcinogenesis does not always result in cancer.[5]

The second stage of carcinogenesis is *promotion*, whereby initiated cells have an increased chance to become malignant. The effects of promoting factors related to their dose and duration of exposure to the cellular host. Unlike of initiation, the effects of promotion are reversible. The latency period

Table 1-1. Glossary of Terms

Epidemiology—The study of the causes of disease and spread of disease in populations incorporating description, prevention, intervention, and evaluation from a public health perspective

MEASURES OF OCCURRENCE

1. Prevalence—The number of people having a specific disease at a single point in time

$$\text{Prevalence} = \frac{\text{Number of people with the disease}}{\text{Number of people at risk}}$$

2. Incidence—The number of people who will develop the disease over a given period of time (e.g., 1 year)

$$\text{Incidence} = \frac{\text{Number of new cases in a fixed time period}}{\text{Number of people at risk}}$$

3. Mortality—The number of people dying of a disease over a given period of time (often calculated as "age-adjusted" rate)

$$\text{Mortality Rate} = \frac{\text{Number of deaths from the disease over a fixed time period}}{\text{Total population}}$$

$$\text{Age-Adjusted Mortality Rate} = \frac{\text{Number of deaths in a particular age range}}{\text{Total number of deaths in a particular age range}}$$

4. Morbidity—The number of people affected by specific complications of a disease over a given period of time (also calculated as a rate)

$$\text{Morbidity} = \frac{\text{Number of people with specific complication of a disease}}{\text{Total number of people with the disease}}$$

5. Survivability—The number of people surviving a disease for a specified period of time. Survivability is calculated either as the "observed" rate, which is the actual rate, or as the "adjusted" rate, which adjusts for normal life expectancy (considering deaths from other factors such as heart disease, accidents, and diseases of old age)

$$\text{Observed Survivability Rate} = \frac{\text{Number of people with a specific disease who remain alive for a specified period of time}}{\text{Number of people with the disease}}$$

MEASURES OF ASSOCIATION

1. Relative Risk—Using exposure as the hallmark, the risk of developing a disease over a specified period of time if exposed (derived from cohort/longitudinal and clinical trial studies)

$$\text{Relative Risk} = \frac{\text{Incidence of disease if exposed}}{\text{Incidence of disease if unexposed}}$$

2. Odds Ratio—Using disease as the hallmark, the odds of having a disease if exposed (derived from case-control studies)

$$\text{Odds Ratio} = \frac{\text{Odds of having disease if exposed}}{\text{Odds of having disease if unexposed}}$$

3. Risk—A loosely used term that encompasses both measures of association, relative risk, and odds ratio. Risk is not static and is only as reliable as the studies that address the exposure and disease in question. Risk status changes with exposure, and risk association changes with increased knowledge of the disease.

MEASURES OF RELIABILITY

1. Sensitivity—A test's ability to correctly identify someone as being positive for a disease or factor (represents a decrease in false-negative rate)

$$\text{Sensitivity} = \frac{\text{Number with the disease who have a positive test}}{\text{Number with the disease}}$$

⋅ᵗᵛ—A test's ability to correctly identify someone as being negative for a disease ⋅presents a decrease in the false-positive rate)

$$\text{ᵗy} = \frac{\text{Number without the disease who have a negative test}}{\text{Number with the disease}}$$

⸌ GR, Blum HM: PDQ Epidemiology. Philadelphia, BC Decker, 1989.

time between exposure to a promoter and development of a malignancy.[5] As cancer evolves, the pathologic changes may become irreversible. Therefore, preventive rather than curative efforts should be the focus of cancer control and health maintenance. This suggests that cancer prevention efforts are most effective when they are aimed at avoidance of promoters rather than at initiators. Indeed, avoiding exposure to promoters, or reducing the dose and duration of exposure, is more likely to lower the probability of malignant expression in initiated cells.[5]

In the final stage of carcinogenesis, *progression*, cancers cause morbidity through local growth, systemic effects, and metastasis to distant organs. *Metastasis* is the ability of malignant tumors to spread from the primary organ site to other locations in the body. This occurs when malignant cells break away from the primary tumor, travel through the body via blood or lymphatic circulation, and then infiltrate organ tissues and grow into new tumor deposits.[5] Metastasis frequently occurs in bone, bone marrow, lymph nodes, brain, liver, and lung tissues.

Each cancer is unique but possesses certain developmental characteristics inherent in all malignancies. By understanding the natural history of the disease and carcinogenesis, it is possible to learn how cancer can be prevented and effectively treated at an early, premetastatic stage, when associated morbidity and mortality are low.

SOURCES OF EPIDEMIOLOGIC INFORMATION

The United States

Currently the United States has no nationwide cancer registry. It is therefore impossible to know exactly how many new cases of cancer are diagnosed annually. Most estimates of the number of new cancer cases expected to be diagnosed in any given year are based on cancer incidence data collected by the National Institutes of Health's Surveillance, Epidemiology, and End Results (SEER) program and on data collected by the United States Census Bureau.[1, 6] The ongoing SEER program tabulates cancer data from nine population-based cancer registries: Connecticut, Hawaii, Iowa, New Mexico, Utah, San Francisco–Oakland, Detroit, Seattle, and Atlanta. Approximately 10% of the U.S. population is covered by these registries, which are useful for monitoring the occurrence of cancer for the nation.[6]

The ACS estimates presented in the tables are based on the best available data sources for the year following the year in which estimates are made. ACS estimates of incidence, probability of developing cancer, and survival are based primarily on SEER data collected between 1979 and 1993. ACS mortality statistics are derived from the underlying cause-of-death data reported by the Division of Vital Statistics, National Center for Health Statistics, U.S. Department of Health and Human Services. Current estimates of cancer deaths are based on cancer mortality data for 1979 through 1993.[1, 6] Information on cancer mortality in minority populations is based on 1992 reported cancer deaths as coded on death certificates for whites, African Americans, Native Americans, Asians and Pacific Islanders, and Hispanics. The number of minority deaths was probably underestimated because of underreporting of Asian, Pacific Islander, Native American, and Hispanic ethnicity on death certificates.[6]

It should be emphasized that it is inappropriate and inaccurate to evaluate cancer incidence and mortality trends using only ACS estimates of new cases and deaths from cancer, since these numbers are only projections and are based on data that are several years old. Rather, these estimates provide the best available measure of the scope of cancer in the United States.[1]

To monitor cancer trends effectively and to identify variations in incidence affected by factors such as age, race or ethnicity, and geographic region, comprehensive, timely, and accurate information about cancer incidence and stage at diagnosis is needed. Data from population-based cancer registries reflect an enormous U.S. cancer burden that varies widely by geographic location and ethnic group. However, few existing state cancer registries ensure minimum standards for quality and completeness of information.[7]

Registries provide a means for collecting important cancer information and may be useful in conducting population-based epidemiologic and biologic research, allocating health resources, and evaluating cancer prevention and control programs.[7] In 1992 the United States Congress enacted the Cancer Registries Amendment Act, authorizing the Centers for Disease Control (CDC) to establish a national program in support of cancer registries. The program's goal is to enhance existing state registries and to help establish additional population-based cancer registries that meet minimum standards for completeness, timeliness, and quality in all 50 states. As of October 1, 1993, nine states had laws authorizing state cancer registries with all essential regulations in place. An additional 29 states had laws authorizing the registries but did not yet have all the essential regulations.[7] Table 1–2 details 20-year trends in U.S. cancer death rates per 100,000 population through 1993.

The World

World Health Organization (WHO) data for 1969 through 1986 are used for site-specific mortality rates.[8] WHO data for 1990 through 1993 are used for ACS estimates of worldwide site-specific cancer incidence in men and women.[1] Where appropriate, estimates using these data are age-adjusted to the WHO standard world population (Table 1–3).[6]

TRENDS IN CANCER EPIDEMIOLOGY

Profile of Cancer in the United States

Anyone can be at risk for cancer. Cancer is primarily age dependent; its incidence rises with age, and in most cases adults are affected in midlife or later. Yet cancer causes more deaths than any other disease among children from birth to 14 years of age. Men have a 50% lifetime probability of developing cancer, and women have a lifetime risk of 33%. It was estimated that more than 1.3 million new cases of cancer would be diagnosed in 1997, exclusive of thousands of cases of carcinoma in situ and almost 900,000 new cases of basal and squamous cell skin cancer. During this same period it was estimated that almost 560,000 Americans would die of cancer—more than 1500 per day. One in every four deaths in the United States is cancer related.[1] Table 1–4 presents ACS 1997 estimates of leading sites of new cancer cases and deaths by sex.

Table 1–2. 20-Year Trends in Cancer Death Rates* per 100,000 Population, 1971–1973 to 1991–1993

SITES	SEX	RATE IN 1971–1973	RATE IN 1991–1993	PERCENT CHANGE	NUMBER OF DEATHS 1973	NUMBER OF DEATHS 1993
All sites	Male	204.5	219.0	7	190,487	279,375
	Female	132.0	142.0	8	159,110	250,529
Brain	Male	4.7	5.1	9	4,650	6,551
	Female	3.2	3.5	9	3,661	5,442
Breast	Male	0.3	0.2	−33	293	355
	Female	26.8	26.4	−1	31,850	43,555
Cervix	Female	5.6	2.9	−48	6,041	4,583
Colon & rectum	Male	25.3	22.3	−12	22,680	28,199
	Female	20.0	15.1	−25	24,823	29,206
Corpus uteri	Female	4.7	3.4	−28	5,686	6,098
Esophagus	Male	5.0	6.2	24	4,768	7,813
	Female	1.4	1.5	7	1,723	2,637
Hodgkin's disease	Male	1.9	0.7	−63	1,732	900
	Female	1.1	0.4	−64	1,188	674
Kidney	Male	4.3	5.1	19	4,004	6,359
	Female	1.9	2.3	21	2,330	3,964
Larynx	Male	2.8	2.5	−11	2,656	3,163
	Female	0.3	0.5	−67	388	818
Leukemia	Male	8.9	8.4	−6	8,262	10,873
	Female	5.3	4.9	−8	6,216	8,834
Liver	Male	3.4	4.6	35	3,013	6,068
	Female	1.8	2.1	17	2,116	3,995
Lung	Male	61.3	73.5	20	59,082	92,493
	Female	12.7	32.9	159	15,706	56,234
Melanoma	Male	2.0	3.2	60	1,964	4,128
	Female	1.3	1.5	15	1,465	2,584
Multiple myeloma	Male	2.8	3.8	36	2,579	4,902
	Female	1.9	2.6	37	2,389	4,939
Non-Hodgkin's lymphoma	Male	5.8	8.1	40	5,473	10,458
	Female	3.9	5.3	36	4,747	10,028
Oral cavity	Male	5.9	4.4	−25	5,553	5,515
	Female	1.9	1.6	−16	2,269	2,726
Ovary	Female	8.6	7.8	−9	9,885	12,870
Pancreas	Male	11.1	10.0	−10	10,380	12,669
	Female	6.7	7.3	9	8,273	13,776
Prostate	Male	21.4	26.8	25	18,830	34,865
Stomach	Male	10.4	6.6	−37	9,178	8,229
	Female	5.0	3.0	−40	6,020	5,621
Testis	Male	0.7	0.2	−71	798	374
Thyroid	Male	0.4	0.3	−25	315	398
	Female	0.5	0.4	−20	657	732
Urinary bladder	Male	7.2	5.7	−21	6,481	7,474
	Female	2.2	1.7	−23	2,855	3,488

*Adjusted to the age distribution of the 1970 US census population. Even though death rates declined or remained stable, the number of deaths increased because the population over 65 years of age has become larger and older. The US population increased 22% from 1973 to 1993.
American Cancer Society Surveillance Research, 1997.
Data source: Vital Statistics of the United States, 1993. © 1997, American Cancer Society, Inc.
From American Cancer Society: Cancer Facts and Figures, 1997. No. 5008.97. Atlanta, American Cancer Society, 1997:7.

Incidence

According to NCI reports, from the mid-1970s to the early 1990s incidence rates for all cancers combined rose among both men and women. The upward trend seemed to affect three groups of malignancies: (1) cancers strongly related to smoking, (2) cancers of the breast and reproductive organs, and (3) a broad grouping of other cancers neither strongly linked to nor unrelated to smoking.[9]

Table 1-3. Cancer Around the World, Age-Adjusted Death Rates* per 100,000 Population by Site for Selected Sites for 48 Countries, 1990–1993

COUNTRY	ALL SITES		BREAST	COLON AND RECTUM		LEUKEMIA		LUNG AND BRONCHUS		ORAL CAVITY AND PHARYNX		PROSTATE	STOMACH		UTERUS
	MALE	FEMALE	FEMALE	MALE	FEMALE	MALE	FEMALE	MALE	FEMALE	MALE	FEMALE	MALE	MALE	FEMALE	FEMALE
United States##	165.3 (27)	111.1 (8)	22.0 (13)	16.5 (23)	11.2 (20)	6.4 (9)	3.9 (11)	57.1 (13)	25.6 (1)	3.6 (35)	1.3 (12)	17.5 (13)	5.0 (48)	2.3 (48)	2.6 (34)
Albania§	96.7 (46)	42.7 (48)	5.2 (46)	2.0 (48)	2.2 (48)	2.7 (47)	1.9 (48)	27.4 (40)	5.0 (39)	4.3 (30)	1.5 (7)	7.0 (38)	14.9 (26)	6.3 (28)	3.2 (27)
Argentina††	153.3 (29)	96.4 (27)	21.3 (16)	13.6 (33)	9.2 (34)	5.2 (27)	3.2 (32)	38.4 (33)	6.0 (35)	4.3 (29)	0.8 (39)	13.6 (24)	11.7 (33)	4.8 (36)	6.4 (5)
Armenia##	137.2 (38)	81.9 (39)	16.5 (29)	9.6 (39)	7.5 (38)	4.3 (38)	3.3 (30)	45.7 (26)	6.4 (33)	2.5 (43)	0.5 (48)	2.8 (46)	20.9 (17)	10.5 (14)	4.2 (20)
Austria	158.5 (28)	100.2 (20)	20.3 (18)	20.2 (10)	13.7 (8)	5.9 (14)	3.8 (13)	40.4 (32)	13.0 (11)	4.5 (25)	1.4 (9)	18.6 (9)	15.5 (25)	7.8 (22)	1.6 (47)
Belarus§§	171.6 (20)	105.6 (16)	21.8 (14)	22.8 (5)	13.7 (9)	5.3 (25)	3.7 (20)	44.6 (27)	9.3 (17)	6.1 (18)	0.9 (30)	17.2 (14)	36.7 (3)	15.1 (5)	4.9 (13)
Bulgaria	199.2 (11)	88.1 (34)	14.4 (38)	15.6 (26)	10.3 (29)	5.7 (21)	3.4 (26)	60.4 (12)	5.0 (41)	8.8 (7)	0.7 (41)	8.0 (35)	19.2 (20)	10.4 (15)	3.9 (22)
Canada##	140.5 (35)	84.6 (37)	15.4 (32)	15.3 (28)	10.7 (25)	4.4 (37)	2.7 (42)	41.2 (30)	6.5 (32)	4.1 (34)	0.7 (44)	8.4 (34)	7.1 (45)	3.2 (46)	6.2 (6)
China†	165.7 (25)	109.1 (9)	23.0 (10)	16.9 (21)	11.2 (21)	6.0 (11)	3.7 (18)	55.1 (17)	21.8 (3)	4.2 (31)	1.3 (13)	17.0 (16)	34.1 (5)	15.7 (4)	2.4 (38)
Costa Rica††	165.7 (26)	89.4 (33)	4.9 (47)	8.1 (41)	6.4 (41)	4.1 (42)	3.2 (33)	38.2 (34)	15.9 (9)	2.6 (41)	1.1 (20)	—	42.5 (1)	10.5 (2)	—
Cuba†	133.3 (39)	94.7 (29)	11.2 (39)	7.4 (42)	7.1 (40)	5.8 (18)	4.6 (2)	14.3 (47)	5.0 (40)	2.8 (39)	1.1 (17)	15.0 (22)	6.6 (47)	3.6 (44)	2.4 (39)
Cyprus	127.4 (41)	93.7 (30)	14.6 (36)	9.7 (38)	11.2 (22)	4.5 (34)	3.9 (10)	37.7 (35)	13.8 (10)	6.0 (19)	1.9 (3)	19.0 (8)	—	—	7.5 (4)
Czech Republic	237.2 (2)	128.0 (3)	21.5 (15)	34.6 (1)	18.1 (3)	7.2 (2)	4.4 (6)	75.3 (2)	10.1 (16)	6.3 (17)	0.9 (29)	15.1 (21)	17.1 (22)	8.0 (20)	5.2 (8)
Denmark	178.7 (17)	138.7 (1)	27.2 (2)	23.0 (4)	17.2 (4)	6.5 (6)	3.9 (12)	50.4 (19)	24.8 (2)	4.2 (32)	1.3 (10)	19.5 (6)	7.1 (44)	3.9 (42)	3.4 (25)
Estonia	211.9 (5)	105.9 (14)	16.6 (27)	18.2 (13)	12.5 (15)	6.5 (5)	3.8 (14)	70.0 (5)	7.5 (24)	8.7 (8)	1.0 (24)	13.0 (27)	28.6 (12)	13.5 (7)	5.1 (10)
Finland	149.9 (31)	89.9 (32)	16.6 (28)	12.4 (35)	8.6 (37)	4.8 (32)	3.2 (34)	46.1 (24)	6.9 (29)	2.3 (45)	0.8 (38)	18.3 (12)	11.5 (34)	6.1 (31)	2.6 (31)
France##	197.4 (13)	86.5 (36)	19.7 (19)	17.4 (18)	10.1 (30)	5.9 (13)	3.6 (23)	47.0 (22)	5.2 (38)	12.9 (3)	1.3 (11)	16.8 (17)	8.2 (43)	3.3 (45)	3.8 (23)
Germany	177.3 (18)	108.2 (11)	22.2 (12)	21.3 (8)	15.1 (6)	5.9 (15)	3.6 (22)	47.9 (21)	8.4 (20)	6.6 (12)	1.1 (18)	16.4 (18)	13.9 (27)	7.3 (24)	3.1 (28)
Greece	145.8 (33)	76.4 (42)	15.1 (33)	7.2 (43)	5.5 (43)	5.6 (23)	3.5 (25)	50.2 (20)	6.9 (28)	1.8 (46)	0.5 (47)	8.7 (33)	9.3 (38)	4.6 (38)	2.6 (35)
Hungary	258.7 (1)	135.2 (2)	23.4 (9)	30.8 (2)	18.5 (2)	7.2 (3)	4.5 (3)	81.6 (1)	16.6 (7)	17.0 (1)	2.2 (2)	15.8 (19)	23.4 (14)	9.9 (16)	5.0 (11)
Ireland##	174.4 (19)	124.3 (6)	26.8 (4)	21.5 (7)	13.8 (7)	5.9 (12)	3.2 (35)	45.8 (25)	17.6 (6)	4.3 (28)	1.0 (23)	18.5 (10)	12.2 (30)	5.9 (33)	2.4 (36)
Israel##	116.9 (43)	101.5 (18)	23.4 (8)	15.3 (29)	12.2 (17)	5.8 (16)	4.5 (4)	25.7 (41)	7.9 (23)	1.4 (48)	0.6 (46)	9.2 (32)	8.7 (41)	4.5 (39)	2.3 (43)
Italy††	189.2 (15)	97.6 (24)	20.7 (17)	15.3 (30)	9.9 (31)	6.5 (7)	4.0 (7)	57.0 (14)	7.3 (25)	6.0 (21)	1.0 (26)	11.6 (29)	16.9 (23)	7.9 (21)	4.6 (18)
Japan	149.8 (32)	75.2 (43)	6.6 (45)	15.7 (25)	9.8 (32)	4.2 (39)	2.7 (43)	30.6 (38)	8.1 (22)	2.4 (44)	0.7 (45)	4.0 (43)	32.8 (6)	14.2 (6)	2.2 (44)

Country															
Kazakhstan	216.8 (4)	105.6 (15)	8.9 (40)	11.9 (36)	8.9 (35)	4.1 (40)	2.5 (46)	68.4 (6)	9.0 (18)	7.4 (10)	1.7 (4)	5.3 (41)	35.6 (4)	15.9 (3)	7.6 (2)
Kyrgyzstan†	140.1 (37)	73.9 (44)	8.7 (41)	8.8 (40)	6.2 (42)	3.6 (45)	2.3 (47)	35.4 (36)	6.1 (34)	4.2 (33)	0.7 (42)	3.7 (44)	29.5 (8)	13.0 (8)	2.8 (29)
Latvia	206.1 (6)	98.7 (23)	16.9 (26)	17.9 (14)	11.6 (18)	6.8 (4)	4.5 (5)	65.4 (8)	6.6 (31)	6.5 (13)	0.7 (40)	12.2 (28)	28.8 (11)	12.3 (10)	5.2 (9)
Lithuania	200.7 (10)	100.2 (19)	17.5 (24)	17.2 (19)	11.1 (23)	7.9 (1)	4.8 (1)	63.1 (9)	5.9 (37)	7.9 (9)	1.0 (27)	13.2 (25)	28.8 (10)	12.3 (11)	4.7 (17)
Mauritius	85.4 (47)	63.8 (46)	7.0 (44)	5.0 (44)	4.6 (44)	2.6 (48)	2.6 (44)	17.2 (44)	4.0 (46)	5.2 (23)	1.4 (8)	7.0 (37)	13.0 (29)	6.4 (27)	8.0 (1)
Mexico	81.6 (48)	77.6 (41)	8.3 (42)	3.3 (47)	3.0 (47)	3.7 (44)	3.0 (39)	15.9 (45)	5.9 (36)	1.8 (47)	0.7 (43)	10.6 (30)	9.9 (37)	7.1 (25)	2.3 (41)
Netherlands##	189.7 (14)	108.5 (10)	26.0 (3)	17.7 (16)	12.8 (14)	5.6 (22)	3.4 (28)	66.9 (7)	10.9 (12)	2.8 (40)	1.0 (21)	18.4 (11)	12.1 (31)	4.7 (37)	2.3 (42)
New Zealand##	170.6 (21)	125.3 (4)	26.0 (5)	26.4 (3)	18.9 (1)	6.4 (8)	3.7 (19)	42.6 (29)	18.0 (5)	3.4 (36)	1.3 (14)	19.0 (7)	9.0 (39)	3.9 (43)	2.7 (30)
Norway##	145.2 (34)	99.4 (22)	18.6 (21)	20.1 (11)	13.5 (11)	4.5 (35)	3.0 (38)	30.9 (37)	10.8 (13)	3.3 (37)	0.9 (35)	22.1 (3)	10.6 (35)	4.9 (34)	2.4 (37)
Poland	204.2 (8)	107.6 (13)	15.9 (31)	15.4 (27)	10.4 (27)	5.8 (19)	3.6 (24)	71.3 (4)	10.2 (15)	6.3 (15)	1.1 (19)	9.9 (31)	21.6 (16)	7.6 (23)	3.9 (21)
Portugal	151.1 (30)	87.6 (35)	18.5 (22)	16.0 (24)	10.4 (28)	5.1 (28)	3.7 (16)	27.9 (39)	4.6 (43)	6.0 (20)	0.9 (31)	15.3 (20)	24.2 (13)	11.5 (13)	4.9 (12)
Romania	140.2 (36)	84.5 (38)	14.8 (35)	10.1 (37)	7.3 (39)	4.4 (36)	3.0 (37)	40.9 (31)	6.6 (30)	6.3 (14)	1.0 (28)	7.6 (28)	17.8 (21)	6.9 (26)	4.2 (19)
Russian Fed.	221.4 (3)	99.9 (21)	14.9 (34)	17.6 (17)	12.3 (16)	5.5 (24)	3.6 (21)	72.8 (3)	7.3 (26)	8.8 (6)	1.0 (22)	6.9 (39)	40.3 (2)	16.9 (2)	4.7 (16)
Singapore##	170.2 (22)	101.8 (17)	14.5 (37)	18.9 (12)	15.5 (5)	5.0 (31)	2.8 (40)	50.5 (18)	16.0 (8)	13.2 (2)	4.0 (1)	4.4 (42)	20.0 (19)	9.3 (19)	2.1 (45)
Slovenia	203.9 (9)	108.0 (12)	22.4 (11)	22.2 (6)	12.9 (13)	5.2 (26)	3.7 (17)	61.0 (11)	8.5 (19)	11.5 (4)	0.9 (34)	14.7 (23)	22.9 (15)	9.4 (18)	4.8 (14)
Spain##	169.8 (23)	80.0 (40)	17.3 (25)	14.6 (32)	9.4 (33)	5.1 (29)	3.4 (27)	46.9 (23)	3.6 (48)	6.9 (11)	0.8 (36)	13.2 (26)	13.7 (28)	6.3 (29)	3.5 (24)
Sweden	128.6 (40)	97.2 (25)	17.7 (23)	14.6 (31)	10.9 (24)	4.8 (33)	3.3 (29)	23.7 (42)	10.6 (14)	2.6 (42)	0.9 (32)	21.1 (4)	8.4 (42)	4.2 (40)	2.6 (33)
Switzerland	167.2 (24)	96.5 (26)	24.0 (7)	17.8 (15)	10.5 (26)	5.8 (17)	3.3 (31)	43.6 (28)	8.3 (21)	6.3 (16)	1.1 (16)	22.5 (2)	8.7 (40)	3.9 (41)	3.2 (26)
Tajikistan‡	100.6 (45)	60.4 (47)	4.4 (48)	4.7 (45)	3.1 (46)	3.7 (43)	2.7 (41)	15.0 (46)	4.4 (44)	4.6 (24)	1.6 (5)	3.5 (45)	29.1 (9)	11.7 (12)	1.8 (46)
Trinidad, Tobago††	120.0 (42)	91.4 (31)	19.6 (20)	12.6 (34)	8.9 (36)	4.1 (41)	3.8 (15)	13.6 (48)	4.0 (47)	4.5 (26)	1.0 (25)	32.9 (1)	10.2 (36)	6.0 (32)	7.5 (3)
Ukraine##	198.4 (12)	95.1 (28)	16.1 (30)	17.0 (20)	11.5 (19)	6.2 (10)	3.9 (9)	63.1 (10)	7.2 (27)	9.4 (5)	0.9 (33)	6.8 (40)	31.3 (7)	12.6 (9)	4.8 (15)
United Kingdom§§	179.1 (16)	124.6 (5)	27.7 (1)	20.3 (9)	13.6 (10)	5.1 (30)	3.1 (36)	55.9 (16)	21.0 (4)	3.0 (38)	1.1 (15)	17.1 (15)	11.8 (32)	4.8 (35)	2.4 (40)
Uruguay†	204.8 (7)	111.7 (7)	25.9 (6)	16.8 (22)	13.3 (12)	5.7 (20)	4.0 (8)	56.1 (15)	4.2 (45)	5.9 (22)	0.8 (37)	21.0 (5)	16.1 (24)	6.1 (30)	6.1 (7)
Uzbekistan‡‡	104.7 (44)	66.9 (45)	7.4 (43)	4.7 (46)	4.3 (45)	3.4 (46)	2.6 (45)	19.7 (43)	4.8 (42)	4.4 (27)	1.5 (6)	1.8 (47)	20.5 (18)	9.4 (17)	2.6 (32)

*Rates are age-adjusted to the World Health Organization world standard population. Ranks within site and sex group are in parentheses.
†1990 only. ‡1991 only. §1992 only. ††1990–1991. ‡‡1991–1992. §§1992–1993. ## 1990–1992.
·Oral cancer mortality rate includes nasopharynx only.
Data source: World Health Organization
From Parker SL, Tong T, Bolden S, Wingo PA: Cancer Statistics, 1997. CA Cancer J Clin 1997;47:5–31.

Table 1–4. Leading Sites of New Cancer Cases and Deaths—1997 Estimates*

CANCER CASES BY SITE AND SEX		CANCER DEATHS BY SITE AND SEX	
MALE	*FEMALE*	*MALE*	*FEMALE*
Prostate 334,500	Breast 180,200	Lung 94,400	Lung 66,000
Lung 98,300	Lung 79,800	Prostate 41,800	Breast 43,900
Colon and rectum 66,400	Colon and rectum 64,800	Colon and rectum 27,000	Colon and rectum 27,900
Urinary bladder 39,500	Corpus uteri 34,900	Pancreas 13,500	Pancreas 14,600
Non-Hodgkin's lymphoma 30,300	Ovary 26,800	Non-Hodgkin's lymphoma 12,400	Ovary 14,200
Melanoma of the skin 22,900	Non-Hodgkin's lymphoma 23,300	Leukemia 11,770	Non-Hodgkin's lymphoma 11,400
Oral cavity 20,900	Melanoma of the skin 17,400	Esophagus 8,700	Leukemia 9,540
Kidney 17,100	Urinary bladder 15,000	Stomach 8,300	Corpus uteri 6,000
Leukemia 15,900	Cervix 14,500	Urinary bladder 7,800	Brain 6,000
Stomach 14,000	Pancreas 14,200	Liver 7,500	Stomach 5,700
All sites 785,800	All sites 596,600	All sites 294,100	All sites 265,900

*Excluding basal and squamous cell skin cancer and in situ carcinomas except bladder.
American Cancer Society Surveillance Research, 1997. © 1997, American Cancer Society, Inc.
From American Cancer Society: Cancer Facts and Figures, 1997. No. 5008.97. Atlanta, American Cancer Society, 1997:9.

Specifically, cancers of the lung, prostate, breast, and colon/rectum account for almost 60% of all new cancer cases. In general, incidence and mortality rates for all cancers tend to be higher among men than women, higher among blacks than whites, and higher among those older than 65 years of age[10] (Tables 1–5 and 1–6).

Mortality

After rising steadily for more than 50 years, cancer mortality rates in the United States are stabilizing. In 1930 the age-adjusted cancer death rate was 13 per 100,000 population. Gradually it rose to 158 per 100,000 in 1950, to 163 per 100,000 in 1970, and to 172 per 100,000 in 1993. This upward trend in cancer mortality can be directly attributed to lung cancer (Figures 1–1 and 1–2). For many other major cancer sites, death rates have leveled off or declined over the last 60 years. In fact, when lung cancer deaths are excluded, cancer mortality between 1950 and 1993 declined by 16%.[1] Although age-adjusted cancer incidence rates continue to increase, educational and screening efforts seem to be having a positive influence on mortality rates. Increased use and improved techniques of cancer detection for breast, colorectal, and prostate cancers are resulting in more of these cancers being detected at earlier stages, when tumors

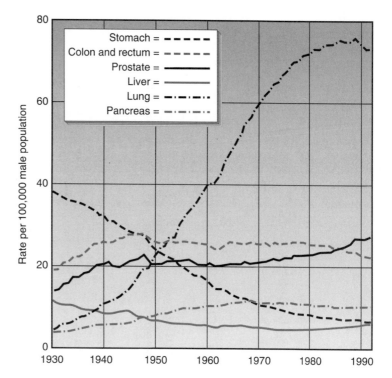

Figure 1-1. Age-adjusted cancer death rates for men by disease site, United States 1930–1993. Rates are age-adjusted to the 1970 US population. (From American Cancer Society: Cancer Facts and Figures 1997. No. 5008.97. Atlanta, American Cancer Society, 1997:2.)

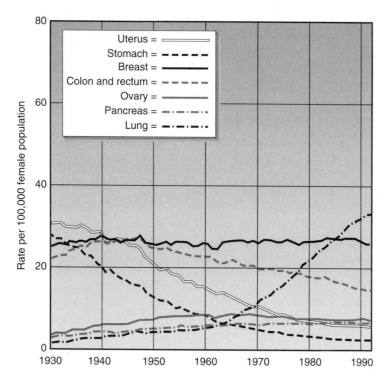

Figure 1-2. Age-adjusted cancer death rates for women by disease site, United States 1930–1993. Reprinted by permission of the American Cancer Society, Inc. Cancer Facts and Figures 1997. No. 5008.97. Atlanta, p. 3. Rates are age-adjusted to the 1970 US population. Uterine cancer rates are for cervix and corpus combined. (From American Cancer Society: Cancer Facts and Figures 1997. No. 5008.97. Atlanta, American Cancer Society, 1997:3.)

Table 1–5. Estimated New Cancer Cases and Deaths by Sex for All Sites, United States, 1997*

	ESTIMATED NEW CASES			ESTIMATED DEATHS		
	BOTH SEXES	**MALE**	**FEMALE**	**BOTH SEXES**	**MALE**	**FEMALE**
All Sites	1,382,400	785,800	596,600	560,000	294,100	265,900
Oral cavity and pharynx	30,750	20,900	9,850	8,440	5,600	2,840
Tongue	6,400	4,200	2,200	1,820	1,200	620
Mouth	11,000	6,700	4,300	2,500	1,400	1,100
Pharynx	8,800	6,400	2,400	2,030	1,500	530
Other oral cavity	4,550	3,600	950	2,090	1,500	590
Digestive system	225,900	120,000	105,900	127,070	67,440	59,630
Esophagus	12,500	9,400	3,100	11,500	8,700	2,800
Stomach	22,400	14,000	8,400	14,000	8,300	5,700
Small intestine	4,900	2,600	2,300	1,140	540	600
Colon	94,100	45,500	48,600	46,600	22,600	24,000
Rectum	37,100	20,900	16,200	8,300	4,400	3,900
Anus, anal canal, and anorectum	3,400	1,400	2,000	410	150	260
Liver	13,600	9,100	4,500	12,400	7,500	4,900
Gallbladder and other biliary	6,900	2,500	4,400	3,500	1,300	2,200
Pancreas	27,600	13,400	14,200	28,100	13,500	14,600
Other digestive organs	3,400	1,200	2,200	1,120	450	670
Respiratory system	194,600	111,400	83,200	165,920	98,490	67,430
Larynx	10,900	8,900	2,000	4,230	3,300	930
Lung	178,100	98,300	79,800	160,400	94,400	66,000
Other respiratory organs	5,600	4,200	1,400	1,290	790	500
Bones and joints	2,500	1,300	1,200	1,410	750	660
Soft tissue (including heart)	6,600	3,700	2,900	4,100	1,900	2,200
Skin (excluding basal and squamous)	54,300	34,900	19,400	9,490	6,100	3,390
Melanomas	40,300	22,900	17,400	7,300	4,600	2,700
Other nonepithelial skin	14,000	12,000	2,000	2,190	1,500	690
Breast	181,600	1,400	180,200	44,190	290	43,900

Site					
Reproductive organs	424,800	343,000	81,800	68,870	42,370	26,500
Cervix uteri	14,500	—	14,500	4,800	—	4,800
Corpus uteri	34,900	—	34,900	6,000	—	6,000
Ovary	26,800	—	26,800	14,200	—	14,200
Vulva	3,300	—	3,300	800	—	800
Vagina and other female genital	2,300	—	2,300	700	—	700
Prostate	334,500	334,500	—	41,800	41,800	—
Testis	7,200	7,200	—	350	350	—
Penis and other male genital	1,300	1,300	—	220	220	—
Urinary system	85,400	58,000	27,400	23,520	15,060	8,460
Urinary bladder	54,500	39,500	15,000	11,700	7,800	3,900
Kidney	28,800	17,100	11,700	11,300	7,000	4,300
Ureter and other urinary organs	2,100	1,400	700	520	260	260
Eye and orbit	2,100	1,100	1,000	250	140	110
Brain	17,600	10,100	7,500	13,200	7,200	6,000
Endocrine system	17,560	5,530	12,030	2,070	870	1,200
Thyroid	16,100	4,700	11,400	1,230	450	780
Other endocrine	1,460	830	630	840	420	420
Lymphoma	61,100	34,200	26,900	25,280	13,220	12,060
Hodgkin's disease	7,500	3,900	3,600	1,480	820	660
Non-Hodgkin's lymphoma	53,600	30,300	23,300	23,800	12,400	11,400
Multiple myeloma	13,800	7,900	5,900	10,900	5,500	5,400
Leukemia	28,300	15,900	12,400	21,310	11,770	9,540
Acute lymphocytic leukemia	3,000	1,600	1,400	1,410	770	640
Chronic lymphocytic leukemia	7,400	4,300	3,100	4,900	2,800	2,100
Acute myelocytic leukemia	9,200	4,700	4,500	6,300	3,400	2,900
Chronic myelocytic leukemia	4,300	2,400	1,900	2,400	1,400	1,000
Other leukemia	4,400	2,900	1,500	6,300	3,400	2,900
Other and unspecified primary sites	35,500	16,500	19,000	34,000	17,400	16,600

*Excludes basal and squamous cell skin cancers and in situ carcinomas except bladder. Carcinoma in situ of the breast accounts for about 30,000 new cases annually, and melanoma/carcinoma in situ accounts for about 17,300 new cases annually. Basal cell and squamous cell skin cancers account for more than 900,000 new cases annually. About 2,100 nonmelanoma skin cancer deaths are included among the deaths from cancer of other and unspecified sites which are expected to occur in 1997.

Estimates of new cases are based on incidence rates from NCI SEER program 1980–1993.

American Cancer Society Surveillance Research, 1997.

Data source: NCI Surveillance, Epidemiology, and End Results Program, 1996. © 1997, American Cancer Society, Inc.

From American Cancer Society: Cancer Facts & Figures, 1997. No. 5008.97. Atlanta, American Cancer Society, 1997:4.

Table 1–6. Percentage of Population (Probability) Developing Invasive Cancers at Certain Ages by Sex, US, 1991–1993

SITE	SEX	BIRTH TO 39	40 TO 59	60 TO 79	BIRTH TO DEATH
All sites°	Male	1.71 (1 in 58)	8.27 (1 in 12)	37.79 (1 in 3)	48.17 (1 in 2)
	Female	1.96 (1 in 51)	9.12 (1 in 11)	22.48 (1 in 4)	38.33 (1 in 3)
Breast	Female	0.46 (1 in 217)	3.92 (1 in 26)	6.94 (1 in 14)	12.61 (1 in 8)
Colon and	Male	0.06 (1 in 1,667)	0.92 (1 in 109)	4.27 (1 in 23)	6.02 (1 in 17)
rectum	Female	0.05 (1 in 2,000)	0.70 (1 in 143)	3.24 (1 in 31)	5.77 (1 in 17)
Lung	Male	0.04 (1 in 2,500)	1.46 (1 in 68)	6.82 (1 in 15)	8.60 (1 in 12)
	Female	0.03 (1 in 3,333)	1.05 (1 in 95)	3.83 (1 in 26)	5.48 (1 in 18)
Prostate	Male	Less than 1 in 10,000	1.58 (1 in 63)	17.04 (1 in 6)	19.84 (1 in 5)

°Excludes basal and squamous cell skin cancers and in situ carcinomas except bladder.
Data source: NCI Surveillance, Epidemiology, and End Results Program, 1996. © 1997, American Cancer Society, Inc.
   From American Cancer Society: Cancer Facts and Figures, 1997. No. 5008.97. Atlanta, American Cancer Society, 1997:11.

are smaller and more amenable to treatment. It is hoped that continuation of such activities will ultimately reduce mortality from cancers at these three sites.[10]

Survivability

Of every 10 Americans who get cancer this year, about 4 will be alive 5 years after diagnosis. By contrast, in the early 20th century few cancer patients had any hope of long-term survival. In the 1930s, fewer than one cancer patient in five survived 5 years; in the 1940s it was one in four; and in the 1960s one in three persons survived 5 years after treatment. Well over half a million people who are diagnosed with cancer this year will be alive in 5 years—a gain of almost 91,000 persons per year over the rate of the 1960s.[1]

The current 40% cancer survival rate (4 in 10) represents the "observed" survival rate. When rates are adjusted for factors such as death from heart disease, accidents, or old age (in other words, normal life expectancy), a "relative" 5-year survival rate can be calculated. The current relative 5-year survival rate in the United States for persons with cancer is 56%. Relative 5-year survival rates include all persons who are alive 5 years after cancer diagnosis, whether in remission, disease-free, or receiving treatment. These relative survival rates are commonly used to monitor progress in early detection and treatment of cancer.[1] Table 1–7 presents relative 5-year survival rates by cancer stage at diagnosis for the period 1986 through 1993.

Caution should be used when interpreting relative 5-year survival rates. Although these rates are reasonable indicators of the average survival experience of cancer patients in a given population, they are less useful for predicting individual prognosis. Interpretation is difficult because the rates are based on patients whose treatment reflected medical practice methods of at least 8 years earlier. In addition, an increase or decrease in survival may be caused by several different factors (such as changes in early detection techniques and treatment strategies) that are not considered in the calculation of the relative 5-year survival rates.[1, 6]

Table 1-7. Five-Year Relative Survival Rates by Stage at Diagnosis*

SITE	ALL STAGES %	LOCAL %	REGIONAL %	DISTANT %
Brain	29	34	32	52
Breast (female)	84	97	76	20
Cervix	69	91	50	9
Colon and rectum	61	91	63	7
Corpus uteri	84	95	66	26
Esophagus	11	22	11	2
Kidney	59	88	60	9
Larynx	66	84	54	40
Liver	6	13	8	2
Lung	14	48	18	2
Melanoma	87	95	61	16
Oral	53	81	42	18
Ovary	46	92	51	25
Pancreas	4	13	5	2
Prostate	87	99	93	30
Stomach	21	61	23	2
Testis	95	99	97	72
Thyroid	95	100	94	47
Urinary bladder	81	93	49	6

*Adjusted for normal life expectancy. This chart is based on cases diagnosed from 1986 to 1992, followed through 1993.

Data source: NCI Surveillance, Epidemiology, and End Results Program, 1996. © 1997, American Cancer Society, Inc.

From American Cancer Society: Cancer Facts & Figures, 1997. No. 5008.97. Atlanta, American Cancer Society, 1997:14.

MAJOR CANCERS WITH RISING INCIDENCE

Breast

The incidence of breast cancer for women of all ages fluctuated during the 1970s but rose steadily each year from 1980 to 1987. Most experts agree that the rising incidence during the early 1980s can be attributed to greater use of mammography by asymptomatic women. Accompanying the rise in breast cancer incidence was the rising trend in diagnosis of smaller lesions (<2 cm) and localized cancers.[10] Although most of the rise in incidence of breast cancer can be associated with earlier detection, other factors (such as the changing prevalence of certain reproductive variables, diet, alcohol consumption, and long-term use of menopausal estrogens) may also contribute to the increase. In recent years there has been a pronounced increase in the number of estrogen receptor-positive tumors detected, particularly among older women.[9]

For decades breast cancer incidence gradually increased while mortality remained stable at about 27 per 100,000 women. Statistics on breast cancer now reveal a true decline in mortality from this disease, most likely as a result of early detection by mammography and diagnosis of the cancer at a localized and curable stage.[10, 11] In addition, the increased survival rate among breast cancer patients has contributed to an overall decrease in mortality rates.[9, 11] Between 1973 and 1990, breast cancer mortality rates rose by 15% in women older than 65 years of age but dropped 6% in women younger than 65. Five-year relative survival rates for breast cancer varied little during the 1970s but rose to about 40% in the 1980s. The 5-year survival rate is now 79% for all breast cancer patients and 93% for those in whom the cancer is diagnosed at an early stage.[10]

Prostate

Prostate cancer is the cancer most commonly diagnosed among men in the United States. Prostate cancer affects primarily older men, with an incidence during the period 1986 through 1990 of 884.1 per 100,000 population for men age 65 and older, compared with 22.7 per 100,000 for men younger than 65 years of age. The incidence of prostate cancer remains higher among black men than white men, perhaps because of early detection practices, yet the race differential has steadily decreased over the last 20 years. In 1970, the incidence of prostate cancer for blacks was 71% higher than for whites; by 1990, the difference had dropped to 27%.[10]

As with breast cancer, the increasing incidence of prostate cancer seems to be related to earlier detection and advances in diagnostic methods. Frequent use of transurethral resections during the 1980s led to increased detection and reporting of clinically occult lesions. Since then the use of transurethral resections has leveled off, but other modes of detection (including serum testing for prostate-specific antigen [PSA], ultrasound-guided needle biopsy, computed tomography, and bone scans) have gained in popularity among clinicians. Although risk factors for prostate cancer are poorly understood, there appears to be a correlation between nutritional practices such as increased consumption of fat and meat and the upward trend in the incidence of this disease.[9]

Mortality rates for prostate cancer also are rising, but at a much slower rate. On average, deaths from prostate cancer have increased at the rate of 1% per year over last 20 years. Age-adjusted prostate cancer mortality rates increased faster for blacks than for whites (40% and 21%, respectively) during the years 1973 through 1990, and the rate differential continues to be almost twice as high for black men.[10] About 58% of all prostate cancers are diagnosed at a localized stage, resulting in a relative 5-year survival rate of 92% for these patients. However, the overall relative 5-year survival rate for invasive prostate cancer is about 78%.[10] Five-year survival rates for men with prostate cancer are rising, partly because of the increased diagnosis of early-stage tumors and perhaps also because of improvements in therapy, although the latter relation is less clear.[9]

Lung

Although for lung cancer there are no effective early diagnostic tests and no curative therapies for advanced disease, a known carcinogen—tobacco—can be targeted effectively through public health initiatives to reverse the rising incidence and mortality of this common cancer. Because of these initiatives and educational efforts, lung cancer incidence has declined in recent years, especially for men younger than 65 years of age, following a decrease in smoking among men that started 20 years ago.[11] Current statistics show that lung cancer mortality is leveling off for men but is still rising for women.[10, 11] Age-adjusted incidence rates reveal, however, that lung cancer incidence continues to increase among older men while it declines substantially among young and middle-aged men. Lung cancer rates are increasing for all women older than 35 years of age.[9] In 1986, lung cancer overtook breast cancer to become the leading cause of cancer death among women, as it continues to be today.[1, 10] For both men and women, lung cancer incidence rates show a strong positive correlation with the age at which smoking began and subsequent smoking prevalence. Therefore, as the effects of reduced smoking prevalence become more evident, the overall age-adjusted lung cancer incidence should begin to decline among men in the 1990s and among women after the year 2000.[9] The impact on cancer mortality would be profound if tobacco were removed from the environment, and past trends for lung cancer could to be reversed.[11]

CANCERS WITH DECREASING INCIDENCE

Colorectal

Colorectal cancer is the third most common cancer among men and women.[1] Between 1973 and 1985, the incidence of colorectal cancer rose 14% overall. Since reaching a peak incidence of 52.8 cases per 100,000 persons in 1985, the age-adjusted incidence rates have decreased by 10%, suggesting that changes in risk factor profiles during the last several decades are lowering rates among men and women.[9, 10] Colorectal cancer rates among black men and women rose steadily from 1973 to 1980, increasing by 26% before leveling off in 1994 to about 52.9 per 100,000 in 1994, a rate 12% higher than that for white men and women.[10]

Age-adjusted mortality rates from colorectal cancer decreased by 14% between 1973 and 1990, to a level of 18.9 deaths per 100,000 persons; this decrease was observed primarily among white men and women. During the same period, colorectal cancer mortality rates for blacks increased by 15%; the rate increased by 33% among black men but only 2% among black women. Since 1974, the overall 5-year survival rate for colorectal cancer has increased to 58.4%, although the rate remains lower for blacks (47.8%) than for whites (59.3%). This positive trend in survival may be attributed to increased use of diagnostic tests, earlier detection of polyps, and refined and improved surgical treatment of the disease.[10]

Uterine

The largest decrease in cancer incidence over the last 20 years has occurred for cancer of the corpus uteri. Uterine cancer incidence rates rose 32% from the late 1960s to 1976, when a fairly abrupt decline in rates began and continued through the 1980s. Today, incidence rates for cancer of the corpus uteri are relatively stable. The sharp increase and subsequent decline in incidence most probably reflect the rise and fall in the use of unopposed menopausal estrogens. In contrast, the incidence of cervical cancer has consistently decreased since the early 1950s, when use of the Pap smear for widespread screening was introduced.[9]

Stomach, Head, and Neck

Other significant decreases in cancer incidence and mortality are seen in cancers of the stomach, oral cavity, pharynx, and larynx. Declines in the incidence of these cancers appear to be related to control of exogenous factors. The decreases in stomach cancer incidence and mortality are probably attributable to improvements in diet, including availability of fresh fruits and vegetables, better methods of food preservation, refrigeration, and a lowered prevalence of *Helicobacter pylori* infection. Declines in the number of new cases and in the number of deaths from head and neck cancers, which are associated with smoking and alcohol intake, suggest benefits from recent decreases in smoking activities, especially among men. However, the rates of oral and pharyngeal cancers are increasing among young men, possibly because of the use of smokeless tobacco, although this relation remains unclear.[10] Tables 1–8 and 1–9 present 1993 reported U.S. deaths for the five leading cancer sites for men and women.

MINORITIES AND THE MEDICALLY UNDERSERVED

Recent estimates suggest that minority groups will make up 51.1% of the total U.S. population early in the 21st century. Although racial and ethnic minority groups have diverse cultures and socioeconomic status, they represent an important part of the undeserved population whose needs must be met.[12] In 1991 the cancer cure rate exceeded 50% for all cancers combined, but for the many Americans living in poverty the survival statistics are less optimistic.[13]

There is substantial evidence to support a relation between rates of cancer incidence and survival and socioeconomic status. In most studies, when adjustments are made for socioeconomic status, mortality and incidence disparities among ethnic groups are reduced or disappear. The challenge to erase health care disparities specifically related to cancer care for minorities and the economically disadvantaged is enormous.[13] To fulfill a major goal of Healthy People 2000, the NCI set as its objective to decrease the cancer mortality rate by 50% by the year 2000. To achieve this goal, it is clear that the issues of access to care, cultural heterogeneity, and development of interventions appropriate to the lifestyles, behaviors, and beliefs of minority groups must be addressed.[9]

In general, cancer incidence rates are about 10% higher for blacks than for whites. In 1992 the incidence rates for all cancers were 465 per 100,000 population for blacks and 419 per 100,000 for whites. Mortality rates for that same year were 227 per 100,000 for blacks and 169 per 100,000 for whites. Cancers of the esophagus, cervix, stomach, liver, prostate, and larynx and multiple myeloma all have significantly higher incidence and mortality rates among blacks than whites. For esophageal cancer, these rates are more than three times higher.[1] Between the years 1986 and 1993, the relative 5-year survival rate for blacks with cancer was about 42%, compared with 58% for whites. Much of this difference in survival can be attributed to a later stage of disease at diagnosis among blacks. Improved early detection and timely treatment can increase survival.[1]

Incidence rates for lung, breast, colorectal, and prostate cancers are lower among Native Americans, Asian and Pacific Islanders, and Hispanics than among whites. For other tumor sites, however, these minority groups have higher incidence and mortality rates than do whites[1, 14] (Tables 1–10 and 1–11).

Clues to the differences in cancer rates between minority and white populations can be found in factors associated with lifestyle and behavior, such as dietary patterns, alcohol use, and sexual and reproductive behaviors. Racial and ethnic groups also vary in their screening behaviors. Belief systems and cultural values embraced by minorities can affect their attitudes about seeking medical

Table 1–8. Reported Deaths for the Five Leading Cancer Sites, Males by Age, United States, 1993

ALL AGES	UNDER 15	15–34	35–54	55–74	75+
All sites	All sites	All sites	All sites	All sites	All sites
279,375	978	3,509	28,782	142,057	104,037
Lung and bronchus	Leukemia	Leukemia	Lung and bronchus	Lung and bronchus	Lung and bronchus
92,493	359	645	8,771	55,421	28,122
Prostate	Brain and ONS	Non-Hodgkin's lymphoma	Colon and rectum	Colon and rectum	Prostate
34,865	255	477	2,508	13,689	22,465
Colon and rectum	Endocrine system	Brain and ONS	Non-Hodgkin's lymphoma	Prostate	Colon and rectum
28,199	113	458	1,699	12,051	11,787
Pancreas	Non-Hodgkin's lymphoma	Colon and rectum	Brain and ONS	Pancreas	Pancreas
12,669	63	209	1,542	6,678	4,580
Leukemia	Soft tissue	Hodgkin's disease	Pancreas	Esophagus	Leukemia
10,873	47	197	1,375	4,661	4,076

ONS = other nervous system
Note: All sites category excludes basal and squamous cell skin cancers and in situ carcinomas except bladder.
Data source: Vital Statistics of the United States, 1996.
From Parker SL, Tong T, Bolden S, Wingo PA. Cancer Statistics, 1997. CA Cancer J Clin 1997;47:5–33.

Table 1-9. Reported Deaths for the Five Leading Cancer Sites, Females by Age, United States, 1993

ALL AGES	UNDER 15	15–34	35–54	55–74	75+
All sites	All sites	All sites	All sites	All sites	All sites
250,529	721	3,308	30,345	111,937	104,203
Lung and bronchus	Leukemia	Breast	Breast	Lung and bronchus	Lung and bronchus
56,234	238	560	9,279	31,803	18,802
Breast	Brain and ONS	Leukemia	Lung and bronchus	Breast	Colon and rectum
43,555	205	441	5,501	18,937	16,137
Colon and rectum	Endocrine system	Brain and ONS	Colon and rectum	Colon and rectum	Breast
29,206	74	326	2,064	10,861	14,778
Pancreas	Bones and joints	Cervix uteri	Ovary	Ovary	Pancreas
13,776	44	323	1,823	6,159	6,909
Ovary	Soft tissue	Non-Hodgkin's lymphoma	Cervix uteri	Pancreas	Non-Hodgkin's lymphoma
12,870	37	214	1,623	5,933	4,854

ONS = other nervous system

Note: All sites category excludes basal and squamous cell skin cancers and in situ carcinomas except bladder.

Data source: Vital Statistics of the United States, 1996.

From Parker SL, Tong T, Bolden S, Wingo PA. Cancer Statistics, 1997. CA Cancer J Clin 1997;47:5–33.

care or following guidelines. Lack of health insurance and lack of transportation are two of the factors that may impede access to care and lead to late diagnosis and poor survival.[1] In the future, interventions designed to encourage cancer prevention and screening behaviors must seek to overcome barriers facing the medically underserved and minority populations in an economically sound and culturally sensitive fashion.[12]

RESEARCH TOPICS AND FUTURE TRENDS

Over the last 30 years, major progress has been made in curing cancers that affect children and young adults. Research has uncovered in great detail many of the processes that transform a normal cell into a malignant one. This knowledge will eventually lead to identification of molecular targets and design of customized prevention and therapeutic strategies. Still, cancer remains a formidable threat to millions of Americans, especially in view of the aging population. Basic epidemiologic research will remain the cornerstone of continued progress in understanding cancer. By increasing the body of knowledge through research, the keys to control and cure cancer are brought within closer reach.[1]

Causes of Cancer

Current and future research into the causes of cancer will focus primarily on the areas of molecular genetics and molecular biology. Molecular genetic research acknowledges that all cancers result from genetic defects—mutations either inherited from a parent or occurring during a person's lifetime as a result of exposure to chemicals or radiation. Genetic abnormalities can initiate cancer in several different kinds of tissue (e.g., breast, lung, prostate, colon). New oncogenes (cancer-causing genes) and tumor suppressor genes are being discovered with regularity.[1]

Epidemiologic studies also continue to investigate the link between suspected exposures to carcinogenic substances and cancer occurrence. The development of new tools to measure a person's levels of exposure and susceptibility is enhanced by a knowledge of molecular biology. Cancer susceptibility genes differ widely among individuals, as do the abilities to handle suspected carcinogens, to respond immunologically, and to repair damaged cellular DNA. Molecular epidemiologic research will reinforce the development of highly specific cancer risk profiles; these will allow susceptible people to avoid certain occupational and environmental exposures.[1]

Prevention

Exciting to the area of cancer prevention research are studies involving chemoprevention and cancer vaccines. A group of highly diverse biologic and chemical agents, including analogs of vitamin A, plant phenolics (green tea), soybeans, antihormones, and drugs such as aspirin, have demonstrated anticancer activity in laboratory investigations. Research involving these agents has the

Table 1–10. Incidence Rates* for the Five Most Frequently Diagnosed Cancers by Race, Ethnicity, and Sex, United States, 1988–1992

MALES

AFRICAN AMERICANS	CHINESE	FILIPINOS	HAWAIIANS	JAPANESE	KOREANS	VIETNAMESE	ALASKA NATIVES	AMERICAN INDIANS	WHITES	HISPANICS†
Prostate 180.6	Lung 52.1	Prostate 69.8	Lung 89.0	Prostate 88.0	Lung 53.2	Lung 70.9	Lung 81.1	Prostate 52.5	Prostate 134.7	Prostate 89.0
Lung 117.0	Prostate 46.0	Lung 52.6	Prostate 57.2	Colon and rectum 64.1	Stomach 48.9	Liver 41.8	Colon and rectum 79.7	Colon and rectum 18.6	Lung 76.0	Lung 41.8
Colon and rectum 60.7	Colon and rectum 44.8	Colon and rectum 35.4	Colon and rectum 42.4	Lung 43.0	Colon and rectum 31.7	Prostate 40.0	Prostate 46.1	Kidney 15.6	Colon and rectum 56.3	Colon and rectum 38.3
Oral 20.4	Liver 20.8	Non-Hodgkin's lymphoma 12.9	Stomach 20.5	Stomach 30.5	Liver 24.8	Colon and rectum 30.5	Stomach 27.2	Lung 14.4	Urinary bladder 31.7	Urinary bladder 15.8
Stomach 17.9	Stomach 15.7	Liver 10.5	Non-Hodgkin's lymphoma 12.5	Urinary bladder 13.7	Prostate 24.2	Stomach 25.8	Kidney† 19.0	Liver† 13.1	Non-Hodgkin's lymphoma 18.7	Stomach 15.3

FEMALES

AFRICAN AMERICANS	CHINESE	FILIPINOS	HAWAIIANS	JAPANESE	KOREANS	VIETNAMESE	ALASKA NATIVES	AMERICAN INDIANS	WHITES	HISPANICS†
Breast 95.4	Breast 55.0	Breast 73.1	Breast 105.6	Breast 82.3	Breast 28.5	Cervix 43.0	Breast 78.9	Breast 31.6	Breast 111.8	Breast 69.8
Colon and rectum 45.5	Colon and rectum 33.6	Colon and rectum 20.9	Lung 43.1	Colon and rectum 39.5	Colon and rectum 21.9	Breast 37.5	Colon and rectum 67.4	Ovary 17.5	Lung 41.5	Colon and rectum 24.7
Lung 44.2	Lung 25.3	Lung 17.5	Colon and rectum 30.5	Stomach 15.3	Stomach 19.1	Lung 31.2	Lung 50.6	Colon and rectum 15.3	Colon and rectum 38.3	Lung 19.5
Corpus uteri 14.4	Corpus uteri 11.6	Thyroid 14.6	Corpus uteri 23.9	Lung 15.2	Lung 16.0	Colon and rectum 27.1	Kidney‡ 16.7	Gallbladder 13.2	Corpus uteri 22.3	Cervix 16.2
Cervix 13.2	Ovary 9.3	Corpus uteri 12.1	Stomach 13.0	Corpus uteri 14.5	Cervix 15.2	Stomach 25.8	Cervix 15.8	Corpus uteri 10.7	Ovary 15.8	Corpus uteri 13.7

*Incidence rates per 100,000, age-adjusted to 1970 US standard population.
†Persons of Hispanic origin may be of any race.
‡Rate is based on fewer than 25 cases and may be subject to greater variability than the other rates which are based on larger numbers.
Data source: NCI Surveillance, Epidemiology, and End Results Program, 1996. © 1997, American Cancer Society, Inc.
From American Cancer Society. Cancer Facts & Figures, 1997. No. 5008.97. Atlanta, American Cancer Society, 1997:20.

Table 1–11. Trends in Cancer Survival by Race and Year of Diagnosis, United States, 1960–1992

RELATIVE 5-YEAR SURVIVAL RATE (%)

SITE	WHITES					AFRICAN AMERICANS				
	1960–63	1970–73	1974–76	1980–82	1986–92	1960–63	1970–73	1974–76	1980–82	1986–92
All sites°	39	43	50	52	59†	27	31	39	40	44†
Brain	18	20	22	25	29†	19	19	27	31	32†
Breast (female)	63	68	75	77	85†	46	51	63	66	70†
Cervix	58	64	69	68	71	47	61	64	61	56†
Colon and rectum	NA	NA	50	55	62†	NA	NA	45	46	53†
Corpus uteri	73	81	89	83	86†	31	44	61	54	56
Esophagus	4	4	5	8	12†	1	4	4	5	8†
Hodgkin's disease	40	67	72	75	82†	NA	NA	69	72	72
Kidney	37	46	52	51	60†	38	44	49	55	55
Larynx	53	62	66	69	68	NA	NA	58	59	52
Leukemia	NA	22	35	39	43†	NA	NA	31	33	34
Liver	NA	NA	4	4	7†	NA	NA	1	2	5†
Lung	8	10	12	14	14†	5	7	11	12	11
Melanoma	60	68	80	83	88†	NA	NA	66‡	60†	72‡
Multiple myeloma	12	19	24	28	28†	NA	NA	27	29	30
Non-Hodgkin's lymphoma	31	41	47	52	52†	NA	NA	48	51	44
Oral	45	43	55	55	55	NA	NA	36	31	33
Ovary	32	36	36	39	46†	32	32	40	39	40
Pancreas	1	2	3	3	4	1	2	3	5	5†
Prostate	50	63	68	75	89†	35	55	58	65	73†
Stomach	11	13	15	16	19†	8	13	17	19	20
Testis	63	72	79	92	95†	NA	NA	76‡	90†	86†
Thyroid gland	83	86	92	94	96†	NA	NA	88	95	90
Urinary bladder	53	61	74	79	82†	24	36	47	59	60†

°Excludes basal and squamous cell skin cancers and in situ carcinomas except bladder.
†The difference in rates between 1974–76 and 1986–92 is statistically significant (p < 0.05).
‡The standard error of the survival rate is greater than 5 percentage points.
NA = not available.
Data source: End Results Group, 1960–1973; NCI Surveillance, Epidemiology, and End Results Program, 1996. © 1997, American Cancer Society, Inc.
From American Cancer Society. Cancer Facts & Figures, 1997. No. 5008.97. Atlanta, American Cancer Society, 1997:16.

potential to extrapolate to cancer prevention in people at high risk. In addition, preventive cancer vaccines are being developed to fight cancers thought to be associated with viruses, including cervical and liver cancers and some lymphomas. Investigators are probing new ways to present tumor-specific proteins, or antigens, that will cause the body's own immune system to respond. Most of the research with cancer vaccines involves malignant melanoma, but therapeutic and potentially preventive vaccines directed at antigens common to many cancers are under development.[1]

The majority of cancer-related expenditures nationally are allocated to early detection and treatment. Current NIH appropriations for cancer research reflect a predominance in the areas of patient treatment and basic research. Present mechanisms for obtaining NIH financial support for cancer-related research underscore this predominant emphasis.[2] To truly change the overall impact of cancer in the United States, monies must be directed not just toward treatment modalities but toward prevention and early detection of cancer and toward the evaluation of interventions to reduce cancer incidence, morbidity, and mortality.

Detection

High-quality mammography, in combination with clinical breast examinations, clearly has influenced reported breast cancer incidence and mortality rates. Widespread use of lower-dose x-rays, digitized computer images, and computer programs to assist in diagnosis will continue to affect early detection. Several new imaging technologies, including magnetic resonance imaging (MRI) and ultrasound, are being developed to assist in breast cancer diagnosis.[1]

A major goal of cancer research is the identification in blood or tissue of genetic or biochemical markers that indicate the earliest changes associated with carcinogenesis. Biomarkers also have the potential to monitor the efficacy of various therapies and preventive interventions. Biomarkers such as gene mutations, hormone receptors, metastasis-inhibiting proteins, and enzymes that metabolize drugs currently are being used to determine the severity and predict the course of certain cancers.[1]

Treatment

Cancer treatment research is centered on gene therapy and on the development of highly specific drugs. Gene therapy is already being evaluated in clinical trials. Several such investigative therapies focus on the use of genes to make cells susceptible to antiviral drugs, genes that increase a patient's immune response, and genes that confer drug resistance to the bone marrow so that higher doses of chemotherapeutic agents can be given. Angiogenesis inhibitors—drugs that block the ability of tumor cells to form blood vessels—are being investigated. Ideally, if angiogenesis could be interrupted, tumors could not grow beyond the size of a pea. Rational drug design is allowing the creation of compounds that will inhibit many factors in the cancer pathway, including oncogene action, hormone receptors, growth factors, metastasis, and angiogenesis. Rational drug design combines the technology of the three-dimensional structure of oncogenes and other molecules with mathematical computer models to design drugs that will interact specifically with cancer molecules.[1]

Psychosocial and Behavioral Research

Lifestyle, cultural factors, and socioeconomic status play significant roles in a person's general health and risk for developing cancer and also influence the person's mental and emotional ability to cope with cancer if it occurs. According to the ACS, as many as 50% of patients who develop fatal cancer could have been saved had they been able to use existing knowledge about smoking, diet, exercise, and means of early detection.[1] Moreover, research on behavioral modification is having a significant impact on management of the symptoms of cancer and cancer treatment. Behavioral modification techniques have proved successful for managing pain, stress, nausea, and vomiting associated with cancer. Several topics are emerging as important for psychosocial and behavioral research, including the responses of both patient and family to the disease, the patient's sexual concerns, rehabilitation, employment, insurance needs, and ways to provide psychosocial support to patients and families.[1]

CONCLUSION

Tremendous progress has been made in the war on cancer. Several major cancers have declined in incidence and mortality, whereas relative 5-year survival rates are rising among certain population groups. Cancers of the lung, breast, and prostate continue to increase in incidence, and statistics for minorities and the medically underserved remain dismal. Although most researchers agree that prevention and early detection of disease have the most definitive impact on cancer incidence, morbidity, and mortality, the preponderance of grant monies is awarded to investigations of treatment and the sequelae of cancer.

Cancer epidemiology seeks to contribute to the interdisciplinary effort to elucidate the causes of cancer by documenting observed differences in disease distribution and by investigating the factors associated with cancer development.[5] Understanding of basic epidemiologic principles is essential for all health care providers so that they can appropriately interpret research and disseminate knowledge about cancer.

REFERENCES

1. American Cancer Society: Cancer Facts and Figures 1997. No. 5008.97. Atlanta, American Cancer Society, 1997.
2. Colditz GA, Gortmaker SL: Cancer prevention strategies for the future: Risk identification and preventive intervention. Milbank Q 1995;73:621–651.
3. Steiner DL, Norman GR, Blum HM: PDQ Epidemiology. Philadelphia, BC Decker, 1989.
4. Vincent B, Mirand A: The nature of cancer. In American Cancer Society (ed): A Cancer Source Book for Nurses. Atlanta, American Cancer Society, 1991.
5. Parkinson DR, Schnipper LE, Weinberg RA: Cancer biology. In American Cancer Society (ed): Cancer Manual. Atlanta, American Cancer Society, 1990.
6. Parker SL, Tong T, Bolden S, Wingo PA: Cancer statistics, 1997. CA Cancer J Clin 1997;47:5–27.
7. Centers for Disease Control: State cancer registries: Status of authorizing legislation and enabling regulations—United States, October 1993. MMWR Morb Mortal Wkly Rep 1994;43:71,74–75.
8. Hoel DG, Davis DL, Miller AB, et al: Trends in cancer mortality in 15 industrialized countries, 1969–1986. J Natl Cancer Inst 1992;84:313–320.
9. Devesa SS, Blot WJ, Stone BJ, et al: Recent cancer trends in the United States. J Natl Cancer Inst 1995;87:175–182.
10. Metropolitan Insurance Companies: Cancer incidence, mortality and survival: Trends in four leading sites. Stat Bull Metrop Insur Co 1994;75:19–27.

11. Lenhard RE: Cancer statistics: A measure of progress. CA Cancer J Clin 1996:46:3–4.
12. Scroggins TG, Bateman M, Allen S, et al: Cancer incidence and mortality among African Americans. J La State Med Soc 1994;146:147–151.
13. Wilkes G, Freeman H, Prout M: Cancer and poverty: Breaking the cycle. Semin Oncol Nurs 1994;10:79–88.
14. Nutting PA, Freeman WL, Risser DR, et al: Cancer incidence among American Indians and Alaska Natives, 1980 through 1987. Am J Public Health 1993;83:1589–1598.

Chapter 2

Tumors of the Central Nervous System

Janet Pinner, MSN, RN,
Paula DeMasi, MSN, RN, CNS, and
Franco DeMonte, MD, FRCS(C), FACS

The brain is a soft mass of nerve and connective tissue attached to the spinal cord. The brain and spinal cord together form the central nervous system (CNS).

The CNS controls personality, memory, speech, emotions, sensation, and movement. Tumors that affect the CNS may originate in the CNS or in other sites with subsequent spread to the CNS. Tumors that originate in the CNS are called primary brain tumors; those that originate in other sites and spread to the CNS are called metastatic tumors.

Tumors that originate in the brain may be classified as benign (slow-growing) or malignant (fast-growing). Although the distinction between benign and malignant is important, either type of tumor can have fatal consequences. The reason for this is that the brain is encased in the closed, unyielding, bony compartment of the skull. Any tumor in the brain that causes a mass or swelling is by its very nature life-threatening. Primary brain tumors typically do not spread outside the brain and spinal cord. This chapter discusses signs and symptoms of brain tumors by location, diagnosis, and the various types of tumors that can occur in the CNS, with incidence, survival, and treatment options. Following that is a discussion of tumors of the spinal cord and column. Finally, an overview of the management of CNS tumors is presented.

BRAIN TUMORS

FACTS AND STATISTICS

The annual incidence rate for all primary brain tumors (benign and malignant) ranges from 4.8 to 19.6 per 100,000, depending on the age group studied. Approximately half of all primary brain tumors are benign and can be treated successfully. On average, 17,500 new cases are diagnosed annually in the United States. Patients with malignant brain tumors treated in clinical trials appear to survive longer than other patients with these tumors.[1]

CAUSES

The cause of primary brain tumors is unknown. It is most likely not a single cause but a combination of factors. Many clinical studies are under way in an attempt to identify possible causes or factors. Current areas of investigation include genetic damage or changes (mutation), inheritance, chance errors in fetal development, ionizing radiation (electromagnetic fields), a weak or defective immune system, viruses, injury, diet, chemicals, hormones, and environmental or occupational factors.[1]

SYMPTOMS

Symptoms of a brain tumor depend on its size and the area of brain it affects. Symptoms are caused both by the tumor and by the swelling or "mass effect" that the tumor produces. The brain is contained within a bony compartment and can tolerate very little increase in mass before rapid increases in pressure occur. One of the most common presenting symptoms of a brain tumor is increased intracranial pressure (ICP). Signs and symptoms of increased ICP include headache, which is worse in the morning and eases during the day; vomiting, which also usually occurs in the morning, with or without nausea; mental status changes such as lethargy and altered level of consciousness; papilledema, which may be associated with decreased visual acuity, visual field defects, or double vision (diplopia); discoordination that manifests as ataxia or clumsiness; focal or generalized seizures; weakness that results in temporary or partial paralysis, sensory loss, or change in sensation; and disturbances in speech and language that may affect expression (verbalization), reception (processing what is heard), or both. ICP also increases as a result of hydrocephalus, which is caused by tumor blocking the normal flow of cerebrospinal fluid (CSF) within the brain.[1-3]

Because various parts of the brain are responsible for specific functions, the symptoms with which a patient presents offer clues about the location of the tumor. The most common symptoms of a tumor of the brain stem (which includes the midbrain [mesencephalon], pons, and medulla oblongata) are vomiting, ataxia, dysphagia, visual changes, dysfunction of the lower cranial nerves, hemiparesis, and unilateral sensory changes. Tumors that occur in the cerebello-pontine angle cause hearing loss, tinnitus, and vertigo.

A tumor of the cerebral hemisphere causes a disruption of the normal functions of the affected lobe. A tumor in the frontal lobe may cause hemiplegia, ataxia, and behavioral changes such as defective memory and impaired judgment.[1] Persons with a tumor of the frontal lobe often complain of headache and slowed thought processes. A constellation of symptoms, collectively referred to as *frontal lobe syndrome*, is common; clinical findings include inappropriate social behavior, indifference, difficulty concentrating, emotional lability, and difficulty with abstract thinking. Tumors that occur at the base of the frontal lobe can cause papilledema and anosmia.

Tumors that occur in the parietal lobe commonly cause seizures and speech disturbances; an inability to recognize objects by feel (astereognosis) and spatial disorientation also occur. If the tumor is in the dominant hemisphere of the parietal lobe (typically the left side), an inability to write (agraphia) is common. Homonymous hemianopia, hypoesthesia or hyperesthesia, and loss of the ability to distinguish between right and left are also noted.

For tumors of the temporal lobe, the most common symptoms are psychomotor seizures, dysphasia, and speech or language disorders. Language disorders include difficulty in understanding and expressing verbal or written language. Homonymous quadrantanopsia, auditory hallucinations, and, sometimes, aggressive behavior are also seen.

Contralateral homonymous hemianopia is the most common symptom resulting from a tumor in the occipital lobe. Visual hallucinations may also occur, and focal or generalized seizures are sometimes seen.

Tumors may also affect the basal ganglia, the pituitary gland, the thalamus, the skull base, the cavernous sinus, or the posterior fossa. Tumors that affect the basal ganglia most commonly cause nonspecific headaches as a result of increased ICP and hydrocephalus. The clinical findings produced by pituitary tumors may include visual loss, diabetes insipidus, and hormonal disturbances that produce amenorrhea, galactorrhea, gigantism, Cushing's syndrome, acromegaly, and hypopituitarism. Common clinical findings of tumors that occur in the posterior fossa (fourth ventricle) include headaches, nausea, papilledema, and ataxia. Tumors in this location may also cause a lack of control over the range of muscular movement (dysmetria), disturbance in gait, and sixth-nerve palsies.

Because of the depth of their location, tumors of the skull base or cavernous sinus often cause paresis of the cranial nerves, which can result in anosmia, loss of visual acuity and portions of the visual field, nystagmus, alteration in pupil response to light and accommodation, inability to open and close the eyelids, facial atrophy and hypoesthesia, facial asymmetry, slurred speech, hearing loss, dysphagia, hoarseness, diminished corneal reflex, tongue fasciculations or atrophy, and decreased size, shape, or strength of the sternocleidomastoid muscles.

DIAGNOSIS OF BRAIN TUMORS

Findings from a patient's complete medical history and physical examination, including a careful neurologic examination, may lead a practitioner to suspect the presence of a brain tumor. The next logical step is to obtain imaging studies, of which magnetic resonance imaging (MRI) is the most useful. The next most useful technique is computed tomography (CT), but CT is less sensitive for imaging of the brain and may not image smaller tumors. Contrast enhancement is required for both MRI and CT if tumor is suspected. An MRI or CT scan without the use of a contrast agent will not provide adequate information and will almost always have to be repeated.

Once a lesion has been identified, other studies may be needed to establish whether it is primary or metastatic. For some tumors, histologic analysis of a tissue sample obtained at biopsy or surgical resection is required for diagnosis. If a lumbar puncture is required, it must be preceded by a CT or MRI scan to determine if hydrocephalus is present or the ICP is increased. In these cases, a lumbar puncture could cause downward herniation of the brain, resulting in compression of the brain stem.

TYPES OF BRAIN TUMORS

PRIMARY BRAIN TUMORS

The most common brain tumors, ranked by incidence, are astrocytomas (including anaplastic astrocytoma and glioblastoma multiforme [GBM]), followed by oligodendroglioma, ependymoma, medulloblastoma, pineal parenchymal tumor, meningioma, germ cell tumor, sarcoma, and hemangioblastoma.

Astrocytoma

Astrocytomas are the most common primary brain tumors and are graded according to their level of malignancy (i.e., low, intermediate, or high). Because astrocytomas often contain cells of different grades, the most malignant or highest grade of cell determines the overall grade of the tumor. Tumor grade is very important for both treatment and prognosis.[3]

Low-grade astrocytomas are often considered benign because they grow very slowly. However, this characteristic is in conflict with this tumor's inherent nature, which is to invade and grow into surrounding areas. Whether to treat low-grade astrocytomas and the type and extent of treatment to use remain controversial issues.[3] If a low-grade astrocytoma is operable, some centers recommend only surgical removal. Other centers recommend that after a definitive diagnosis is made from tissue specimens obtained at biopsy or surgical resection, the patient should undergo radiation therapy of the involved area and periodic follow-up with serial MRI or CT scans. The prognosis of low-grade astrocytoma depends on the tumor's location, the patient's age, the extent of resection, and the patient's functional status after surgery.

Middle-grade astrocytomas, also called anaplastic astrocytomas or malignant astrocytomas, are, as the name implies, infiltrating, malignant tumors.[1, 3] These tumors grow more rapidly and recur more quickly than do low-grade astrocytomas; sometimes they recur as higher-grade tumors.[1] Their treatment is based on the location of the tumor and on the general health and age of the patient. Surgery followed by radiation therapy and chemotherapy is usually recommended.[1, 3]

The high-grade astrocytomas include GBM, gliosarcoma, and giant cell glioblastoma.[1] High-grade astrocytomas are the most common primary brain tumors to occur in middle-aged adults, and they account for about 30% of all primary brain tumors and 50% of all astrocytomas.[3] High-grade astrocytomas are grade 4 tumors; they are more common in men than in women. These are the most malignant of brain tumors.[1, 3] A GBM can double in size every 10 to 15 days. Most symptoms of GBM (e.g., seizures, headaches, behavior changes) are caused by increased ICP. Treatment depends on tumor location, extent of disease, and the patient's age at onset. The prognosis depends on tumor location, extent of resection, and the patient's functional status after surgery. The treatment of choice is surgery followed by irradiation and chemotherapy.[4] Among adults with GBM who undergo surgery and radiation therapy, 25% to 50% survive 1 year, 10% survive 2 years, and 1% survive 5 years or longer. Many clinical trials are currently under way to investigate the use of gene therapy, monoclonal antibodies, biologic response modifiers, and chemotherapeutic agents for GBM. New treatments are being investigated constantly for this most frequently occurring astrocytoma.[2, 3]

Ependymoma

Ependymoma is the next most common primary brain tumor. These tumors arise from the ependymal cells that line the ventricles and the central canal of the spinal cord. They comprise 6% of all primary brain tumors and 10% of brain tumors in children. The majority (70%) of ependymomas occur in the posterior fossa; the rest are found in the supratentorium and the spinal cord. Ependymomas can be infiltrative or noninfiltrative and can occur in people of all ages. Benign, low-grade ependymomas occur more often than do malignant, high-grade ependymomas. The malignant form, called anaplastic ependymoma, represents about 10% of these tumors and can seed to other locations in the CNS via the CSF.

The treatment of choice for these tumors is surgical excision followed by irradiation of the brain and spinal cord. Frequently, a ventriculoperitoneal shunt is required to relieve the increased ICP caused by an ependymoma.[4] Chemotherapy may be used for recurrent ependymoma. Other treatments such as gene therapy are being investigated. These tumors recur if all cells are not removed or killed by treatment. Recurrence is usually in the area of the original tumor or in the CNS. For patients with ependymomas, 5-year survival rates range from 20% to 60%, depending on tumor site, grade, and completeness of excision.[1, 3]

Oligodendroglioma

The next most prevalent primary brain tumor is oligodendroglioma. These tumors arise from the supportive brain tissue and typically arise in the white matter and infiltrate the cortex.[3] Oligodendroglioma is most likely to occur in the cerebral hemisphere of a middle-aged adult, but it is not uncommon in children. Men are affected more often than women.[1] These tumors may be present for years before their diagnosis. Oligodendrogliomas account for 5% of all primary brain tumors and for 10% to 15% of gliomas.

Tumors recur when cells that have not been removed by surgery or killed by other treatments multiply. An oligodendroglioma may recur as a higher-grade tumor.[1] Surgical resection followed by irradiation is the recommended treatment. This type of glioma is more chemosensitive than astrocytoma, and the combination of procarbazine, lomustine, and vincristine (PCV) has been found to be effective treatment.[1]

Choroid Plexus Papilloma

Choroid plexus papilloma is a rare, benign tumor that most frequently occurs in the lateral ventricles. It is most common in children younger than 12 years of age and represents about 4% of primary brain tumors in that age group. In adults, this tumor is commonly located in the fourth ventricle and represents 1% of primary brain tumors. Choroid plexus papillomas grow slowly within the ventricles and eventually block the flow of CSF, resulting in increased ICP and hydrocephalus. As with most brain tumors, the treatment of choice is surgery. Some patients require a ventriculoperitoneal shunt in addition to surgical resection to control their hydrocephalus. Choroid plexus papilloma is resistant to radiation therapy; however, irradiation may be recommended for resistant or residual tumors.[1]

Medulloblastoma

Medulloblastoma is the most common primary brain tumor in children, although 20% of these tumors occur in adults.[1] This malignant, rapidly growing tumor accounts for 15% to 20% of pediatric brain tumors and is always located in the cerebellum.[1] Medulloblastoma is invasive and spreads to other parts of the CNS via the CSF. Because this type of brain tumor is relatively radiosensitive, therapy consists of surgical excision followed by irradiation of the brain and spinal cord. Very young children may be treated with surgery followed by chemotherapy, with radiation therapy delayed until they are older. This tumor is very responsive to treatment. Patients with residual tumor after surgery or with a tumor involving the brain stem receive adjunctive chemotherapy. Medulloblastomas do recur and require repeat surgery followed by chemotherapy. Clinical trials of therapies for this tumor are being conducted at specialty centers.

Pineal Region Tumors

Pineal region tumors represent fewer than 1% of all primary brain tumors, although 5% to 8% of childhood brain tumors occur in this area.[1] The most common tumor to occur in the pineal region is a germinoma. Germinomas account for more than one third of the tumors in this region, and they occur most commonly in teenagers.

Pinealocytoma is a slow-growing, low-grade tumor. The malignant, more aggressive form is called a pinealoblastoma. The presenting symptoms of pineal region tumors typically are caused by obstructive hydrocephalus. Surgical resection or biopsy for diagnosis (if a resection is not possible) is recommended, followed by irradiation, which may be either conventional radiotherapy or radiosurgery. Chemotherapy is also employed if the tumor is a pinealoblastoma. A ventriculoperitoneal shunt may be required if the hydrocephalus cannot be controlled with steroids.

Meningiomas

Meningiomas typically are benign and slow-growing tumors, but 5% to 10% of them are malignant and aggressive. This tumor, which represents 15% to 20% of all primary brain tumors, occurs more frequently in middle-aged adults and is more common in women.[1] Benign meningiomas are slow growing, with distinct borders. Typically, meningiomas compress rather than invade nearby structures; for this reason, the tumor can become quite large before it causes symptoms.[5] Atypical meningiomas are faster growing and tend to recur. Anaplastic meningiomas and hemangiopericytomas are malignant and tend to invade brain tissues.[5] The more malignant meningiomas are difficult to eliminate by surgery alone; therefore, postoperative radiation therapy may be given. Several clinical trials currently under way are exploring chemotherapy and hormone-modulating drugs for the treatment of this tumor.[1, 12, 13]

Hemangioblastoma

Hemangioblastoma is a benign, tumor-like mass that occurs in the cerebellum and accounts for 2% of all primary brain tumors. Hemangioblastoma typically occurs in people between the ages of 35 and 45 years. When it occurs in the blood vessels of the cerebellum, the most common site, this tumor is usually cystic. Polycythemia may be present in 20% of patients owing to the tumor's ability to secrete erythropoietin.[1] Hemangioblastoma can also occur in the retina or spinal cord. An autosomal dominant form of hemangioblastoma is associated with the genetic syndrome known as von Hippel-Lindau disease.

These tumors are slow growing and do not metastasize. Surgery is the treatment of choice. Hemangioblastomas that occur in the brain stem can be treated with stereotactic radiosurgery. The prognosis is good with complete removal of the tumor. Radiation therapy is indicated if the tumor recurs.[1-3]

Pituitary Adenoma

Pituitary adenomas account for 15% of all primary brain tumors. Although rarely diagnosed before puberty, they occur in every age group. Pituitary tumors are classified according to the hormone they secrete, their histologic characteristics, and their size. Pituitary tumors smaller than 10 mm in diameter are called microadenomas; larger ones are called macroadenomas.[1, 7] In general, symptoms include visual disorders, headache, and hormone abnormalities. Specifically, prolactin-secreting tumors produce amenorrhea, galactorrhea, impotence, infertility, and, in the long term, osteoporosis.

Growth hormone–producing tumors represent 20% of all pituitary adenomas, are more common in men, and often are macroadenomas at the time of diagnosis. These tumors produce gigantism, acromegaly, and decreased initiative.

Adrenocorticotropic hormone–producing adenomas make up 14% of pituitary adenomas and occur most often in women. Symptoms of these tumors are related to the excess cortisol, which causes Cushing's syndrome, "moon face," myopathy, hypertension, and glucose intolerance.

Nonsecreting pituitary tumors, which account for 25% of all pituitary adenomas, are usually macroadenomas, and the diagnosis and presenting symptoms are related to the size of the tumor. The symptoms include visual loss, headache, panhypopituitarism, weakness, fatigue, and loss of sexual function.

Depending on the hormone secreted, medical therapy may be indicated. The most common example is treatment of prolactin-secreting tumors with bromocriptine. Therapy for pituitary tumors depends on hormonal activity of the tumor, size and location of the lesion, and age and overall health of the patient. The goals of treatment include complete surgical removal of the tumor, reduction in tumor size if complete excision is not possible, and rebalancing of hormone levels. Radiation therapy is sometimes employed for resistant tumors. Microadenomas have a high cure rate when treated surgically and typically do not recur. Macroadenomas may require additional surgery combined with radiation or drug therapy, or both.[1,7]

METASTATIC BRAIN TUMORS

Metastatic brain tumors are tumors that originated elsewhere in the body and spread to the brain. Tumors can metastasize to any area of the brain, spinal cord, or spinal column. The cancers that most frequently spread to the brain are lung, breast, colon, and kidney cancers and melanoma. Cancers that metastasize to the bones of the spinal column include breast, prostate, lung, and kidney cancers and melanoma. Metastasis to the spinal cord is extremely rare but can occur from melanoma or cervical, breast, or lung cancers.[8-11]

Most cerebral metastases (80%) occur within the cerebral hemispheres, with lesser numbers found in the cerebellum and brain stem. Metastases have a marked propensity to produce extensive edema in surrounding brain tissues. Frequently, there is rapid neurologic deterioration and dysfunction.[9] In considering treatment, many factors must be evaluated, including tumor size, site, and histology; the patient's age, overall status, and neurologic condition; and the extent of systemic disease. A poor prognosis accompanies disseminated cancer; more than 50% of these patients have uncontrolled systemic disease. Resection of metastases in the brain is performed to maintain or improve the patient's quality of life and/or to allow more time for further therapy such as chemotherapy.[8–10]

TUMORS OF THE SPINAL CORD AND COLUMN

As in the brain, tumors of the spinal cord may be primary or metastatic, benign or malignant. Common tumor types include metastatic tumors (from breast, prostate, lung, kidney, and melanoma), chordomas, schwannomas, meningiomas, astrocytomas, and ependymomas. Primary spinal cord tumors are most often intradural and extramedullary.[1, 2] Malignant tumors that invade the bones of the spinal column result in bone destruction, vertebral collapse, pain, and spinal cord compression.[1]

Metastatic disease in the spine and spinal cord compression are major causes of morbidity and mortality in cancer patients. The skeletal system is the third most common site of metastatic involvement, after the lung and the liver. Within the skeletal system, the spinal column is the most common site of metastatic disease.[14] Treatment of metastatic disease to the spine frequently requires surgical decompression, reconstruction, and stabilization in addition to radiation therapy and chemotherapy.[11]

Many symptoms of spinal tumors are caused by compression of the spinal cord and have a gradual onset. Pain, muscle weakness, sensory changes, and bowel or bladder dysfunction or incontinence are the most common presenting symptoms. Pain and paresis are dictated by the level of spinal cord involvement. Tumors in the cervical spine cause paresis or paralysis of the upper and lower extremities. Those at the thoracic and lumbar levels cause paresis of the lower extremities, sensory changes, sexual dysfunction, and changes in bowel or bladder function.

Surgery is the treatment of choice for spinal tumors, with irradiation recommended for malignant or partially resected tumors. In cases of spinal cord compression, time is of the utmost importance. Treatment, whether surgery or radiation, must by instituted within 72 hours of compression to avoid complete and irreversible paralysis. Steroids may be given to protect spinal cord function, but this is only a temporary measure. Radical removal of spinal tumors is now possible because of the availability of an apparatus for spinal reconstruction.[1, 10, 11, 14]

Metastasis to the intradural extramedullary compartment of the spine is rare. Only 5% of cases of metastatic disease involve this area.[10] Pain, weakness, and sensory changes are presenting symptoms. Surgical excision is the recommended treatment if it is possible, with irradiation and chemotherapy for inaccessible tumors.[10]

TUMOR MANAGEMENT

As indicated by the descriptions of individual tumors, surgery is the treatment of choice for tumors that occur in the CNS. The goals of surgery may include

(1) removal of all visible tumor; (2) removal of at least part of the tumor in order to provide relief of symptoms, improve the patient's quality of life, and reduce the tumor burden, thereby allowing the tumor to be treated with other modalities; (3) establishment of an exact diagnosis to guide future therapies; and (4) stabilization of the spine and protection of spinal cord function. Many benign tumors are treated by surgical excision alone.

Because many tumor cells are radiosensitive, radiation therapy (to the whole brain, focal field, or craniospinal axis; stereotactic radiosurgery or brachytherapy) may be used depending on the tumor type and location. Use of radiation therapy is limited by the most sensitive structure in the planned radiation field. Only a limited amount of radiation can be delivered to a given area in a lifetime; in the case of the brain, whole-brain irradiation can be delivered only once.[2–5]

Chemotherapy is available for some CNS tumors, but the structure of the CNS makes the use of this modality difficult. The brain and spine are areas of sanctuary from toxic substances. The blood-brain barrier, which protects the CNS from many diseases, also prevents many systemic chemotherapy regimens from being very effective. Some chemotherapy regimens can cross the blood-brain barrier, but their use is limited by the size and type of the tumor. Chemotherapy may be delivered intrathecally through an Ommaya reservoir or by means of a lumbar puncture. It may also be given intra-arterially or intraoperatively directly to the tumor site. In addition, large cancer centers offer investigational protocols and therapies, which may be beneficial.

Steroids are frequently used to control swelling and edema in the tissues of the brain and spinal cord. Dexamethasone and prednisone are examples of commonly used steroids. These are given in the perioperative period and during radiation therapy. Their long-term use is not recommended because of their side effects, which include psychosis, muscle atrophy, gastric ulceration, excess fat deposition, osteoporosis, and Cushing's syndrome. Steroid administration is tapered off rather than abruptly stopped. This is because steroids cause adrenal suppression and the abrupt cessation of steroid administration may put the patient into an adrenal crisis, which can be life-threatening.[2]

Finally, the use of biologic response modifiers to treat CNS tumors is under investigation at large cancer centers, with available protocols depending on tumor type.[13]

Several national organizations offer additional information on CNS tumors. These include the American Brain Tumor Association, the National Brain Tumor Foundation, the American Cancer Society, and the Anderson Network of The University of Texas M.D. Anderson Cancer Center.[*]

---

[*]American Brain Tumor Association, 1-800-886-2282; National Brain Tumor Foundation, 1-800-934-CURE; American Cancer Society, 1-800-227-2345; Anderson Network of the University of Texas M.D. Anderson Cancer Center, 1-800-345-6324.

REFERENCES

1. Thapar K, Laws ER Jr: Tumors of the central nervous system. In Murphy GP, Lawrence W Jr, Lenhard RE Jr (eds): American Cancer Society Textbook of Clinical Oncology, 2nd ed. Atlanta, American Cancer Society, 1995:378–410.
2. Hickey J: The Clinical Practice of Neurological and Neurosurgical Nursing, 3rd ed. Philadelphia, JB Lippincott, 1992.
3. Levin VA (ed): Cancer in the Nervous System. New York, Churchill-Livingstone, 1996.
4. Rengachary S, Wilkins R (eds): Principles of Neurosurgery. London, Wolfe, 1994,
5. What You Need to Know About Brain Tumors. NIH publication no. 93-1558. Washington, DC, National Cancer Institute, 1992.

6. Cheek WM (ed): Pediatric Neurosurgery, 3rd ed. Philadelphia, WB Saunders, 1989.
7. Soo EW, Galindo EG, Levin VA: Brain tumors. In Pazdur R (ed): Medical Oncology: A Comprehensive Review, 2nd ed. Huntington, NY, PRR Inc, 1995.
8. Sawaya R, Ligon L, Flowers A, et al: Management of metastatic brain tumors: A review. Neurosurgery Quarterly 1994;3:140.
9. Bindal R, Sawaya R, Leavens M, et al: Surgical treatment of multiple brain metastases. J Neurosurg 1994;79:210.
10. Chow TS, McCutcheon IE: The surgical treatment of metastatic spinal tumors within the intradural extramedullary compartment. J Neurosurg 1996;85:225–230.
11. Gokaslan ZL: Spine surgery for cancer. Curr Opin Oncol 1996;8:178–181.
12. DeMonte F, Al-Mefty O: Meningioma. In Kaye AH, Laws ER (eds): Brain Tumors. Edinburgh, Churchill-Livingstone, 1995:675–704.
13. Kaba S, DeMonte F, et al: The treatment of unresectable and malignant meningiomas with interferon alpha 2B. Neurosurgery 1997;40(2):271–275.
14. Akeyson E, McCutcheon IE: Single-stage posterior vertebrectomy and replacement combined with posterior instrumentation for spinal metastasis. J Neurosurg 1996;85:211–220.

Chapter 3

Head and Neck Cancer

Debra S. Foreman, BS, PA-C, and
David L. Callender, MD, MBA

Cancers of the head and neck develop between the base of the skull and the thorax. Many organ systems are closely integrated in this space, each with its characteristic function and interdependent with all the others. The organ systems of the head and neck region are the upper respiratory and digestive tracts, the eyes, the cranial nerves, and important vascular trunks including the internal and external jugular veins, the internal and external carotid arteries, vertebral arteries, and lymph vessels. Also part of the system are the ears, the thyroid, and the skin. The area has 50 potential sites for the origin of primary tumors.

Head and neck cancers represent only a small percentage of malignancies, but their impact and that of associated treatments are a significant component of total cancer morbidity and mortality. The effects include loss of speech and swallowing, loss of vision, and significant cosmetic deformity. Because of the myriad of primary sites and tissues involved, it is important to divide the head and neck into manageable sections for study. This chapter discusses the lips and oral cavity; oropharynx and hypopharynx; nasal cavity, nasopharynx, and paranasal sinus; larynx; salivary glands; neck; and ears. Thyroid and skin cancers are discussed in other chapters. Primary ophthalmic tumors are rare and are not discussed here, except to note that the orbit and its contents may be invaded by other malignancies of the head and neck.

EPIDEMIOLOGY

Cancers of the head and neck comprise approximately 4% of all cancers diagnosed in the United States.[1] In 1997, 41,650 new cases of head and neck cancer and 16,100 thyroid cancers were documented in the United States, with approximately 12,670 deaths.[1] Worldwide, 500,000 new head and neck cancers are projected to occur annually.[2] These cancers strike men predominantly, but an increased incidence has been noted in women. The cancers occur generally during the fifth to sixth decades of life, although an increased incidence in the third to fourth decades of life has been noted for cancers of the oral cavity and tongue.[2] At 15-fold higher risk are long-term users of alcohol, tobacco, and betel nut.[2] In Utah, the incidence and mortality rates for head and neck cancer are one half those of the United States as a whole. This is probably a result of the Mormon religious practice of an alcohol- and tobacco-free lifestyle. New Jersey, in contrast, has one of the highest rates of head and neck cancer in the country.[1]

The fact that head and neck cancers are diagnosed and treated more effectively in whites than in blacks is believed to be related to the limited access to health care of people of low socioeconomic status.[1] Furthermore, 5% to 10% of those who present with a head and neck cancer have a malignancy in another nearby area.[2]

Certain regions of the world report a higher prevalence of head and neck cancer. In Hong Kong and South China, nasopharyngeal cancer is prevalent and may be linked to genetic and viral causes and to a diet rich in nitrosamines.[2] In Bombay, India, a higher incidence of oral cavity and base-of-tongue cancers is associated with the practice of reverse smoking—that is, smoking with the lighted end of the cigarette in the oral cavity.[3]

In addition to heavy, long-term alcohol abuse, the abuse of tobacco products such as smokeless tobacco, snuff, cigarettes, pipe tobacco, and cigars and marijuana increases the risk of head and neck cancer.[3] More than 30 carcinogens are associated with a 20 pack-year history of smoking.[1]

Diet is an important risk factor in head and neck cancer. A diet high in nitrosamines and one deficient in vitamin C, riboflavin, and iodine contributes to the risk, as does the poor nutritional state commonly found in chronic alcoholics. Also at risk are patients with Plummer-Vinson syndrome, which usually occurs in middle-aged women with hypochromic anemia.[2]

The genetic diseases associated with head and neck cancers include Bloom syndrome and Li-Fraumeni syndrome. Associated viral diseases include those caused by the human papilloma and Epstein-Barr viruses.[2]

Many environmental factors have been associated with head and neck cancer. Woodworking, furniture manufacturing, and nickel refining are occupations associated with increased risk. Exposure to asbestos, textile fiber, or leather refinishing carries such a risk, as does exposure to coke ovens, polycyclic hydrocarbons, or radiochemicals.[1]

Head and neck irradiation is a strong risk factor in the development of head and neck cancer.[1] In the past, patients underwent external beam irradiation for acne, tonsils, adenoids, thymus enlargement, and psoriasis, treatments that predispose to carcinoma of the head and neck. Today these problems are treated with other methods.

Other risk factors include poor oral hygiene and irritation from ill-fitting dentures and appliances.[4] Prolonged ultraviolet light exposure from outdoor occupations, tanning beds, and psoriasis treatments has also been linked to cancer of the head and neck. Other risk factors are chronic sinusitis, syphilis, and the chronic immunosuppression that organ transplantation patients must undergo as part of their treatment.

GENETICS

Two autosomal dominant growth disorders already mentioned, Bloom and Li-Fraumeni syndromes, are associated with head and neck cancers in patients who have had minimal exposure to tobacco.[2]

Some patients with head and neck cancer seem to be more sensitive than others to the mutagenic effects of bleomycin; theirs may be a mutagen sensitivity.[2] Xeroderma pigmentosum, a hereditary condition that begins in early childhood with the appearance of skin cancers, is also associated with head and neck cancers. Affected patients usually die in early puberty.

PRESENTING HISTORY AND PHYSICAL EXAMINATION

The physical examination should be thorough, with emphasis on the head and neck region. It should include visual inspection as well as manual palpation. Such an examination may reveal ulcerative lesions, exophytic lesions, pigmented lesions, a firm mass, cranial nerve deficits (abnormal tongue protrusion or abnormal palatal elevation), leukoplakia (white plaques that do not rub off with swab), or erythroplakia (red, velvety lesions).

First, a visual examination of the skin (scalp, face, ears, and neck) should be conducted. Then, in concise and logical order, the following examination should be done:

1. Visually inspect the lips and oral cavity with tongue blades. Evaluate all mucosal surfaces—gingiva, tongue,

lingual tonsils, anterior tonsillar pillar, retromolar trigone, alveolar ridges, hard and soft palate, uvula, and floor of mouth. A proper head and neck examination is always performed without the patient's dentures or other dental appliances.

2. Position the patient properly for examination of the nasal cavity. Ask the patient to sit upright with legs uncrossed in a "sniffing" position (head slightly extended with nose in a sniffing position). Visually inspect the nares and anterior nasal cavity with the nasal speculum.

3. Place the patient in a proper position to begin the mirror examination of the nasopharynx, oropharynx, hypopharynx, and larynx. Fiberoptic examination of these sites may be appropriate as well. The nasopharyngeal and laryngeal mirrors must be warmed in advance of the examination to avoid fogging of the mirror. Testing the mirror on the back of the examiner's hand will prevent inadvertent burns to the patient's mucosa.

   a. To examine the nasopharynx, place a tongue blade on the patient's tongue and insert the nasopharyngeal mirror posteriorly behind the uvula. Ask the patient to breathe slowly through the nose to facilitate this examination.

   b. Examination of the oropharynx, hypopharynx, and larynx requires the examiner to be patient and practiced. Ask the patient to protrude the tongue; then grasp the tongue with gauze. Apply a firm and steady pull while the warmed mirror is inserted posteriorly. Ask the patient to keep eyes open and to pant-breathe. Visualization of the vocal cords in respiration and vocalization is imperative.

4. With a gloved hand, palpate the oral cavity, floor of mouth, base of tongue, and oropharynx.

5. Visually examine the external auditory canals and tympanic membranes with the otoscope.

6. Visually inspect and palpate the neck at all nodal stations and the thyroid gland. Evaluate any masses, tenderness, or skin lesions.

7. Inspect all cranial nerve functions for deficits.

LIPS AND ORAL CAVITY

This region includes the oral tongue, buccal mucosa, lips, alveolar ridges, floor of mouth, tonsils, hard and soft palate, and uvula (Fig. 3–1). The patient's presenting history may include painful or painless ulcer or recurrent sore or blister that bleeds and does not heal, exophytic mass, referred otalgia, oral bleeding, difficulty chewing or swallowing, ill-fitting dentures, slurred speech,

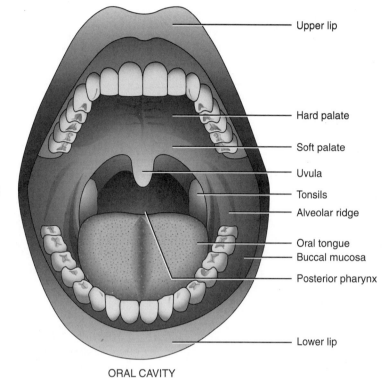

Figure 3–1. Region of lips and oral cavity.

ORAL CAVITY

mass, sore throat, weight loss, or neck mass. All of these complaints must be addressed to obtain an accurate picture of the patient's chief complaint.

OROPHARYNX AND HYPOPHARYNX

This region includes the anterior tonsillar pillar, faucial arch, tonsillar fossa, soft palate, base of tongue, pharyngeal wall, and pyriform sinus (Fig. 3–2). A

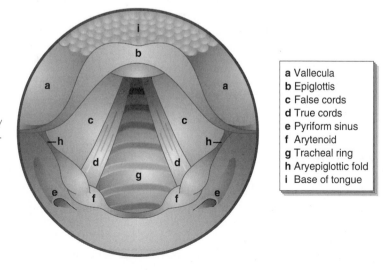

Figure 3–2. Region of oropharynx/hypopharynx as seen by direct/indirect laryngoscopy.

a Vallecula
b Epiglottis
c False cords
d True cords
e Pyriform sinus
f Arytenoid
g Tracheal ring
h Aryepiglottic fold
i Base of tongue

history should be obtained of the following complaints: odynophagia or pain with swallowing, sore throat, globus sensation, local pain, otalgia, dysphagia, trismus, bleeding, weight loss, neck mass, aspiration, chronic cough, dental changes, ulcer, and hoarseness.

A thorough physical examination that includes visual evaluation and palpation as well as an indirect mirror or fiberoptic examination may reveal ulcerative lesions, exophytic lesions, induration, mass, or cranial nerve deficits.

NASAL CAVITY, NASOPHARYNX, AND PARANASAL SINUS

This region includes the anterior nares, nasopharynx, septum, turbinates, and frontal, maxillary, ethmoid, and sphenoid sinuses. A thorough history may suggest nasal obstruction, mass, rhinorrhea, postnasal drip, epistaxis, dental changes (loose teeth, pain), proptosis, diplopia, bulging cheek mass, lateral rectus muscle paralysis, visual changes, pain, headache, unilateral hearing loss, sore throat, sensory nerve changes (hyperesthesia of infraorbital nerve, numbness over cheek), trismus, or halitosis.

A complete physical examination of this region should include a visual inspection with the indirect mirror or fiberoptic endoscope, nasopharyngoscopy, otoscopy, anterior nasal inspection, and direct laryngoscopy. This examination may reveal ulcerative bleeding or exophytic mass, polypoid mass, pigmented lesion, or edematous membranes.

LARYNX

This region is composed of the supraglottic, glottic, and subglottic larynx. The supraglottic larynx includes the area from the tip of the epiglottis to the true cords. It also includes the false cords, the ventricles, the arytenoid cartilage, and aryepiglottic folds. The glottis is considered the plane that incorporates the true vocal cords; the subglottic area is below the true vocal cords. A complete history of this region should include questions concerning sore throat, otalgia, dysphagia, odynophagia, cough, aspiration, shortness of breath, stridor, weight loss, neck mass, globus sensation, or hemoptysis.

A thorough physical examination requires visual inspection with indirect laryngoscopy, fiberoptic laryngoscopy, or both to check for polyps, leukoplakia, mass (ulcerative or exophytic, submucosal), paralysis of one or both of the true or false vocal cords, pooling of secretions in the pyriform sinus, papillomas, laryngocele, or cord edema with abnormal mucosal waves.

MAJOR AND MINOR SALIVARY GLANDS

The major salivary glands include the paired parotid glands, the sublingual glands, and the submaxillary glands. A history should include questions regarding any painless mass, cranial nerve VII palsy, otalgia, ulcer, exophytic mass, or neck mass.

Physical examination should include visual and bimanual examination of the

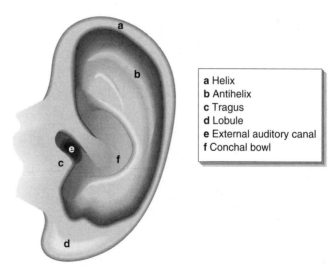

a Helix
b Antihelix
c Tragus
d Lobule
e External auditory canal
f Conchal bowl

Figure 3–3. Ear region. Auricle (pinna).

major salivary glands and their associated ducts. This may reveal a firm, fixed or nonfixed mass, ductal occlusion, facial nerve paralysis, or ulcerative lesions.

NECK

The neck is a conduit for many of the major organ systems of the human body. Careful attention to the regional anatomy of all associated organ systems may reveal a mass (firm, fixed or nonfixed), decreased range of motion, or pulsatile mass with bruit.

EARS

This region includes the external ear or pinna, the external auditory canal, the middle ear, and the inner ear (Fig. 3–3). A careful history should include questions concerning lesions (painless, ulcerative, bleeding, exophytic), decreased hearing, otalgia, otorrhea, tinnitus, and vertigo.

Physical examination of the region should include otoscopy, pneumatic otoscopy, visual inspection, and palpation. Examination findings may include lesions (exophytic, ulcerative, bleeding, indurated, exudative), hearing loss (conductive or sensorineural), or an obstructed canal (firm mass or ulcerative lesion).

PATHOLOGY AND RADIOLOGIC EVALUATION

LIPS AND ORAL CAVITY

Benign tumors in this area include hemangiomas, which are tumors of endothelial cell origin. Also found are lymphangiomas, which are benign congenital malformations of lymphatic tissue, and papillomas, which are benign epithelial tumors.[3]

Ninety-five percent of cancers in this region are squamous cell carcinomas, but other malignant tumors may be present, among them minor salivary gland tumor, melanoma, lymphoma, primary bone tumor, basal cell carcinoma, and epidermoid carcinoma.[3]

Diagnostic radiology is of little use in primary cancer of the lip unless distant or local metastasis has occurred at the time of presentation. Computed tomography (CT) and magnetic resonance imaging (MRI) are useful for detecting soft tissue and bone invasion and lesions that represent metastasis from the neck. Panographic radiograph evaluation of the mandible may be useful for assessing bony invasion.

OROPHARYNX AND HYPOPHARYNX

Benign tumors found in this region include hemangioma, lymphangioma, lipoma (tumor of fat), fibroma (tumor of connective tissue), pleomorphic adenoma (glandular epithelial tumor), myxoma (tumor formed of mucous connective tissue), chondroma (cartilaginous tumor), neurinoma (tumor of peripheral nerves), papilloma (tumor of epithelium), and keratoacanthoma (papular lesion filled with keratin plug).[3]

Malignant tumors in this region, other than squamous cell carcinoma, may include lymphoepithelioma (poorly differentiated squamous cell carcinoma variant), verrucous carcinoma (well-differentiated carcinoma), minor salivary gland tumor, lymphoma, sarcoma, and melanoma.[3]

Radiologic evaluation of this region should include CT or MRI. These are valuable for assessing lymphadenopathy, bone invasion, vessel involvement, and perineural spread. A panographic radiograph of the mandible may be useful for assessing bony involvement.

NASAL CAVITY, NASOPHARYNX, AND PARANASAL SINUS

Benign tumors of this region may include osteoma (bony tumor), fibrous dysplasia (fibro-osseous tumor), papilloma, hemangioma, lymphangioma, glioma (tumor composed of neuroglial cells), nasopharyngeal angiofibroma (the most common benign tumor), chordoma (a rare tumor of embryonic nerve tissue), teratoma (embryonic tumor), fibroma, or lipoma.[3] Because of the proximity of organ systems in the head and neck, treatment of a benign mass may not prevent disfigurement or impairment of function. The course of benign masses may be as aggressive as or more so than that of malignant ones.

Malignant tumors of the nasopharyngeal area include basal cell carcinoma, squamous cell carcinoma, melanoma, adenoid cystic carcinoma (a type of salivary gland carcinoma), adenocarcinoma, sarcoma (rare), lymphoma (rare), histiocytosis X, and rhabdomyosarcoma.[3]

Because vascular tumors may be present in the head and neck, all masses should be screened before a random biopsy is performed. If a vascular tumor is suspected, angiography should be performed before a tissue diagnosis is obtained. Radiologic evaluation of this region should include MRI of the head, base of skull, pharynx, and neck. Arteriography is essential in the diagnosis and evaluation of potential vascular tumors.

LARYNX

Benign lesions of the larynx may include laryngocele, papilloma, vocal cord polyp, Reinke edema (edema of the true vocal cords), retention cyst, and chondroma.[5]

Ninety percent of malignant tumors of the larynx are squamous cell carcinomas. Other malignant tumors of the larynx include verrucous carcinoma, adenocarcinoma, carcinosarcoma, fibrosarcoma, and chondrosarcoma.

Radiologic evaluation should include CT or MRI and a chest radiograph to rule out metastatic lesions.

SALIVARY GLANDS

Benign tumors of the salivary glands include adenoma, pleomorphic adenoma, hemangioma, lymphangioma, and Warthin tumor, the last usually appearing as a unilateral mass.

Twenty-five percent to 30% of major salivary gland tumors are malignant.[6] Mucoepidermoid carcinomas make up 34% of salivary gland tumors.[3] Other malignant tumors of the salivary glands include acinic cell, squamous cell, and adenoid cystic carcinomas, adenocarcinoma, carcinoma ex pleomorphic adenoma, and lymphoma.

Radiologic evaluation of this region should include CT or MRI of the head and neck.

NECK

The neck can be a primary site of tumor origin, but usually it is the site of local metastasis. Here, again, benign tumors may act as aggressively as malignant ones, so their risk of morbidity and mortality may be as significant as that of malignant tumors. Benign tumors found in the neck include hemangioma, lymphangioma (cystic hygroma), aneurysm, carotid body tumor (chemodectoma), lipoma, neurofibroma, schwannoma, and leiomyoma (smooth-muscle tumor).

Malignant masses in the neck include angiosarcoma and hemangiopericytoma. Other malignant tumors of the neck are leiomyosarcoma, liposarcoma, Hodgkin's lymphoma, and non-Hodgkin's lymphoma. Most metastatic lesions of the neck originate in a head and neck primary tumor.

Radiologic evaluation of this region includes CT and MRI. If a vascular lesion is suspected, arteriography should be performed.

EARS

The region of the ear may include benign lesions such as keloid masses, hemangioma, lymphangioma, dermoid tumor, papilloma, keratoma, lipoma, nevus (a congenital skin lesion), and chemodectoma (a benign, chromaffin-negative tumor of the chemoreceptor system).

Malignant lesions include basal cell carcinoma, squamous cell carcinoma, and melanoma. Precancerous lesions include Bowen's disease (a squamous cell carcinoma in situ, sometimes on mucous membranes), keratoacanthoma (a locally destructive epithelial tumor), and actinic keratosis.

Radiologic evaluation of this region should include CT and MRI if cervical metastasis is suspected and arteriography if a vascular lesion is suspected.

DIFFERENTIAL DIAGNOSIS AND DECISION ALGORITHMS

The TNM staging classification (based on the primary *tumor*, regional lymph *nodes*, and distant *metastasis*) must be used in planning treatment[7] (Tables 3–1 and 3–2). This abbreviated classification system gives the primary care practitioner an overview of the patient's condition. Even in the case of a benign lesion, the patient may require resection or other treatment to preserve life or organ function. The diagnosis of a benign lesion does not always bring with it a guarantee of definitive treatment.

OVERVIEW OF TREATMENT AND REFERRAL

LIPS AND ORAL CAVITY

Treatment of tumors of the lips and oral cavity is determined by the location and stage of the primary tumor (Fig. 3–4). Small lesions (T1 and some T2) may

---

Table 3–1. TNM Classifications of Head and Neck Tumors

Primary tumor
T_0	No evidence of primary tumor
Tis	Carcinoma in situ
T1	T_1–T_4 tumor classifications are site dependent—see Table 3–2
T2	
T3	
T4	

Cervical lymph nodes
Nx	Cannot be assessed
N0	No clinically positive nodes
N1	Single clinically positive node, ipsilateral, ≤3 cm
N2	Single ipsilateral node >3 cm and <6 cm, or multiple ipsilateral nodes none >6 cm, or bilateral or contralateral nodes none >6 cm
N2a	Single ipsilateral node >3 cm and <6 cm
N2b	Multiple ipsilateral nodes, none >6 cm
N2c	Bilateral or contralateral nodes, none >6 cm
N3	Node >6 cm

Distant metastasis
M0	No known metastasis
M1	Distant metastasis

Stages
I	T1 N0 M0
II	T2 N0 M0
III	T3 N0 M0, T1–3 N1 M0
IV	T4 N0–1 M0, any T N2–3 M0, any T any N M1

TNM, staging system for primary tumor (T), regional lymph nodes (N), and distant metastasis (M).
Data from Robbins KT (ed): Pocket Guide to Neck Dissection Classification and TNM Staging of Head and Neck Cancer. Alexandria, VA, American Academy of Otolaryngology–Head and Neck Surgery, 1991.

Table 3–2. TNM Staging of Tumors of the Head and Neck

Lips and oral cavity
    T1   ≤2 cm
    T2   >2 cm and <4 cm
    T3   >4 cm
    T4   >4 cm with deep invasion
Oropharynx and hypopharynx
    T1   ≤2 cm, confined to site of origin
    T2   >2 cm and <4 cm, extending to adjacent site without fixation of hemilarynx
    T3   >4 cm, extension to adjacent site with fixation of hemilarynx
    T4   >4 cm with invasion of bone or soft tissue
Nasal cavity, nasopharynx, and paranasal sinus
    T1   In situ or positive biopsy only
    T2   Two sites, posterosuperior and lateral walls
    T3   Extension to nasal cavity, nasopharynx, or oropharynx
    T4   Skull invasion, cranial nerve involvement
Larynx
    T1   Site of origin, normal mobility
    T2   Adjacent site without fixation
    T3   Limited to larynx with fixation
    T4   Extension beyond larynx
Major and minor salivary glands
    T1   <2 cm
    T2   2–4 cm
    T3   4–6 cm
    T4   >6 cm
           (a) No local extension
           (b) Local extension

TMN, staging system for primary tumor (T), regional lymph nodes (N), and distant metastasis (M).
Data from Robbins KT (ed): Pocket Guide to Neck Dissection Classification and TNM Staging of Head and Neck Cancer. Alexandria, VA, American Academy of Otolaryngology–Head and Neck Surgery, 1991.

be treated adequately by surgical excision or radiotherapy. Small tumors may also be well treated with an interstitial implant (brachytherapy). Combined surgical excision and postoperative radiotherapy are used for T3 and T4 lesions (Fig. 3–5). Clinically positive neck nodes are best treated with selective neck dissection and postoperative external beam radiation therapy, as are positive nodes of the mouth floor (Figs. 3–6 and 3–7). Chemotherapy is not a primary treatment modality for these areas.

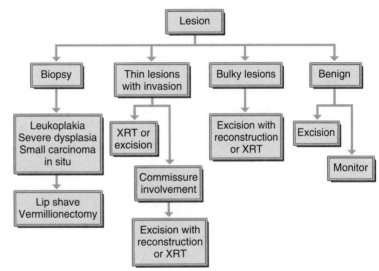

Figure 3–4. Treatment algorithm for cancer of lips and oral cavity. T, tumor; XRT, radiotherapy.

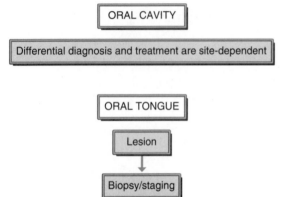

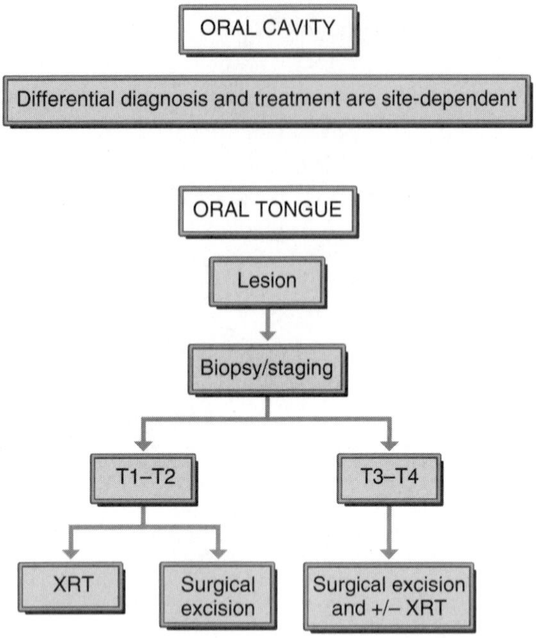

Figure 3–5. Treatment algorithm for cancer of oral cavity. XRT, radiotherapy.

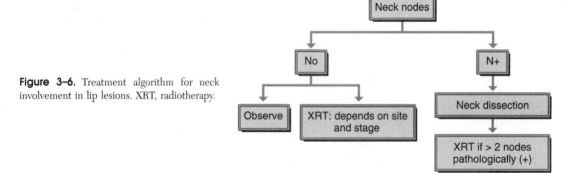

Figure 3–6. Treatment algorithm for neck involvement in lip lesions. XRT, radiotherapy.

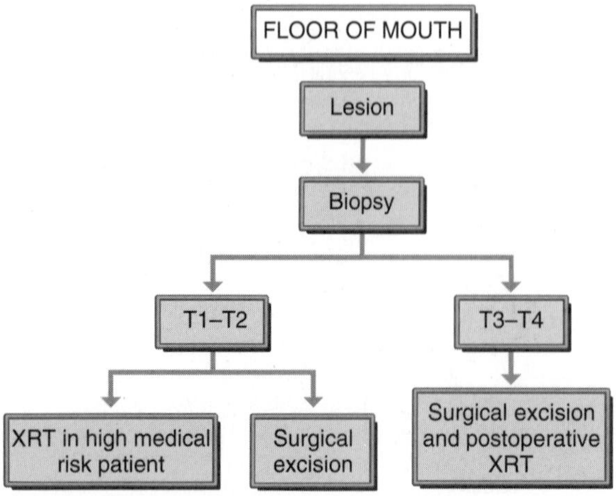

Figure 3–7. Treatment algorithm for cancer of floor of mouth. XRT, radiotherapy.

OROPHARYNX AND HYPOPHARYNX

Small lesions of the oropharynx and hypopharynx usually respond well to external beam primary radiation therapy. Site and extent of tumor are the two most important factors in determining treatment modality. Treatment options include surgical resection, external beam radiation therapy, combined surgery and radiotherapy, chemotherapy with or without combined therapy, and palliative care. Other factors to consider when planning treatment include the location, size, and extent of tumor, the patient's performance status, and the availability of proper treatment facilities. Chemotherapy is not considered a primary treatment modality for this region.

NASAL CAVITY, NASOPHARYNX, AND PARANASAL SINUS

External beam radiation is the primary modality for treatment of carcinoma of the nasopharynx. Small nasal skin lesions and lesions of the nasal vestibule or septa may be surgically excised. Tumors of the paranasal sinus are primarily treated with surgical resection. Postoperative radiation of paranasal sinus carcinomas depends on the size and extension of the tumor as well as its perineural or perivascular invasion. Chemotherapy is not a primary treatment for this cancer, but it may play a palliative role for patients whose tumors are deemed surgically unresectable.

LARYNX

The goal of treatment of laryngeal cancer is to preserve the patient's life and vocal function. As is the case for all carcinomas, the possibility of a cure is the first priority. Small T1 or T2 lesions may be treated with primary external beam radiation therapy. The tumor's location may dictate a supraglottic or vertical hemilaryngectomy. T3 and T4 lesions usually are best treated with total laryngectomy. Physicians in several cancer centers are investigating the effectiveness of chemotherapy and radiotherapy in preserving the laryngeal function of patients undergoing treatment for laryngeal cancer.

MAJOR AND MINOR SALIVARY GLANDS

Surgical excision is the primary treatment for benign or malignant salivary gland tumors. Postoperative radiation therapy is indicated for certain histologic types, including high-grade mucoepidermoid carcinoma, adenocarcinoma, malignant mixed tumor, squamous cell carcinoma, and adenoid cystic carcinoma.

Perineural or perivascular involvement, positive lymph nodes, and skin involvement are also indicators for postoperative radiation therapy. Although it is controversial, neck dissection with concurrent surgical salivary gland resection remains the treatment of choice for these tumors. Chemotherapy is not the primary treatment in these cases.

NECK

Surgical resection of primary tumors of the neck is the preferred treatment. Metastatic nodes usually are removed in a neck dissection, followed by postoperative radiation therapy. These treatment modalities are still a subject of debate.

EARS

Surgical resection is the treatment of choice for lesions of the pinna. Electrodesiccation and cautery may be used to resect basal cell carcinoma of the pinna, and Moh's technique of serial excision may be considered for small lesions. As an alternative to resection, external beam irradiation may be used for larger basal cell and squamous cell carcinomas of the ear.

Some practitioners reserve chemotherapy for patients with massive primary tumors or unresectable disease and those whose performance status does not permit extensive surgical resection. Carcinomas of the external auditory canal, middle ear, and temporal bone are treated primarily with surgical resection. Small basal cell and squamous cell carcinomas in the external auditory canal may respond well to external beam radiation therapy. Postoperative radiation usually is employed in conjunction with resection. Chemotherapy usually is reserved for unresectable carcinomas or palliative care.

REFERRAL

Patients with head and neck carcinomas are best managed by a multidisciplinary team consisting of a head and neck surgeon, head and neck radiation oncologist, head and neck oncologist, reconstructive surgeon, speech pathologist, neurosurgeon, social worker, and dentist. Not all of these specialists are always needed, but they should be available for consultation.

AFTER-TREATMENT SURVEILLANCE

A thorough head and neck examination with visual inspection, indirect or direct laryngoscopy, otoscopy, and manual palpation is mandatory at all patient visits. A careful physical examination includes areas most likely to be involved in local or regional metastasis. Lungs are evaluated by auscultation and percussion. The patient is questioned carefully about bone pain and decreased range of motion. Neurologic changes, mental status changes, dizziness, vertigo, and cranial nerve deficits are documented.

The frequency of examinations may vary. A general schedule of return visits after treatment consists of examinations every 3 months for the first 2 years, every 6 months for the second 2 years, and annually after 5 years. A high level of suspicion is always maintained for detecting a second primary tumor.

Laboratory studies, an integral part of the posttreatment examination, include complete blood count, chemistry survey, liver function studies, and thyroid studies if the thyroid was irradiated or resected or if the patient is otherwise symptomatic.

Radiologic examinations include annual chest radiographs. MRI and CT examinations are essential for evaluating the nasopharynx or the middle ear or to rule out recurrence. Postsurgical sequelae should be addressed for their influence on the patient's quality of life. The patient may have significant cosmetic deformities that require reconstructive surgery. Cranial nerve deficits may also be present. Speech and deglutition deficits require the aid of a speech pathologist skilled in the care of cancer patients. For patients who require help because of hearing deficits or to maintain good nutrition, audiologists and nutritionists are valuable members of the treatment team.

Radiation-induced sequelae, including those from external beam radiotherapy and brachytherapy, are difficult to manage and require a team approach. Radiation fibrosis, xerostomia, and trismus are vexing problems. Hypothyroidism and hypopituitarism are also postirradiation sequelae and should be assessed as needed. Osteoradionecrosis and chondroradionecrosis, severe side effects of external beam radiation therapy, require vigilant surveillance to prevent significant morbidity.

The Lhermitte sign, a complication of radiation therapy that resembles sudden feelings of electric shock when the patient flexes his or her head, must be distinguished from possible cord involvement. Frey syndrome is another postirradiation problem that is manifested by localized flushing and sweating of the ear and cheek region in response to eating. It may occur after parotidectomy and is believed to be caused by reinnervation of sweat glands by parasympathetic fibers. It usually is a minor problem.

Among patients who receive chemotherapy for head and neck tumors, sequelae may include hearing loss, ototoxicity, decreased renal and hepatic function, cardiomyopathy, and fibrosis of lung parenchyma. Care must be taken to address these life-threatening complications.

CANCER PREVENTION AND EARLY DETECTION

Screening examinations for head and neck cancers should include dental checkups every 6 months to 1 year, especially if the patient wears a dental appliance or dentures. Regular skin examinations are done to check for new lesions and to evaluate changes in previous lesions.

The prevention of head and neck cancer depends on the avoidance of tobacco products—cigarettes, pipes, cigars, snuff, and smokeless tobacco—and betel nut. Also recommended is abstinence from or moderate use of alcohol, proper oral hygiene, and avoidance of foods with high concentrations of nitrosamines. Wearing proper protective wear when working in furniture manufacturing, in leather production, and with radiation may also be helpful. A balanced diet and proper skin care that includes avoidance of prolonged sun exposure and peak sunlight hours and the use of sunscreen, protective clothing, sunglasses, and hats may also help in the effort to prevent head and neck cancer.

SELF-SCREENING EXAMINATION FOR HEAD AND NECK CANCER

Visually inspect the skin for lesions, ulcers, changes in pigmentation, hair loss, and masses.

Visually inspect the oral cavity for lesions, ulcers, changes in pigmentation, asymmetry, abnormal elevation of the palate, and tongue protrusions.

Notice changes such as hoarseness, sore throat, pain or difficulty in swallowing, ear pain, double vision, visual acuity changes, hearing changes, and changes in sensation.

REFERENCES

1. Parker SL, Tong T, Bolden S, Wingo P: Cancer statistics, 1997. CA Cancer J Clin 1997;47:5–27.
2. Murphy G, Lawrence W Jr, Lenhard RE Jr (eds): American Cancer Society Textbook of Clinical Oncology, 2nd ed. Atlanta, American Cancer Society, 1995.
3. Myers E, Suen J (eds.): Cancer of the Head and Neck, 2nd ed. New York, Churchill Livingstone, 1989.
4. Casciato DA, Lowitz BB (eds.): Manual of Clinical Oncology, 2nd ed. Boston, Little, Brown, 1988.
5. Becker W, Naumann HH, Pfaltz CR: Larynx, hypopharynx and trachea. In Buckingham RA (ed): Ear, Nose, and Throat Diseases, 2nd rev. ed. New York, Thieme Medical Publishing, 1994.
6. Bergaer DH, Feig BW, Furhman GM: The M.D. Anderson Surgical Oncology Handbook. Boston, Little, Brown, 1995.
7. Robbins KT (ed): Pocket Guide to Neck Dissection Classification and TNM Staging of Head and Neck Cancer. Alexandria, VA, American Academy of Otolaryngology–Head and Neck Surgery, 1991.

Chapter 4

Lung Cancer

Sandra C. Henke, MSN, RN, CS, ANP, and
Frank Fossella, MD

Lung cancer, once a rare disease, is now the leading cause of cancer death for both men and women in the United States.[1] In 1997, there were an estimated 178,100 new lung cancer cases diagnosed, with 160,400 lung cancer-related deaths.[2] This increase in morbidity and mortality from lung cancer has occurred despite advances in diagnostic techniques, surgical procedures, and medical management of this disease. Lung cancer presents a frustrating problem. There are no effective screening methods or early diagnostic tests for lung cancer, and there are no curative therapies for advanced disease. However, the cause of lung cancer is well known. If recommendations for eliminating tobacco use were followed, the result would be a decrease in the incidence of lung cancer followed by a decrease in mortality.[2] It is most discouraging, then, that the efforts and expense connected with medical and surgical diagnosis, treatment, and research are still unsuccessful against a disease that in most cases is considered to be preventable.

EPIDEMIOLOGY

The 5-year survival rate for all patients diagnosed with lung cancer is 13%.[3] Most persons diagnosed with lung cancer die as a direct result of the disease or indirectly from one of its many complications. This statistic holds true regardless of the type of lung cancer, the stage of disease, or the method of treatment. As with all cancers, the earlier this disease is diagnosed and successfully treated, the more favorable the prognosis. However, 75% of all patients newly diagnosed with lung cancer are found to have extensive disease at the time of initial assessment. Of the remaining 25%—those considered to have "early disease"—only 20% are found to have truly limited disease at the time of surgery. Fewer than 15% of all new cases, then, can be classified as local disease.[2] Even in this select group, "cure" is still not certain even with successful surgical resection and close medical monitoring. The 5-year survival rate after surgical resection for patients with limited disease is reported to be 40% to 70%[2] (Fig. 4–1). These are grim statistics overall for a disease that is considered preventable in the majority of cases.

Although prostate cancer remains the most prevalent cancer among men and breast cancer among women, cancer of the lung is the leading cause of cancer death for both men and women in the United States[1] (Fig. 4–2). There are several explanations for this fact. First, breast and prostate cancers are associated with relatively long survival times. Lung cancer, by comparison, is associated with an overall survival time of 6 to 12 months. Second, effective screening tools are available that make early detection of prostate and breast cancers possible. In patients at high risk for lung cancer, regular chest radiographs and sputum collection have not been found to be effective means of early detection and have not improved overall survival rates. In addition, these are expensive screening tools with an overall low yield of detected cancers. Early detection by identification of physical symptoms of the disease also is not effective. Patients with lung cancer typically are asymptomatic in the early stages, and the disease is often advanced before symptoms prompting medical attention develop or before lung cancer is included in the differential diagnosis. Finally, effective treatments are available for breast and prostate cancers. Current medical management is often ineffective in arresting lung cancer or controlling and preventing lung cancer metastases for any length of time.

The peak incidence of lung cancer occurs in the age range of 50 to 75 years.

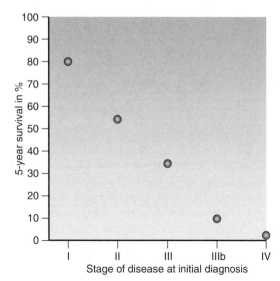

Figure 4-1. Five-year survival after surgical resection of lung cancer. (Data from Friedland DM: Perioperative therapy of lung cancer. Semin Oncol 1995; 22:571.)

The mean age at diagnosis is 65 years.[1] Lung cancer may be diagnosed in much younger people, but typically only in those with a significant smoking history. Fewer than 5% of all lung cancer patients are younger than 30 years of age.[3]

Race does not appear to be a predisposing factor in the development of lung cancer. In women, the number of lung cancer-related deaths among nonwhites is similar to that among whites. In men, the mortality rate for nonwhites has surpassed that for whites; however, this may be related to a decrease in the prevalence of smoking among white men.[1]

RISK FACTORS

The relation between tobacco use and lung cancer has been the basis of much political and social controversy. Only recently have researchers presented

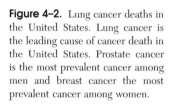

Figure 4-2. Lung cancer deaths in the United States. Lung cancer is the leading cause of cancer death in the United States. Prostate cancer is the most prevalent cancer among men and breast cancer the most prevalent cancer among women.

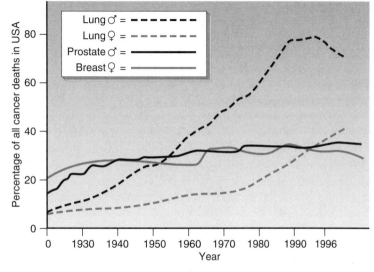

conclusive evidence that tobacco is the major causative agent for the development of lung cancer, providing data to support what has long been considered a strong correlation with this disease.[4] Eighty percent to 85% of all patients diagnosed with lung cancer are long-term cigarette or tobacco users. The remaining 15% to 20% of cases not related to tobacco use are believed to be the "true" lung cancer cases. These statistics demonstrate how rare lung cancer would be without the use of tobacco. Tobacco use alone does not "guarantee" that a person will develop lung cancer. Only about 10% of all smokers develop this disease.[5] However, given the correlation between tobacco use and lung cancer, lung cancer should be considered in the differential diagnosis when the patient is a current or former tobacco user.

Environmental or occupational chemical exposure is also a risk factor for the development of some lung cancers. Chemicals in the environment that lead to the development of lung cancer include the following: (1) asbestos, which affects miners, millers, and those who work with building materials; (2) benzene, which is commonly used in the shipping industry; and (3) radon or other elements produced by the decay of radioactive substances.[6]

GENETICS

In lung cancer, the contribution of environmental factors seems to be greater than that of genetic factors, although both environmental and genetic factors usually interact in causing the disease. At present, there are no reliable means of identifying people who are more or less likely to develop lung cancer in response to tobacco smoke or other environmental factors. Researchers are attempting to identify a gene or trait that would predict increased risk for the development of lung cancer.[4] If there were a clear causal relation between tobacco smoke and lung cancer, then all smokers would develop this disease. One major research question is why only 10% of the cigarette smokers in the United States develop lung cancer. One possible explanation is that there is a genetic tendency toward the development of lung cancer in some persons who are exposed to the most significant risk factor (i.e., tobacco chemicals). Those with have a family history of cancer, particularly lung cancer, should be considered to be at increased risk for development of this disease.[4]

PHYSICAL ASSESSMENT

HISTORY

A key component of the pertinent medical evaluation is the tobacco history. The smoking history includes the age when the patient started smoking, the average number of packs smoked per day, and the number of years smoked. Although it is now known that tobacco use is a major risk factor for the development of lung cancer, it has not been determined how much smoking is necessary before lung cancer develops. Generally, there is no "safe" amount. Any smoking history is relevant. Even if a former user discontinued tobacco use many years previously, there remains a risk for development of lung cancer. A latency period of 20 years before the smoker develops lung cancer is considered standard. Conversely, a period of approximately 20 years is needed before the former smoker reaches the lowest possible risk for the development of lung cancer. Even after this period, a former smoker is still at a higher risk than a person who has never smoked[2] (Fig. 4–3). All forms of inhaled tobacco, including pipe smoke and cigar smoke, should be included in the history, because inhaled tobacco from any source can contribute to the development of lung cancer.

Exposure to chemicals in the home or at work, particularly those chemicals mentioned in the section on risk factors, should be included in the history. The duration of specific chemical exposures should also be included in the assessment.

Any cancer diagnoses among first-degree relatives should be further investigated. A strong pattern of any type of cancer among first-degree relatives should alert the care provider that a genetic tendency toward the development of cancer is possible.

SYMPTOMS

CHIEF COMPLAINT

The evaluation of the chief complaint and the findings on physical examination are key to alerting the care provider to consider lung cancer in the differential diagnosis. A variety of symptoms may be present in the patient with lung cancer. In many cases, the symptoms and complaints seem unrelated to each other, but frequently they represent manifestations of advanced disease. The signs and symptoms of lung cancer can be divided into three categories: pulmonary (intrathoracic), metastatic (extrathoracic), and general (paraneoplastic).[5]

PULMONARY (INTRATHORACIC) SYMPTOMS

Cough, the most common complaint, occurs in 75% of patients diagnosed with lung cancer.[7] Usually this is a nonspecific symptom. The patient with undiagnosed lung cancer is usually 55 to 65 years old and a cigarette smoker of long duration; frequently the patient also has chronic obstructive pulmonary

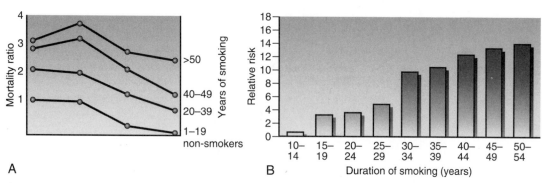

Figure 4–3. **(A)** Risk of lung cancer after discontinuing tobacco use. (Data from Turner-Warwick M, Hodson M: Lung Cancer. London, Gower Medical Publishing, 1991.) **(B)** Relative risk of developing lung cancer among smokers. (Data from Aisner J, Arriagada R, Green MR, et al (eds): Comprehensive Textbook of Thoracic Oncology. Baltimore, Williams and Wilkins, 1996.)

disease. A cough is not necessarily a new symptom in such a patient. Often the patient seeks medical attention only when the cough becomes irritating and disrupts some aspect of a normal lifestyle, such as sleep. Characteristics that should be evaluated include (1) recent change in the character of the cough, (2) change in the quality or quantity of sputum, (3) sudden onset of paroxysms of hacking dry cough, and (4) any change that does not resolve over a short period of time. Dyspnea is also a frequently unreported and nonspecific symptom in lung cancer. Again, many of these patients have been diagnosed with chronic obstructive pulmonary disease secondary to prolonged tobacco use, and they may have gradually altered their lifestyles to accommodate the decreased pulmonary function. Such patients are often unaware of their decreasing lung capacity until it becomes quite advanced and interferes with routine activities. Increasing dyspnea on exertion, orthopnea, and paroxysmal nocturnal dyspnea may be mentioned as presenting or associated complaints.

Hemoptysis, as opposed to cough and dyspnea, usually prompts patients to seek immediate medical evaluation. In most cases, hemoptysis is caused by ulceration of the bronchial mucosa; therefore, the amount of blood seen in the sputum is minimal. The mass may be within the lung, compressing the airway externally, or it may be located within the airway itself, causing direct irritation of the bronchial wall (Fig. 4–4). Hemoptysis is not a common finding: many patients diagnosed with lung cancer never experience an episode of hemoptysis. Conversely, hemoptysis in and of itself is not necessarily indicative of lung cancer. Hemoptysis is frequently seen in bacterial pneumonia and bronchitis.

Hoarseness is a cause for concern in the patient who is being evaluated for lung cancer. This symptom develops when tumor invasion causes entrapment of the recurrent laryngeal nerve. This is usually noted in patients who are found to have a left upper lobe lung mass. The recurrent laryngeal nerve is in a more anterior position on the left and therefore is more easily affected by a mass. No pain, erythema, or inflammation of the throat should be associated with hoarseness. Hoarseness in a patient diagnosed with lung cancer indicates extensive metastatic disease.

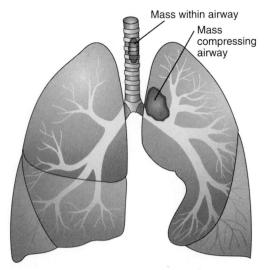

Mass within airway

Mass compressing airway

Figure 4–4. Hemoptysis as a symptom in lung cancer. In most cases, hemoptysis is caused by ulceration of the bronchial mucosa. The mass may be within the lung itself, compressing the airway externally, or it may be within the airway, causing direct irritation of the bronchial wall.

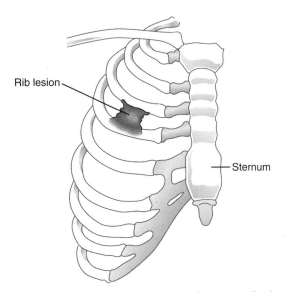

Rib lesion

Sternum

Figure 4–5. Chest pain as a symptom in lung cancer develops as a result of a mass located peripherally in the thoracic cavity, compressing or invading the nerves of the ribs and chest wall.

Chest pain occurs in approximately 50% of patients with lung cancer.[7] It develops when a mass located peripherally in the thoracic cavity compresses or invades the nerves of the ribs and chest wall (Fig. 4–5). The patient usually presents with the symptom of nonradiating chest pain of some duration. A chest radiograph as part of the initial evaluation often identifies in the periphery of the lung the mass responsible for the pain.

METASTATIC (EXTRATHORACIC) SYMPTOMS

Seizures, confusion, and persistent headaches are manifestations of brain metastases. A patient who presents with seizures should be treated on an emergency basis and given immediate medical attention. Often, however, the patient presents with complaints of a persistent headache unrelieved by conventional medication. Patients may mention a feeling of dizziness causing unsteadiness of gait. Symptoms and physical findings resembling those of stroke are common in patients with undiagnosed brain metastases.[7]

Complaints of persistent and gradually increasing bone pain are often an indication of bone metastases. A precise location of pain over a bony area should be palpable. Pain located over a weight-bearing area such as the pelvis may indicate an impending fracture. Although analgesics may control the pain temporarily, the dose and frequency must be increased regularly until specific treatment for the cancer and the metastases is initiated.[7]

GENERAL (PARANEOPLASTIC) SYMPTOMS

Paraneoplastic symptoms are general symptoms caused by the cancer process and not by direct invasion of the tumor itself. These symptoms are vague and are rarely described by the patient unless the examiner specifically mentions them. These symptoms do not necessarily indicate extensive or metastatic disease.

The most common presenting symptoms are weight loss, fatigue, and night sweats. Weight loss usually is indicative of a neoplastic process and often is accompanied by a general decrease in appetite. A weight loss of more than 10% of the total body weight is considered to be a poor prognostic indicator. Fatigue and general malaise also are usually associated with a neoplastic process. The patient usually attributes the fatigue to other symptoms, such as weight loss, decreased appetite, or the flu. Patients with night sweats may state that they wake up and have literally "soaked the sheets with perspiration." This symptom may indicate metastasis, specifically to the liver.[8]

PHYSICAL EXAMINATION

PULMONARY EXAMINATION

Patients who present with complaints of cough, dyspnea, shortness of breath, or respiratory changes should undergo an examination of the pulmonary system. The examiner should not automatically expect to hear abnormal breath sounds in the patient with a lung mass. In fact, it is common for patients diagnosed with lung cancer to have normal breath sounds and entirely unremarkable findings on pulmonary examination. In addition, abnormal findings such as distant breath sounds or expiratory wheezing often are present as a result of the chronic obstructive process brought on by long-term tobacco abuse.

Wheezing that is new is a cause for concern. The wheezing may be inspiratory or expiratory. The presence of wheezes indicates an obstructive process, and in the case of lung cancer it indicates an obstruction of one of the major bronchi. Stridor is heard only over the upper airways. It usually is audible without the use of a stethoscope. Stridor is considered a medical emergency and requires immediate attention. It is caused by a partial obstruction of the trachea, either by tumor inside the trachea (intrinsic compression) or by tumor that is growing outside the trachea, in the lung itself, and compressing the trachea (extrinsic compression).

Absent breath sounds are often noted on pulmonary examination. Surprisingly, the patient may have absence of breath sounds over a large area of one lung and not complain of anything more than mild shortness of breath. The absence of breath sounds at the base of one lung is often caused by a pleural effusion. Pleural effusions result when fluid produced by inflammation of the tumor or by the tumor itself cannot be cleared and is allowed to collect within the pleural space. Pleural effusions are not always present in the patient diagnosed with lung cancer. Percussion of the involved area produces a hyperresonant sound just above the effusion and a dull sound in the location of the effusion. A pleural effusion associated with lung cancer is usually unilateral. Bilateral effusions may indicate other medical processes, such as congestive heart failure.[5]

NEUROLOGIC EXAMINATION

Complaints of persistent headaches, vertigo, or dizziness should prompt a neurologic examination. Physical findings may include miosis of the pupils and specific motor deficits similar to those produced by a stroke. However, as with the pulmonary examination, findings on the neurologic examination may be entirely unremarkable in patients with early metastatic disease. Abnormal findings also may be caused by electrolyte imbalances resulting from an underlying cancer diagnosis. Imbalances such as hyponatremia and hypercalcemia often are present in patients with certain types of lung cancer.

ABDOMINAL EXAMINATION

The findings on abdominal examination may be entirely benign even in the presence of metastatic disease. All lung cancer cell types have the potential to metastasize to the liver and the adrenal glands. The liver can be very heavily involved with disease before it becomes enlarged or the patient appears jaundiced. In fact, liver enlargement and jaundice usually appear in the terminal period of this disease. However, enlargement or palpable nodularity of the liver may be noted during the physical examination and should be investigated.

Additional components of the physical examination may produce some related findings. Clubbing of the nail beds is frequently present. Although it is more indicative of chronic obstructive pulmonary disease secondary to long-term tobacco use, clubbing may also indicate pulmonary hypertension resulting from tumor obstruction in the lung. Skin metastases may be present as newly developed, firm, tender nodules over the body. Lung cancer has the potential to metastasize to any area, so any new complaint in a patient already diagnosed with lung cancer should be addressed.[7]

HISTOLOGIC FINDINGS

Decisions regarding appropriate treatment for lung cancer are based on findings of the diagnostic workup. This workup is focused on determining the tumor's size and precise location in the chest, the presence and extent of metastatic spread, and the histologic type of the carcinoma based on its cellular features. There are four histologic types of lung cancer: small cell carcinoma (also known as oat cell carcinoma); squamous cell carcinoma; adenocarcinoma; and large cell carcinoma.[8]

SMALL CELL LUNG CANCER

Small cell (oat cell) lung carcinoma comprises about 20% of all lung cancers.[9] The most striking difference between small cell lung cancer and the other lung cancer types is its aggressiveness. With a doubling time of only 30 days, small cell lung cancer almost always metastasizes to regional lymph nodes or to a distant location before symptoms develop. If small cell lung cancer is suspected, referral becomes urgent because treatment must begin quickly. Left untreated, small cell lung cancer leads to death within 3 to 4 weeks. However, with expeditious diagnosis and the initiation of treatment, patients may survive as long as 2 years. In cases of limited disease, cure is possible.

Small cell lung cancer occurs almost exclusively in persons with a significant

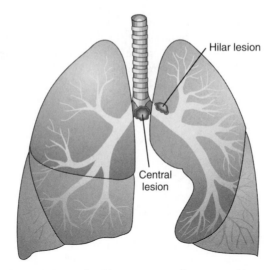

Figure 4–6. Small cell lung cancer usually is a central lesion, originating near a major bronchus or the hilum.

smoking history. This type of cancer usually occurs as a central lesion; that is, it originates around a major bronchus or the hilum (Fig. 4–6). With this type of presentation, the clinician would expect symptoms related to pulmonary compression or obstruction. The patient often presents with a new or persistent cough. Because the mass is located near the major airways, it may irritate the bronchial mucosa, resulting in hemoptysis. If there is compression of the bronchus, the patient should experience increased dyspnea with exertion and shortness of breath.

Although the presenting complaint may be pulmonary or intrathoracic, symptoms suggestive of extrathoracic metastasis often give clues that an aggressive neoplastic process is present. General symptoms of decreased appetite, weight loss, and malaise are frequently uncovered during the initial evaluation.

NON–SMALL CELL LUNG CANCER

The remaining three histologic types (squamous cell carcinoma, adenocarcinoma, and large cell carcinoma) can be classified under the broad heading of non–small cell lung cancers. Although there are major differences among these three cancer types, there are some general characteristics common to them: (1) they have a doubling time of approximately 100 days, much longer than that of small cell lung cancer; (2) at the time of diagnosis, they are more likely to be local than to have metastasized to distant areas; and (3) when the disease is metastatic at presentation, the prognosis is approximately 6 to 12 months with or without treatment.[10]

Squamous cell lung cancer now comprises almost 25% of lung cancer cases. Like small cell lung cancer, it is almost always associated with a significant smoking history. Squamous cell lung cancer also often occurs as a central pulmonary lesion. Frequently, the mass grows so large in this central location that it begins to cavitate (Fig. 4–7). Because of the location of the mass, patients often present with intrathoracic symptoms, primarily a productive cough, shortness of breath, and dyspnea.[10]

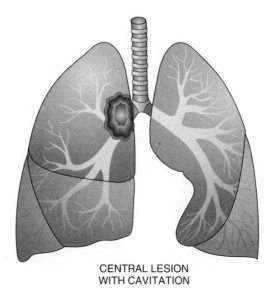

CENTRAL LESION
WITH CAVITATION

Figure 4–7. Squamous cell lung cancer often is a central pulmonary lesion with cavitation.

Adenocarcinoma has recently become the most common type of lung cancer, comprising almost 40% of all cases. More women than men are diagnosed with this type. Adenocarcinoma is the most common histologic type in patients who have never smoked and in those who smoked for only a short time and quit smoking many years before their diagnosis. Patients with adenocarcinoma characteristically present with a peripheral lung lesion (Fig. 4–8). Instead of pulmonary symptoms, the patient complains of chest or rib pain. Adenocarcinoma is more likely than the other lung cancer types to metastasize to the brain, and neurologic symptoms often are present.[10]

Large cell carcinoma comprises the remaining 15% of lung cancer cases. Large cell carcinoma can occur as either a central or a peripheral lesion, so symptoms may be of any category[10] (Fig. 4–9).

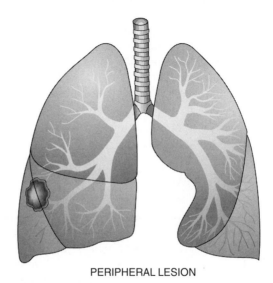

PERIPHERAL LESION

Figure 4–8. Adenocarcinoma of the lung is characteristically a peripheral lesion.

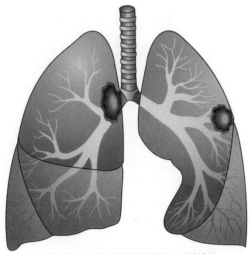

CENTRAL OR PERIPHERAL LESION

Figure 4–9. Large cell carcinoma of the lung can be either a central or a peripheral lesion.

METASTATIC DISEASE SITES

When a diagnosis of lung cancer is suspected, the physical examination should address all probable sites for metastasis (Fig. 4–10). These are described in the following sections.

BONE

Bone metastasis is common among all histologic types. The symptom that indicates bone metastasis is a specific localized area of pain over a bony structure. Although analgesics are helpful, the pain eventually intensifies, necessitating larger and more frequent doses of pain medication. The situation of greatest concern is bone metastasis involving a weight-bearing structure such as the pelvis or the head of the femur. In this setting, the patient is at risk for a pathologic fracture. A pathologic fracture occurs when there is no apparent trauma or cause of injury. The patient may simply be performing a routine activity and feel a deep pain; subsequent radiographs confirm the fracture.[7]

CENTRAL NERVOUS SYSTEM

Neurologic changes, including confusion, seizures, loss of consciousness, and symptoms resembling those of a cerebrovascular accident, will almost always prompt a patient to seek medical care. Subtle symptoms include persistent headache unrelieved by analgesics, vertigo, and mild dizziness. The findings on neurologic examination may be entirely unremarkable, or there may be specific findings of neurologic deficits.[7]

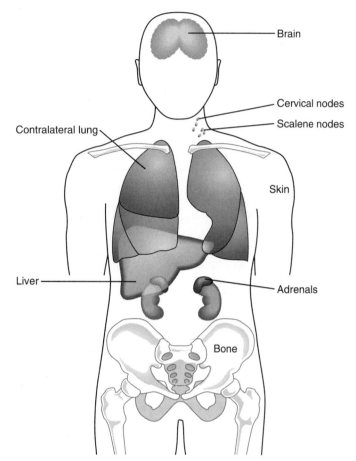

Figure 4–10. Common sites of metastasis for lung cancer.

ABDOMEN

The most common sites for abdominal metastases are the liver and the adrenal glands. Abdominal metastasis can be confirmed only by computed tomography (CT) of the abdomen. Although bone and brain metastases most frequently occur with correlating physical symptoms, abdominal sites may be heavily involved with disease without any symptoms. Abdominal examination should include percussion and palpation of the liver, but an enlarged liver does not definitively indicate metastasis, and benign findings on examination do not exclude metastasis.[7]

LYMPH NODES

The lymph nodes are commonly evaluated for the presence of metastasis. Supraclavicular lymph nodes that are easily palpable on examination indicate possible metastatic disease. Other lymph node sites usually are not amenable to physical examination. Mediastinal and hilar lymph nodes, which are the ones most frequently involved, can be evaluated only with technological diagnostic tools. These nodes are often first visualized and considered to be enlarged on chest radiographs or CT scans. Confirmation is then made by a surgical mediastinoscopy. This procedure requires tissue sampling of the lymph nodes,

Table 4–1. Lung Cancer Stages

STAGE	TUMOR (T)	NODAL INVOLVEMENT (N)	METASTASIS (M)
I	3.0 cm or larger	No	No
II	3.0 cm or larger	Peribronchial or ipsilateral hilar	No
III	Tumor of any size Extension to chest wall or pericardium	May include contralateral mediastinal lymph nodes	No
	Does not invade pericardium, heart, or carina		No
IV	Any size	Any involvement	Yes

which are then submitted for pathologic evaluation to confirm metastatic involvement.[7]

STAGES OF LUNG CANCER

The stage of lung cancer is determined by (1) the size of the tumor and the extent of invasion into adjacent structures such as the chest wall, trachea, or any of the vessels; (2) the extent of mediastinal lymph node involvement; and (3) the presence of metastatic disease (Table 4–1). Lung cancer stages range from stage I (earliest stage) to stage IV (metastatic disease).[11]

Stage I and stage II disease carry the best prognosis. These stages are associated with relatively small tumors and either no nodal disease or very limited mediastinal nodal involvement. Patients diagnosed to have stage I or II disease are considered for surgical resection of the tumor.[12]

Stage III disease is diagnosed by the extent of nodal involvement. Typically, patients with highly suspicious mediastinal lymphadenopathy on chest CT scan undergo mediastinoscopy to evaluate for nodal disease. Patients with stage III disease have an estimated 5-year survival rate of 17%.[11]

Stage IV lung cancer refers to metastatic disease at the time of diagnosis. Approximately 75% of all newly diagnosed patients are considered to have extensive disease. Evaluation of the patient with suspected lung cancer must include a workup for metastatic disease, because the signs and symptoms of metastasis frequently are present at initial examination.

MEDICAL EVALUATION AND DIAGNOSTIC WORKUP

The medical evaluation begins at the time of the patient's presentation to the care provider. The patient usually seeks attention for one of the nonspecific symptoms (e.g., cough). There may also be associated symptoms such as fever, decreased appetite, and malaise. Prolonged use of tobacco is noted in the history. A prescription for an antibiotic is given for treatment of "chronic bronchitis," but the symptoms do not resolve and perhaps even intensify. The patient returns again for the same complaint. At this point, a chest radiograph should be considered.

The chest radiograph provides the first hint of the diagnosis of lung cancer. Although the chest radiograph cannot diagnose a cancer, it can provide reason for further investigation and referral to an oncology specialist. The patient who has any abnormality noted on chest radiography, a significant smoking history, and corresponding symptoms should be considered for referral (Fig. 4–11).

The specialist initiates the appropriate diagnostic workup. This includes a CT scan of the chest to provide information about the size and location of the abnormality and the presence of any related mediastinal adenopathy. The metastatic workup includes radiographic studies of the bones, brain, and abdomen to confirm disease spread to any of these areas. The next important step is to determine the histologic type of the cancer. The radiographic evaluation can help the care provider determine the most expeditious method of obtaining cells or tissue for histologic examination. When the mass is centrally located in or near a major airway, the patient has complained of an increase in the frequency of cough, and the cough is productive, diagnosis may be attempted by sputum cytology. The cancer cells may be close enough to the airway to slough off and be expectorated for analysis. When the cough is not productive but the tumor mass is still centrally located, a bronchoscopy may be indicated. Bronchoscopy is most likely to yield results when the mass is centrally located. A bronchoscope can be passed only through the trachea, the bronchi, and the major portion of the bronchioles. Beyond that point, the airways become too small to allow passage to obtain adequate specimens for diagnosis.[13] Peripheral lesions are diagnosed by fine-needle aspiration. The lesion is visualized under fluoroscopy or by CT, and a needle is inserted into the tumor mass. A specimen is then aspirated and sent to the pathologist for diagnosis.

Only by direct tissue examination can a diagnosis of lung cancer be made.

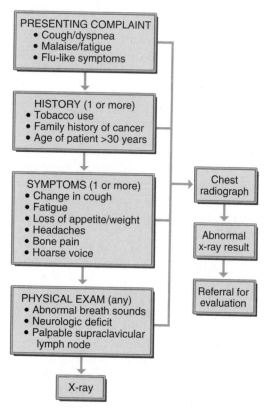

Figure 4–11. Algorithm for medical evaluation and diagnostic workup for lung cancer.

Even though there are radiographic cues that prompt the interpreter to suggest malignancy, only a pathologist can make the actual diagnosis. Spiculated or coin-like lesions on the radiograph, central lesions or peripheral lesions, and correlation with a history and physical examination may tempt the clinician to predict malignancy and histologic type. However, such speculation should not be shared with the patient, because it is confusing to the patient and could easily prove incorrect.

TREATMENT MODALITIES

Treatment for lung cancer is determined and managed by the specialist. This section provides an overview of the available treatment options.

SURGERY

In the patient who is diagnosed with stage I, II, or IIIA lung cancer, surgery is always considered first because it carries the best chance for long-term survival. However, only 25% of all patients diagnosed with lung cancer are eligible for complete surgical resection.

Surgery involves complete resection of the entire anatomic structure in which the cancer is located. A lesion confined to one lobe requires a lobectomy. If the mass involves more than one lobe because it crosses the fissure that separates two or more lobes, surgery must include removal of all affected lobes. If the tumor is at the hilum, complete pneumonectomy is considered for surgical management; this approach allows the most complete resection and the greatest chance for long-term survival.[12] Often, the patient believes that only the tumor and a small amount of lung must be removed, but such treatment allows a much higher risk of tumor recurrence. Because a major portion of lung is removed with surgery, special attention is given to the patient's underlying medical condition. Because 80% to 85% of all patients diagnosed with lung cancer are long-term tobacco users, chronic obstructive pulmonary disease is a common finding and concern. Patients may be considered ineligible for surgery because of poor pulmonary function. Surgical excision of a major portion of lung could significantly compromise the patient's pulmonary status and increase the risk of major morbidity and mortality with surgery.

Cardiac status is another important consideration, especially in older patients with a significant smoking history, and it should be evaluated before the patient is considered for general anesthesia and surgical resection.

Surgical candidacy for primary lung cancer is also determined by additional factors. Patients with small cell lung cancer are almost always ineligible for surgery because of the aggressive and metastatic nature of this histologic type. For all types of lung cancer, metastatic disease is an automatic exclusion criterion for resection. Metastasis to any site indicates that the disease has probably spread to another location as well. The surgery itself is quite extensive and is associated with a long recovery time. Any other treatment must be delayed until recovery from surgery is complete. Therefore, patients with stage IIIB or stage IV disease are not considered candidates for surgery.[12]

RADIATION THERAPY

The second major treatment for lung cancer is radiation therapy.[14] Radiation therapy is recommended as primary management for patients with stage III disease and for those with stage I or stage II disease who are not surgical candidates because of medical contraindications. The treatment is aggressive, requiring approximately 6 weeks of daily irradiation targeted to the primary tumor and the mediastinum to include nodal disease. The survival rate for patients with stage I or II disease treated with irradiation is approximately 30%.

Radiation therapy has certain side effects. Radiation produces a "burn" to the area and causes an inflammatory response in the treated sites. Such inflammation in a lung can result in shortness of breath and long-term pulmonary fibrosis. The esophagus is also included in the radiation field because it is adjacent to the lungs. The side effects of irradiation of the esophagus range from mild dysphagia to severe esophagitis requiring nutritional support. These toxic effects can be short or long term and mild or severe.[14]

CHEMOTHERAPY

Chemotherapy is reserved for patients with small cell lung cancer or extensive non-small cell lung cancer; it is given either as a single modality or in conjunction with radiation therapy. Disease that has already spread to even one distant site may also be present at other locations. Chemotherapy given intravenously should provide treatment to all potential and probable affected sites of disease. Chemotherapy is highly effective against small cell lung cancer. Responses frequently are seen after only one course of therapy and include significant reductions in the size of the tumor and improvement in the patient's presenting symptoms. However, cure is not likely in patients with metastatic disease. Eventually the tumor stops responding to the therapy and again begins to grow and metastasize.[9]

Chemotherapy is not an effective primary therapy for non–small cell lung cancers. It is useful in preventing further metastasis and growth of the primary mass, but long-term survival is not significantly improved with the use of chemotherapy alone as the primary treatment.[9]

COMBINED-MODALITY THERAPY

Combinations of surgery, radiation therapy, and chemotherapy as treatment for lung cancer are the focus of much current research.[14] For patients undergoing radiation therapy, standard treatment includes concomitant chemotherapy. Chemotherapy increases the sensitivity of the tumor cells to radiation and has been shown to result in prolonged survival and more complete tumor control.[10]

TREATMENT FOLLOW-UP

Follow-up guidelines are outlined and managed by the specialist and tailored to the individual patient. The histologic type and the extent of disease not only help determine the treatment but also provide clues as to how the patient should be monitored during treatment and how the disease may progress.

Recurrence is always the major concern after surgery. It is currently recommended that patients be monitored with a chest radiograph every 6 months for a period of at least 5 years.[12] If the disease recurs, it usually recurs first in the lung and can be identified on the radiograph. Monitoring for metastasis then becomes a clinical matter. Knowledge of the probable sites of metastasis (bone, brain, liver, and adrenal glands) and the correlating symptoms is most important. Identification of persistent pain and development of neurologic symptoms should be reported to a specialist for further evaluation.

Progression of the primary disease is also monitored by the specialist. When a patient is receiving chemotherapy or radiation therapy, the specialist monitors the primary lesion, usually by chest radiography, for response. If the tumor shrinks or stabilizes, the recommended treatment is continued. If the tumor grows or a new site of metastatic disease is identified, treatment is discontinued, and an alternative treatment plan may be developed.

In most cases, a point is reached beyond which no further treatment can be given. The disease may be so widespread and may have so severely weakened the patient that he or she can no longer tolerate additional therapy. At some point, palliative or supportive care may be considered and discussed with the patient. A common concern among patients treated for lung cancer is the fear of recurrence or progression. The patient may fear that any new complaint is related to cancer. The midlevel care provider should be aware of the key symptoms to be monitored and refer the patient to the specialist when appropriate. The specialist usually depends on the primary care provider to perform routine follow-up and to differentiate between symptoms of recurrence or progression of lung cancer and new, unrelated health problems. Each new symptom must be evaluated separately from the primary cancer diagnosis and treated accordingly. Care providers often just want to refer the patient back to the specialist for any new-onset health care problems, but an investigation of the chief complaint and a brief physical examination to ensure stabilization of the patient is the minimum needed for follow-up.

PREVENTION AND EARLY DETECTION

Prevention of lung cancer rests with tobacco control. The following steps should be taken with every patient.

- Talk to the patient about smoking cessation. Even though lung cancer carries an extremely poor prognosis, discontinuation of tobacco use will help the patient to tolerate the treatment and its side effects.
- Encourage family members to quit smoking. There is a genetic correlation such that when cancer is diagnosed in a family, the other family members are at increased risk for development of a cancer if they are exposed to the predominant risk factors.
- Discuss smoking cessation aids with the patient. Nicotine gum and patches are available over the counter. Nicotine is a very addictive drug, and patients often need assistance when attempting to eliminate nicotine from their lifestyles.

Many health care professionals fail to talk to patients about smoking cessation. They think that the patient will not be able to quit or that quitting will not change the outcome. It is the job of the health care professional to tell patients that smoking is harmful and to officially recommend that they quit. Eighty-five percent of lung cancers in the United States could potentially be eliminated if people quit smoking. Other cancers such as those of the head and neck, esophagus, and bladder also are more prevalent in smokers, as are heart disease and other pulmonary diseases. It is important and necessary to instruct patients and their families to quit smoking.

There are no easy or cost-effective methods of screening for lung cancer. Researchers are still attempting to identify a serum marker correlated with lung cancer, but none has been found so far. Screening of the high-risk population with serial chest radiographs has proved to be costly and to have a low yield in early diagnosis. Currently, prevention of tobacco use and skilled observation of patients at risk for lung cancer are the only tools available to the health care service that may help reduce incidence of lung cancer.

REFERENCES

1. Parker SL, Tong T, Bolden S, Wingo PA: Cancer statistics, 1997. CA Cancer J Clin.
2. Gilliland FD, Samet JM: Lung cancer. In Sidebottom E (ed): Trends in Cancer Incidence and Mortality, vol 19/20. Cold Spring Harbor, NY, Cold Spring Harbor Laboratory Press, 1995.
3. Schottenfeld D: Epidemiology of Lung Cancer. In Pass HI, Mitchell JB, Johnson DH, et al (eds): Lung Cancer Principles and Practice. Philadelphia, Lippincott-Raven, 1995.
4. Davidson BJ, Hsu TC, Schantz SP: The genetics of tobacco-induced malignancy. Arch Otolaryngol Head Neck Surg 1993;119:1198–1205.
5. Snider GL: History and physical examination. In Barker LR, Burton JR, Zieve PD (eds): Principles of Ambulatory Medicine, 4th ed. Baltimore, Williams & Wilkins, 1994.
6. Barr L, Smith PL: Lung cancer. In Barker LR, Burton JR, Zieve PD (eds): Principles of Ambulatory Medicine, 4th ed. Baltimore, Williams & Wilkins, 1994:678.
7. Midthum DE, Jett JR: Clinical presentation of lung cancer. In Pass HI, Mitchell JB, Johnson DH, et al (eds): Lung Cancer Principles and Practice. Philadelphia, Lippincott-Raven, 1994.
8. Salazar OM, McDonald S, Van Houtte P, et al: Lung cancer. In Rubin P (ed): Clinical Oncology: A Multidisciplinary Approach for Physicians and Students, 7th ed. Philadelphia, WB Saunders, 1996.
9. De Lima MJG, Khouri IF, Glisson BS: Small cell lung cancer. In Pazdur R (ed): Medical Oncology: A Comprehensive Review, 2nd ed. Huntington, NY, PRR, 1995.
10. Diamandidis D, Huber M, Pisters K: Non-small cell lung cancer. In Pazdur R (ed): Medical Oncology: A Comprehensive Review, 2nd ed. Huntington, NY, PRR, 1996.
11. Mountain CF: Staging of lung cancer. In Roth JA, Cox JD, Hong WK (eds): Lung Cancer. Boston, Blackwell Scientific Publications, 1992.
12. Martini N, Ginsberg RJ: Treatment of stage I and II disease. In Aisner J, Arriagada R, Green MR, et al (eds): Comprehensive Textbook of Thoracic Oncology. Baltimore, Williams & Wilkins, 1996.
13. Heelan RT, Larson S: Imaging of thoracic neoplasms. In Aisner J, Arriagada R, Green MR, et al (eds): Comprehensive Textbook of Thoracic Oncology. Baltimore, Williams & Wilkins, 1996.
14. Klastersky J: Therapy of non-small cell lung cancer. Lung Cancer 1995;12(suppl):S133–S145.

Chapter 5

Cancer of the Breast

*Alice F. Judkins, MS, RN, and
S. Eva Singletary, MD*

In the United States, breast cancer is the most common cancer in women. There were an estimated 180,300 new cases of invasive breast cancer documented in 1998.[1] Breast cancer crosses all socioeconomic, racial, and cultural lines. Ninety-nine percent of patients diagnosed with breast cancer are women, and only 1% are men. Breast cancers in men are of the same histologic types as breast cancers in women, and surgical treatment is the same for both sexes.

Because of myths surrounding breast cancer, many women newly diagnosed with the disease are confused about the consequences of treatment, including lifestyle changes, and about the risk of dying of their disease. Women also experience an array of other psychological and psychosocial dilemmas, including those related to sexuality and body image. The midlevel practitioner plays a very important role in educating women about breast cancer risk and screening and in helping women diagnosed with breast cancer to fully understand their disease and their treatment options.

RISK FACTORS

Known and suspected breast cancer risk factors are described in this section and summarized in Table 5–1. However, most women diagnosed with breast cancer have no documented risk factors; their only risk factor is that they are female. No woman is free of the risk of developing breast cancer. Regardless of her history or age, if a woman presents with a questionable change on a physical examination or mammogram, it should never be ignored or dismissed without a thorough evaluation.

AGE

The risk of developing breast cancer increases with age. Women in their 50s have eight times the breast cancer risk of women in their 30s; the breast cancer risk of a 70-year-old woman is three times that of a 50-year-old woman.[2]

PERSONAL HISTORY OF CANCER

Women diagnosed with breast cancer in one breast have an increased risk of developing primary breast cancer in the other breast. Women with a personal history of endometrial, ovarian, or colon cancer also have an increased risk of developing breast cancer.

Table 5–1. Risk Factors for Breast Cancer

Age older than 50 years
Personal history of breast cancer
Family history of breast cancer, particularly in premenopausal relatives
Personal history of endometrial, ovarian, or colon cancer
Early menarche
Late menopause
Age older than 30 years at first full-term pregnancy

FAMILY HISTORY OF BREAST CANCER

Women with a history of breast cancer in a first-degree relative (mother, sister, or daughter) have an increased risk of developing breast cancer. This risk is higher if the relative's breast cancer developed before menopause or if the relative had bilateral breast cancer.

GENETIC PREDISPOSITION

The genes *BRCA1* and *BRCA2* have been linked to breast cancer. Women who inherit either of these genes have an increased risk of breast cancer. However, these genes are thought to account for only a small proportion of breast cancer cases.

REPRODUCTIVE FACTORS

A number of reproductive factors increase the risk of breast cancer. These include early menarche and late menopause. Women who have never been pregnant and women who were older than 30 years of age when they first give birth are also at increased risk for the development of breast cancer.

ESTROGEN REPLACEMENT THERAPY

Whether hormones used for estrogen replacement therapy in postmenopausal women increase the risk of breast cancer has been a subject of controversy for many years. Although there are conflicting data about the risk of estrogen replacement therapy,[3-5] it is advisable to review the dosage and duration of therapy with the patient's health care provider on an annual basis. The benefits of estrogen replacement therapy in postmenopausal women must also be considered. Estrogen has been found to lower the risks of heart disease and osteoporosis. The reduced risk of hip fractures usually outweighs the possible increased risk of developing breast cancer.

SCREENING EXAMINATIONS

The earlier a breast cancer is detected, the better the prognosis. Therefore, women should be encouraged to have regular mammograms and professional breast examinations and to practice regular breast self-examination. Recommendations for these screening examinations are summarized in Table 5–2.

PHYSICAL EXAMINATION OF THE BREASTS

A physical examination of the breasts should always begin with an update of the woman's medical history. Ask whether there has been any change in her personal history of breast lumps or her family history of breast cancer. Any

Table 5–2. Recommended Screening Examinations

EXAMINATION	AGE TO PERFORM	FREQUENCY
Breast self-examination	Begin by age 20 years	Monthly
Breast examination by a doctor or nurse	Begin by 20–30 years	Annually
Mammography	40–49 years	Every 1–2 years depending on physical findings and family history
	50 years or older	Annually

breast surgery since the last visit should also be noted. Review and discuss any unusual findings from the previous breast examinations.

Physical examination of the breasts should be done in a well-lighted, private area with the patient sitting and disrobed from the waist up. It is important to evaluate the symmetry of the breasts. Most women have one breast that is slightly larger than the other, and when questioned, most women can describe their normal breast size. The presence of prominent unilateral veins should be noted because this could be an indication of an underlying tumor. Any discoloration of the breast, particularly erythema, may have significance. Puckering, dimpling, or retraction of the skin or nipple-areola complex is often indicative of an underlying tumor (Fig. 5–1). When examining the nipples, evaluate

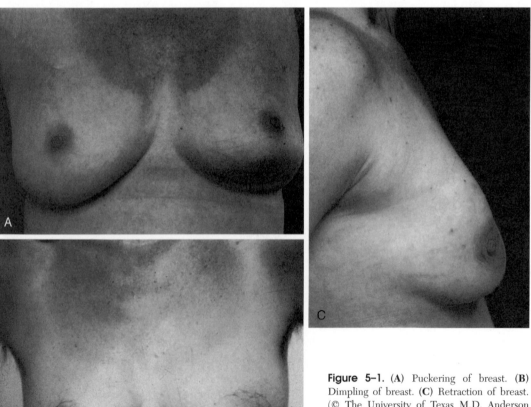

Figure 5–1. (A) Puckering of breast. **(B)** Dimpling of breast. **(C)** Retraction of breast. (© The University of Texas M.D. Anderson Cancer Center.)

whether they are retracted either unilaterally or bilaterally. If there is any unusual finding on the visual examination, ask the woman whether it represents a change in her physical presentation or has always existed.

After the visual examination, carefully palpate the breasts, chest, and axillary areas while the woman sits on the end of the examining table. Sweep your hands down the chest wall, beginning at the supraclavicular area and moving down to the nipple-areola complex. Support the opposite breast while performing the palpation-and-sweeping technique. Gently compress the nipple to check for discharge. If discharge is present, carefully evaluate whether it is from a single duct or multiple ducts within the nipple. Note the color and amount of the discharge. Fluid from a cyst is usually clear, green, or amber.

After examining both breasts, the chest wall, and the supraclavicular areas, examine the axillary areas. With one hand, gently support the woman's elbow and forearm. With your other hand, carefully palpate the entire axillary area. Repeat the procedure for the opposite axilla.

Next, ask the patient to lie down on the examining table. Place the arm of the side being examined behind the patient's head to evenly spread the breast tissue over the chest wall. Very systematically palpate the area around the breast mound, beginning at the outer perimeters and moving toward the center. Be sure to cover the entire area, and end by palpating the nipple-areola complex. Some health care providers prefer to use sweeping motions instead of circular motions. Either pattern is acceptable so long as a consistent technique is used. To complete the examination, repeat these steps on the opposite breast. It is better to move to the opposite side of the table than to reach over the woman to examine the contralateral side.

DOCUMENTATION OF THE PHYSICAL EXAMINATION

When documenting a breast examination, it is important to describe the physical appearance of the breasts, starting with symmetry. Be specific when describing changes or abnormalities: note the quadrant of the breast in which the abnormality is found, the exact location of the abnormality, and the size of the abnormality in centimeters or millimeters. Also describe the shape, consistency, and mobility of the abnormality. Is it oval, round, or elongated? Is it hard, nodular, or smooth? Is it fixed to the skin or underlying tissue, or is it freely movable? Examples of appropriate documentation are "breasts are symmetric without discrete palpable masses" and "diffuse cystic tissue noted." The latter description would be used in the case of areas of increased fibrocystic tissue.

For purposes of documentation, breasts are divided into four quadrants and a central area. The majority of breast cancers are found in the upper outer quadrant of the breast; the second most common site is the center of the breasts beneath the nipple-areola complex. This is one of the reasons that it is extremely important to depress the nipple during the part of the examination when the patient is lying down.

Physical examinations and mammograms go hand in hand. A mammogram should not be the only mechanism to detect abnormalities in a patient's breasts. Physical examinations complement mammograms because they add extra clinical information, allowing the radiologist to better evaluate findings on the mammogram. Approximately 10% to 15% of breast cancers identified on a physical examination are not detected on a mammogram. Often women themselves observe a difference in the feel or presentation of their breasts. However subtle, this too can be detected during a professional physical examination.

If a woman has been treated for breast cancer, document any changes in her treated breast or on the chest wall. In most cases, these changes are sequelae of treatment and not signs of recurrence. Examination of the patient with a history of breast cancer is discussed in the section on follow-up care.

MAMMOGRAPHY

Mammography should accompany a woman's physical examinations beginning at age 40 years. Mammography should be performed annually or semiannually between the ages of 40 and 49 and annually beginning at age 50. Women who have never been treated for breast cancer are generally candidates for screening mammography, which includes a two-view study (from top to bottom and sideways) of each breast. Diagnostic mammograms, which include an additional oblique view, are important for women with previously documented breast abnormalities.

BREAST SELF-EXAMINATION

After puberty, all women should begin practicing breast self-examination. Breast self-examination should be encouraged as a lifetime habit along with regular dental care, exercise, and Papanicolaou (Pap) smears. The proper technique for breast self-examination is illustrated in Figure 5–2.

A good technique for teaching breast self-examination is to incorporate the teaching into the professional physical examination. While examining a woman's breasts, explain what is being looked for, what is being felt, and why certain areas are being examined. In this manner, the physical examination can be turned into a breast self-examination lesson.

Breast self-examination for the woman with a history of breast cancer is discussed in the section on follow-up care.

DIAGNOSIS

If an abnormality is detected on physical examination or mammography, the next step is to determine whether the abnormality represents a benign condition or breast cancer (Figs. 5–3 and 5–4). Frequently, breast cancers go undiagnosed in women younger than 40 years of age because changes in their breasts are assumed to be benign fibrocystic changes. Any palpable breast mass or abnormality should be fully evaluated regardless of the woman's age. In premenopausal women, a mass is most likely a fibroadenoma or a cyst.

FIBROADENOMAS

A fibroadenoma is a round, smooth, rubbery, benign nodule. If a fibroadenoma has been documented on physical examination and ultrasonography and shown

MONTHLY BREAST SELF-EXAMINATION

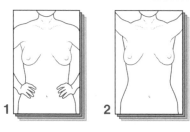

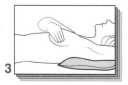

In front of a mirror

1 Place your hands on hips, turn from side to side. Press shoulders inward and bend forward. Gently squeeze each nipple to look for discharge.

2 Place your hands behind your head and press forward, turning from side to side.

Look for:
- Changes in breast size, shape, skin texture or color, redness, dimpling, or puckering.
- Nipple changes such as discharge, scaliness, a pulling to one side or a change in direction.

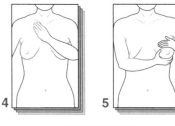

Lying flat

3 Place a small pillow or towel under your left shoulder. Put your right hand at the top of the left breast, keeping fingers together and flat. Move your fingers in a circle around the breast, moving inward in smaller circles until you have examined the entire breast. Repeat exam on the other breast.

> Feel for lumps, thickening, or any changes from one self-exam to the next.

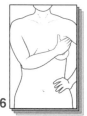

In the shower

4 Feel for lumps above and below the collarbone. From the collarbone, rub down firmly with a soapy hand to the nipple of one breast. Feel for any lumps, thickening, or changes.

5 Support the breast with one hand while the other hand and fingers slide across the top of the breast.

6 Check for lumps under your arm while relaxing your arm at your side. Keep fingers together and flat.

Repeat exam on other breast. Report any changes to your health care provider immediately.

Figure 5–2. Technique of breast self-examination. (© The University of Texas M.D. Anderson Cancer Center.)

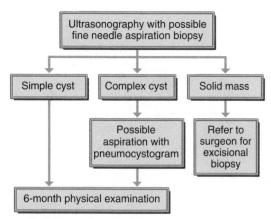

Figure 5–3. Diagnostic decisions for the patient with abnormal findings on physical examination but a normal mammogram.

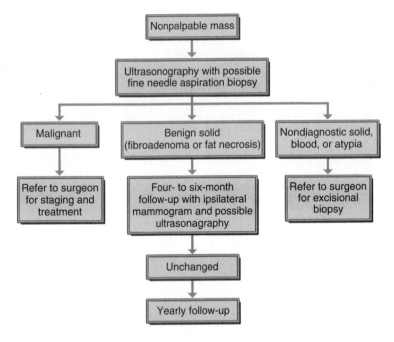

Figure 5–4. Diagnostic decisions for the patient with normal findings on physical examination but an abnormal mammogram.

to be stable, it usually is not surgically excised. However, should it begin increasing in size, surgical excision is recommended.

CYSTS

A cyst is a round, smooth, mobile, fluid-filled mass. Cysts can become quite large and hard. Benign simple cysts identified on ultrasonography can be observed without the need for biopsy. If a cyst causes symptoms or if concern exists over the correct diagnosis, the cyst may be aspirated by inserting a needle (usually 20 or 23 gauge) directly into the cyst and gently withdrawing the fluid. For cysts deep in the breast, the needle is inserted under ultrasound guidance. These procedures usually are not painful to the woman and provide relief from discomfort.

Typically, cyst fluid is clear, green, or amber. If the fluid is bloody or contains pus, it should be sent to the laboratory for cytologic evaluation. A cancer within a cyst is unusual: fewer than 1% of all breast cancers are intracystic carcinomas. It usually is not recommended that women have repeat excisional biopsies to remove cysts, because this leads to the development of scar tissue, which tends to make subsequent physical examinations more difficult. Cysts are not a precursor of breast cancer.

ULTRASONOGRAPHY

A sonogram of the breast is valuable in further evaluating palpable abnormalities that do not correspond with mammographic findings. Ultrasonography, which uses sound waves to produce images, can differentiate between cysts and solid masses. If a dominant mass is palpated on a physical examination, ultrasonography may be helpful in further evaluation (see Fig. 5–3).

BIOPSY

A number of different biopsy techniques can be used to obtain tissue or cells for pathologic examination.

FINE-NEEDLE ASPIRATION

If a solid or suspicious mass is detected on ultrasonography, fine-needle aspiration (FNA) performed under ultrasound guidance is an efficient method of obtaining cells for cytologic diagnosis. FNA is done on an outpatient basis with little or no local anesthesia. The preliminary results of FNA can be obtained within 2 to 3 hours. A suspicious mass with a negative FNA result should be surgically excised.

The disadvantage of FNA is its inability to distinguish infiltrating or invasive cancers from noninvasive cancers. If this information is needed before surgery (e.g., to determine whether preoperative chemotherapy should be given), a core biopsy should be performed.

CORE BIOPSY

Core biopsy requires the use of a larger-gauge needle than that used for FNA and allows removal of a greater portion of tissue. Core biopsy also allows the pathologist to evaluate the specimen in greater detail and give a more complete diagnosis. A diagnosis usually is available within 48 hours. If a woman has previously been treated with radiation, core biopsy must be used instead of FNA because of radiation-induced changes in the breast tissue.

STEREOTACTIC CORE BIOPSY

With the use of screening mammography, microcalcifications are frequently diagnosed (Fig. 5–5). In most cases, microcalcifications do not indicate a malignant or premalignant process. However, when calcifications increase in number, appear in clusters, or change their configuration, they may be an indication of early cancer such as ductal carcinoma in situ (DCIS). In such cases, a stereotactic core biopsy may be performed. In a stereotactic core biopsy, the radiologist uses a computer-driven needle to remove a core of tissue containing the calcifications. Core biopsy is an outpatient procedure performed under local anesthesia. It takes a pathologist 2 to 3 days to complete the diagnosis.

The stereotactic core biopsy needle has a throw of approximately 2 cm. Therefore, this type of biopsy is contraindicated in women with small breasts and for calcifications located near the chest wall because of the risk of puncturing

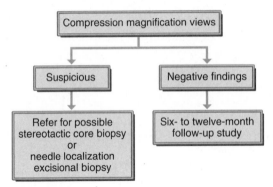

Figure 5–5. Diagnostic decisions for the patient with microcalcifications on mammogram.

a lung. When stereotactic core biopsy is contraindicated, needle localization biopsy is required.

NEEDLE LOCALIZATION BIOPSY

In a needle localization biopsy, the radiologist takes a radiograph of the breast and inserts a small needle into the center of the calcifications. The needle is temporarily taped in place. The woman then goes to the surgical suite for an excisional biopsy performed under local or monitored anesthesia with intravenous sedation. A mammogram of the surgical specimen should be obtained to ensure that the calcifications identified on the prebiopsy mammogram are the same as the calcifications that were removed. The specimen should be submitted for permanent section evaluation because the pathologist is working with microscopic tissue rather than a solid mass. A definitive diagnosis is available in approximately 48 to 72 hours.

EXCISIONAL BIOPSY

When a diagnosis cannot be obtained by FNA or core biopsy, an excisional biopsy is performed. In an excisional biopsy, the suspicious mass is surgically removed along with a margin of normal tissue. The surgeon should ink the margins of the mass so that the margin status can be determined if the mass is malignant. Excisional biopsies are performed on an outpatient basis under local or monitored anesthesia. In most cases, the surgical specimen is evaluated in the operating room by frozen section techniques, and a preliminary diagnosis is available immediately after the surgical procedure. Immediate diagnosis enables the woman, her surgeon, and her support group to begin discussing treatment options if the tumor is malignant.

TYPES OF BREAST CANCER

There are various types of breast cancer, each with its own prognosis and treatment options. Many times when a woman is told that she has breast cancer, her mind immediately leaps ahead to stories of a friend's, neighbor's, or colleague's experience with the disease. It is important to help the patient thoroughly understand her diagnosis and the treatment options available for her particular situation.

LOBULAR CARCINOMA IN SITU

Lobular carcinoma in situ (LCIS) is currently thought to be a marker of increased risk as opposed to a true cancer. LCIS is usually detected as an incidental finding when a woman undergoes an excisional biopsy for another condition. Pathologists refer to LCIS as a lobular neoplasm, indicating that these are cell changes within the breast lobules, not breast cancer. The risk of developing a subsequent breast cancer after a diagnosis of LCIS is approximately 20% to 30% over a woman's lifetime. However, this risk is equally divided between the breasts (10% to 15% for each breast).[6]

DUCTAL CARCINOMA IN SITU

DCIS is a noninvasive breast cancer that is being diagnosed with increasing frequency with the aid of regular screening mammography. DCIS is often detected on a mammogram as calcifications, which may or may not be associated with a mass. If DCIS is not surgically removed, it may progress to an invasive, life-threatening breast cancer. There are two subtypes of DCIS: comedo and noncomedo. The comedo subtype is associated with a higher proliferative rate and a greater risk of progression to invasive breast cancer.

INVASIVE BREAST CANCER

Invasive (also called infiltrating) breast cancer grows beyond the confines of the ducts or lobules and is potentially life-threatening. Invasive breast cancers are classified as ductal or lobular according to the part of the breast in which they arise. The majority of invasive breast cancers are ductal. However, there are several special subtypes of invasive cancer—tubular, medullary, mucinous, and papillary—which generally have a more favorable prognosis than invasive ductal breast cancer.

Invasive lobular carcinomas are less common. They are more difficult to diagnose because they often occur as a thickening rather than a firm nodule on physical examination. Invasive lobular carcinoma often is not detected by mammography.

STAGING OF BREAST CANCER

Once a breast cancer is diagnosed, the next step is to determine its stage. The stage is based on the size of the mass, skin changes such as edema, the presence of adenopathy in the axilla or supraclavicular areas, and the presence of distant metastasis (Table 5–3). The stage of the disease is the determining factor for treatment options.

Clinical staging is done at the time of the physical examination before any treatment. Breast cancer cells can metastasize to lung, bones, or liver. A staging workup should include a chest radiograph, a bone scan, and an ultrasound or computed tomography scan of the abdomen. Laboratory tests should include a complete blood count and measurement of serum lactate dehydrogenase and serum alkaline phosphatase. After surgery, pathologic staging is done. In many cases, the clinical and pathologic stage are different.

Factors that affect the prognosis of breast cancer include not only the size of the tumor but whether the cancer has metastasized to axillary nodes or any other part of the body. Survival is linked to the number of nodes that are involved with metastatic disease. Overall, women with node-negative tumors on pathologic staging have a better prognosis than do women with node-positive tumors. Patients with more than 10 positive nodes have a higher incidence of recurrence or metastatic disease. The hormone receptor status also affects prognosis. If the tumor is estrogen receptor-positive, meaning the tumor requires the presence of estrogen to nurture the cancer cells, there is the additional advantage of antiestrogen therapy as adjuvant treatment. High-nuclear-grade tumors such as Black's nuclear grade I (poorly differentiated) tumors and tumors

Table 5–3. TNM Breast Cancer Classification System

Primary tumor (T)			
Tx	Primary tumor cannot be assessed		
T0	No evidence of primary tumor		
Tis	Carcinoma in situ or Paget disease of the nipple with no associated tumor		
T1	Tumor ≤2 cm, in greatest dimension		
T2	Tumor >2 cm but ≤5 cm in greatest dimension		
T3	Tumor >5 cm in greatest dimension		
T4	Tumor of any size with direct extension to chest wall or skin		
Regional lymph node (N)			
Nx	Regional lymph nodes cannot be assessed		
N0	No regional lymph node metastasis		
N1	Metastasis to ipsilateral axillary lymph nodes		
N2	Metastasis to ipsilateral axillary node(s) fixed to one another or other structures		
N3	Metastasis to ipsilateral internal mammary lymph node(s)		
Distant metastasis (M)			
Mx	Presence of distant metastasis cannot be assessed		
M0	No distant metastasis		
M1	Distant metastasis (includes metastasis to supraclavicular lymph nodes)		
Stage grouping			
Stage 0	Tis	N0	M0
Stage I	T1	N0	M0
Stage IIA	T0	N1	M0
	T1	N1	M0
	T2	N0	M0
Stage IIB	T2	N1	M0
	T3	N0	M0
Stage IIIA	T0	N2	M0
	T1	N2	M0
	T2	N2	M0
	T3	N1, N2	M0
Stage IIIB	T4	Any N	M0
	Any T	N3	M0
Stage IV	Any T	Any N	M1

Reprinted with permission from Lippincott-Raven from Balch C, Singletary SE, Bland KI: Clinical decision-making in early breast cancer. Annals of Surgery, Volume 217, No. 3, March 1993, pp. 207–225.

with a high S-phase fraction (high proliferative rate) are more aggressive and have a poorer prognosis.

TREATMENT OPTIONS

When discussing treatment options with a woman diagnosed with breast cancer, it is important to ensure that she understands her particular kind of breast cancer (i.e., invasive versus noninvasive, lobular versus ductal). The patient should be given the opportunity to ask questions about the various treatment options available to her and to be an active participant in choosing the final treatment plan.

LOBULAR CARCINOMA IN SITU

Since LCIS usually is an incidental finding when a biopsy is performed for another condition, no further surgery is required. Regular follow-up with physical examinations and mammograms on a yearly basis is considered appropriate treatment for this risk marker.

DUCTAL CARCINOMA IN SITU

Treatment of DCIS includes excision of the calcifications (usually by needle localization excisional biopsy), followed by radiation therapy to the breast mound to destroy any remaining cancer cells. A radiograph of the surgical specimen is obtained to ensure that the calcifications removed are those identified on the mammogram, and the specimen is examined by a pathologist to ensure that the margins are clear. Axillary lymph node dissection usually is not required with a pathologic diagnosis of DCIS, because the risk of any cells traveling to the axilla is very small.

INVASIVE BREAST CANCER

All invasive breast cancers are treated with the same surgical options: breast-conserving therapy or modified radical mastectomy (with or without breast reconstruction). Women with tumors that are small in relation to breast size usually are candidates for breast-conserving therapy. Women with tumors that are very large in relation to the size of the breast mound and women with multicentric cancer (cancer in more than one quadrant of the breast) are not candidates for segmental mastectomy because the extent of the surgery would yield an unacceptable cosmetic result.

Age should not be a factor in the choice of treatment options. Many women in their seventh or eighth decade of life choose breast-conserving therapy instead of modified radical mastectomy. Conversely, some women in their fourth or fifth decade may opt for a modified radical mastectomy even without breast reconstruction. The woman's personal preference, her activities, and her level of comfort with the treatment options are extremely important and must be considered when guiding her to a suitable surgical treatment option.

BREAST-CONSERVING THERAPY

Breast-conserving therapy consists of a segmental mastectomy and axillary node dissection followed by irradiation of the remaining breast tissue (Fig. 5–6). The axillary node dissection is performed not for therapeutic benefit but for staging purposes—it reveals whether metastatic disease is present in the axillary nodes.

Women usually stay in the hospital overnight after surgery. Drains are placed in the wound at the time of surgery and are left in place for approximately 7 to 10 days while healing takes place. The drains do not prevent a woman from carrying out minimal activities and are easily managed by the patient or family members.

Most women are able to return to work 3 to 5 weeks after surgery. Radiation treatments begin approximately 2 weeks after the drains are removed and continue Monday through Friday for 5 to 6 weeks. Radiation treatments are performed on an outpatient basis. This allows the woman to continue her lifestyle as it was before diagnosis.

MODIFIED RADICAL MASTECTOMY

An alternative to breast conservation is a modified radical mastectomy. A modified radical mastectomy consists of removal of the breast mound, including the nipple-areola complex, and a level I and II axillary node dissection (removal of the fatty tissue containing lymph nodes under the pectoralis major and minor muscles below the axillary vein and in front of the latissimus dorsi muscle) (Fig. 5–7). As with breast-conserving surgery, the axillary node dissection is performed for the purpose of histologic staging. The pectoral muscles are left intact. The final result of modified radical mastectomy without breast reconstruction is a

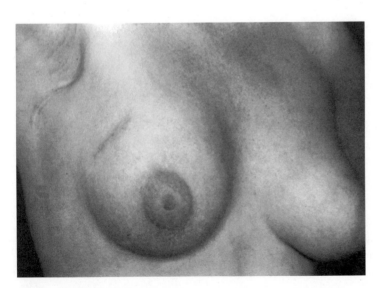

Figure 5–6. Breast conservation. Segmental mastectomy and axillary node dissection. (© The University of Texas M.D. Anderson Cancer Center.)

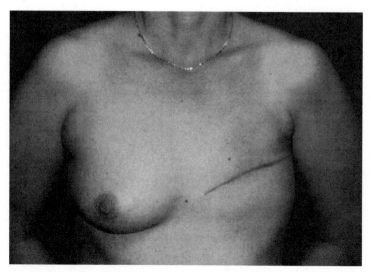

Figure 5-7. Modified radical mastectomy. (© The University of Texas M.D. Anderson Cancer Center.)

smooth, flat chest wall with a scar that runs diagonally across the chest area, slanting slightly upward toward the axilla.

BREAST RECONSTRUCTION

Many women treated with modified radical mastectomy choose to undergo breast reconstruction, either at the time of their mastectomy (immediate reconstruction) or at a later time. If immediate reconstruction is chosen, a skin-sparing mastectomy is performed. A skin-sparing mastectomy is similar to a modified radical mastectomy except the majority of the breast-mound skin is preserved. Breasts can be reconstructed using either a saline implant/tissue expander or the patient's own tissue taken from a different part of the body (Fig. 5–8). The most common tissue flap for breast reconstruction is the transverse rectus abdominis myocutaneous flap (the "TRAM flap") (Fig. 5–9). The goal of breast reconstruction is to achieve symmetry between the reconstructed breast mound and the

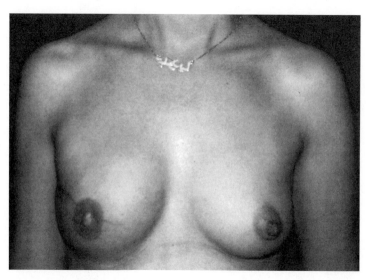

Figure 5-8. Implant reconstruction. (© The University of Texas M.D. Anderson Cancer Center.)

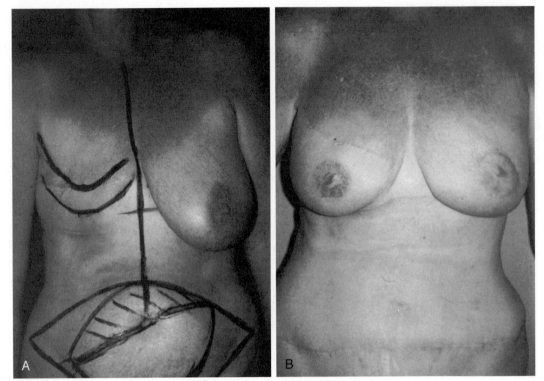

Figure 5–9. **(A)** Skin markings before TRAM reconstruction. **(B)** TRAM reconstruction. (© The University of Texas M.D. Anderson Cancer Center.)

contralateral breast. The nipple-areola complex is reconstructed by a plastic surgeon at a later date. Although the reconstructed breast provides symmetry and balance, it does not have the same sensations as the natural breast.

SYSTEMIC THERAPY

The use of chemotherapy or hormone therapy in the treatment of breast cancer depends on the clinical and pathologic stage of the disease. Systemic therapy is not indicated for DCIS or LCIS. Adjuvant chemotherapy and hormone therapy after surgery improve the overall survival in selected patients with node-negative tumors larger than 1 cm. All women with positive nodes should be considered candidates for systemic therapy.

If a woman who has undergone breast-conserving therapy requires radiation to complete her treatment, the optimal sequence of systemic therapy and radiation therapy is unclear. Most oncologists prefer to delay radiation therapy until after completion of the chemotherapy.

For premenopausal women, combination chemotherapy is usually administered regardless of the estrogen receptor status. For postmenopausal women with tumors that are estrogen receptor-positive, an estrogen antagonist such as tamoxifen is used. For postmenopausal women with estrogen receptor-negative tumors, adjuvant chemotherapy is the better choice.

FOLLOW-UP CARE

Women who have been treated for breast cancer should have regular physical examinations to check for signs of recurrence.[7] The risk of recurrence is greatest during the first 2 years after treatment and decreases thereafter. The 5-year disease-free anniversary after diagnosis and treatment of breast cancer is considered a milestone because the incidence of recurrence is significantly decreased beyond this point.

INVASIVE BREAST CANCER

Women who have been treated for invasive breast cancer should be examined every 4 months for the first 2 years after treatment, every 6 months for years 3 through 5, and annually thereafter. The examination should include a physical examination, a chest radiograph if the patient had breast radiation, and mammography of nonreconstructed breasts. At each visit, the patient's medical history, including risk factors, should be updated, and the health care provider and patient should discuss the future plan of care.

Studies have indicated that bone scans, computed tomography scans, and extensive laboratory evaluations are not beneficial in detecting early recurrence.[8–10] These tests should be ordered on an individual basis depending on presenting symptoms. It is important to incorporate regular breast self-examination into the plan of care, so that the patient can note any changes and report these to her health care provider at the next visit.

NONINVASIVE BREAST CANCER

Because the risk of recurrence for noninvasive breast cancers is low, women who have been treated for noninvasive breast cancer require only annual physical examinations and mammograms. Breast self-examination should be incorporated into the follow-up program.

PSYCHOLOGICAL SUPPORT

Psychological support is also necessary to help women rebuild their lives after treatment for breast cancer. One great difficulty women face after treatment for this disease is the fear of recurrence. Changes in the treated breast or chest wall or any changes in the body may cause a woman to become alarmed and immediately suspect that cancer has metastasized or recurred. It is important to help the patient realize that although changes may be a sign of a recurrence, they may also be a sign of normal physical aging or other unrelated medical conditions.

An experience with breast cancer is not something that can be tucked away in a woman's memory and relived only at physical examinations. It is something that permeates the fabric of her life and being. She lives with it every day as she bathes, dresses, experiences the growth of new hair after chemotherapy, or endures hot flashes because she cannot take estrogens. These experiences color her life and change her physically, emotionally, and spiritually. Follow-up programs should offer women hope, self-esteem, and satisfaction in the care they are receiving.

EXOGENOUS ESTROGENS AFTER BREAST CANCER TREATMENT

Women treated for breast cancer should consult their physician before taking exogenous estrogens in the form of estrogen replacement therapy or oral contraceptives. Although there is no definitive answer as to the advisability of estrogen replacement therapy after treatment of breast cancer, women should be evaluated on an individual basis to determine whether the benefit of estrogen replacement therapy outweighs the theoretic risk of recurrence.

BREAST SELF-EXAMINATION AFTER BREAST CANCER TREATMENT

Women who have had a segmental mastectomy should perform breast self-examination in the same manner as women who have not had a mastectomy. Women who have had radiation therapy after a segmental mastectomy may notice a change in the texture of the breast. It may feel firmer and have a slightly altered contour. Dimpling may also be noticed in the scar area. It is important to note whether this has occurred as a result of the surgery.

Women who have had a modified radical mastectomy should examine their untreated breast in the normal manner (see Fig. 5–2). The chest wall on the treated side is examined by applying a smooth pressure over the entire area, beginning at the clavicle and extending down toward the abdomen. Local recurrences usually are located in the skin or subcutaneous tissue of the mastectomy flap.

CONCLUSION

Continual surveillance against breast cancer is a must for every woman. Regular breast examinations by a health care provider in conjunction with mammography and breast self-examination lead to earlier detection of abnormalities. The advanced care practitioner can be instrumental in educating and encouraging women to become involved in their health care. Should a cancer be detected, early diagnosis and referral for treatment can result in a better prognosis and a greater range of treatment options.

REFERENCES

1. Landis SH, Murray T, Bolden S, Wingo PA, et al: Cancer Statistics 1998;65:6–31.
2. Vogel V, Yeomans A: Evaluation of risk and preventive approaches to breast cancer. The Cancer Bulletin 1993;45:489–494.

3. Hulka BS: Hormone-replacement therapy and the risk of breast cancer. CA Cancer J Clin 1990;40:289–296.
4. Steinberg KK, Thacker SB, Smith SJ, et al: A meta-analysis of the effect of estrogen replacement therapy on the risk of breast cancer. JAMA 1991;265:1985–1990.
5. Grady D, Rubin SM, Petitti DB, et al: Hormone therapy to prevent disease and prolong life in postmenopausal women. Ann Intern Med 1992;117:1016–1037.
6. Singletary SE: Lobular carcinoma in situ of the breast: A 31-year experience at The University of Texas M.D. Anderson Cancer Center. Breast Disease 1994;7:157–163.
7. Judkins AF, Peterson SK, Singletary SE: Satisfaction of breast cancer patients with a nonphysician-provider model of long-term follow-up care. Breast Disease 1996;9:139–144.
8. Yeh KA, Fortunato L, Ridge JA, et al: Routine bone scanning in patients with T1 and T2 breast cancer: A waste of money. Ann Surg Oncol 1995;2:319–324.
9. The GIVIO Investigators: Impact of follow-up testing on survival and health-related quality of life in breast cancer patients: A multicenter randomized controlled trial. JAMA 1994;271:1587–1592.
10. Del Turco MR, Palli D, Cariddi A, et al: Intensive diagnostic follow-up after treatment of primary breast cancer: A randomized trial. JAMA 1994;271:1593–1597.

Endocrine Cancer: The Thyroid, Parathyroid, Adrenal Glands, and Pancreas

Pamela A. Stanford, MN, RN, OCN, and Douglas B. Evans, MD

THE THYROID GLAND

The largest endocrine gland in the body, the thyroid gland produces two hormones, thyroxine and triiodothyronine, which are active in the body's metabolism. The two lateral lobes of the thyroid are joined by the isthmus, which lies across the trachea below the cricoid cartilage. Each lobe is covered anteriorly by the sternocleidomastoid muscles. The thyroid is affixed to the trachea and larynx so that it ascends with these structures when a person swallows. This movement helps clinicians to distinguish thyroid nodules from other masses in the neck. The superior and inferior thyroid arteries supply the highly vascular gland. The recurrent laryngeal nerves are close to the gland's posterior surface. Lymphatic drainage of the thyroid to the regional cervical lymph nodes is extensive.[1, 2]

Malignant disease of the thyroid is uncommon, and it is one of the cancers described as potentially "curable" by surgical resection. Cancer of the thyroid may occur in the very young and in the elderly. Age at presentation is a prognostic factor, because in an elderly person thyroid cancer is a more serious condition. Overall, few patients with thyroid malignancy die as a result of the disease.[2–4]

EPIDEMIOLOGY AND RISK FACTORS

An estimated 16,100 new cases of thyroid cancer occurred in 1997, with an estimated 1230 deaths. Women, in whom the disease is more prominent, accounted for an estimated 11,400 new cases, and there were an estimated 4700 new cases in men. About 90% of all endocrine gland malignancies occur in the thyroid.[2, 4, 5]

Low-dose irradiation of the head and neck is an established risk factor, with a latency period of 5 to 35 years.[6] Such low-dose irradiation is now uncommon but was used many years ago for acne, tonsillitis, or thymic enlargement. When evaluating a patient who presents with a thyroid nodule, it is important to determine whether he or she has been exposed to radiation, especially in childhood.[8] Treatment with radioactive iodine for goiter carries little, if any, risk. According to one study, patients who have undergone mantle irradiation for Hodgkin's disease have a 16 times higher risk of developing thyroid cancer.[2] When the radiation dose is greater than 2000 rads, however, the risk of thyroid cancer decreases. Lower radiation doses damage the DNA of the thyroid epithelial cells. The radiation-induced cellular damage results in increased release of thyroid-stimulating hormone (TSH), which is believed to play a role in promoting the development of cancer.[2–4]

The contribution of radiation exposure to thyroid cancer was underscored by the dramatic increase in thyroid cancers in children exposed to ionizing radiation from the Chernobyl nuclear disaster in the Ukraine in 1986. Reports describe more than 100 cases of pediatric thyroid cancer in the Gomel region of Belarus since 1989, in an area where no more than one or two pediatric thyroid cancers per year had been reported. An unusual aspect of the Chernobyl experience is how rapidly thyroid cancer developed in these children.[3, 7]

Factors in the development of papillary or follicular thyroid cancer include iodine deficiency and autoimmune thyroid disease. Iodine deficiency has been implicated in the development of goiter (thyroid enlargement) and a rising incidence of follicular cancer. The iodination of salt in the United States has decreased the incidence of follicular cancer, making papillary cancer the predominant cellular type.[2-4]

Thyroiditis does not seem to predispose to cancer. Patients with a history of severe Hashimoto's thyroiditis, however, have an increased incidence of lymphoma of the thyroid. Eighty percent of patients with anaplastic thyroid cancer have a history of nodular goiter.[2, 4]

PATHOLOGY AND HISTOLOGY

Primary cancer of the thyroid may be classified as differentiated (papillary or follicular), medullary, or undifferentiated (anaplastic). Other, less common types are lymphoma, sarcoma, and squamous cell cancer. The thyroid may be a site of metastasis from cancer of the lung, breast, or kidney or melanoma.

The prognosis of papillary and follicular thyroid cancer is based largely on the patient's age at diagnosis (unlike the prognosis for other solid tumors) and on the size and extent of disease.[2-4]

PAPILLARY AND FOLLICULAR CANCERS

Approximately 75% to 80% of all thyroid cancers are papillary and mixed papillary-follicular cancers, with no difference in prognosis based on cell type. Pathologic review shows multifocality in 30% to 80% of these tumors; psammoma bodies and lymphatic invasion are common. Metastasis to regional lymph nodes does not adversely affect prognosis in young patients without lung or bone metastases. The lungs are a common site of metastatic spread.[2-4] Indicators for poor prognosis include a tumor larger than 4 cm and extrathyroidal tumor invasion.

Approximately 10% of all thyroid cancers are follicular cancers, which are characterized by vascular invasion and hematogenous spread. The diagnosis of follicular cancer is established by histologic review, as the criterion for malignancy is vascular or capsular invasion.[2, 4, 9]

Approximately 2% to 4% of all thyroid cancers are Hürthle cell or oxyphil cell tumors, which are derived from follicular cells. As is the case for other follicular neoplasms, the criterion for malignancy is histologic evidence of capsular or vascular invasion.[2, 4, 9]

Recently, genetic factors have been ascribed a role in a small percentage of papillary and follicular thyroid cancers. Gardner's syndrome (familial colonic polyposis) and Cowden's disease (familial goiter and skin hamartomas) are known to be associated with well-differentiated thyroid cancers. Papillary thyroid cancer is reported to occur with increased frequency in families with breast, ovarian, renal, or central nervous system malignancies.[3]

The identification of cancer-causing genes has progressed in the last 5 years. The *RET* proto-oncogene has been identified in the genesis of malignant transformation in both papillary and medullary thyroid cancer. Two different mutational mechanisms have been implicated in the genesis of these tumors.[3, 4]

MEDULLARY CARCINOMA

Medullary thyroid cancer (MTC) occurs either as a sporadic event or secondary to an autosomal dominant pattern of inheritance. Familial MTC may occur as part of multiple endocrine neoplasia type 2A (MEN-2A), which includes MTC, pheochromocytoma, and parathyroid hyperplasia, or as part of MEN-2B (MTC, pheochromocytoma, mucosal and alimentary neuromas, and marfanoid habitus), or it may occur without other endocrinopathies (familial nonMEN MTC). Until recently, patients who were known members of a familial MTC kindred were screened at specialty medical centers by measurement of their serum levels of pentagastrin-stimulated calcitonin. An abnormal calcitonin response to pentagastrin stimulation indicated the need for thyroidectomy in an attempt to remove the thyroid prior to the development of invasive cancer. Since the *RET* proto-oncogene on chromosome 10 was discovered to be responsible for all forms of familial MTC, DNA mapping has been used to identify single-point mutations; this procedure is now available in most laboratories.[3, 7, 8]

Indicators of high risk of tumor recurrence are age older than 40 years, male sex, extension of cervical disease to the mediastinum, extranodal tumor extension, incomplete surgical resection of the primary tumor, and adjacent lymph node metastases.

Like the prognosis of papillary and follicular cancers, the prognosis of MTC depends on the extent of disease. MTC associated with MEN-2B denotes a more aggressive form of disease. Because MTC is characterized by early spread to regional lymph nodes, the majority of patients with invasive MTC are likely to have metastasis to regional lymph nodes at the time of diagnosis.[2, 4, 8] Distant metastases occur in liver, lung, bone, and occasionally brain.[2, 7]

ANAPLASTIC (UNDIFFERENTIATED) CANCER

Anaplastic thyroid cancer is characterized by progressive dedifferentiation of malignant tissue with increasing age. These thyroid cancers respond poorly to therapy. Anaplastic thyroid cancer often is characterized at diagnosis by locally invasive disease. The prognosis is dismal, with most studies showing a 2-year survival rate of zero.[2, 4] Airway control usually requires tracheostomy. Treatment is with combined chemotherapy and irradiation.

CLINICAL PRESENTATION AND PHYSICAL EXAMINATION

The clinical presentation often provides some clues for differentiating malignant from benign thyroid nodules. The patient's history of radiation exposure and a family history of thyroid malignancy are important. Recent change in voice may signify palsy of the recurrent laryngeal nerve, suggesting malignancy.[2–4, 6, 8]

However, most patients with thyroid cancer have an asymptomatic thyroid nodule discovered during a routine physical examination. An estimated 4% to 7% of the population have thyroid nodules, of which fewer than 5% are malignant. Thyroid malignancy may rarely occur as a dominant nodule in a multinodular goiter. Not infrequently in adults, and especially in children, the initial manifestation of thyroid cancer is a palpable lymph node in the neck.[2, 4, 9]

Diarrhea may be a presenting symptom of MTC, which may be accompanied by other hormonal syndromes including excessive production of corticotropin (ACTH). Other findings suggestive of MEN include pheochromocytoma and hypercalcemia. Cushing's syndrome is a rare presentation of MTC.[4, 6, 10]

Anaplastic cancer may be seen as a fixed or rapidly enlarging neck mass. Associated symptoms may include hoarseness, dysphagia, stridor, or neck pain. These symptoms should prompt immediate airway evaluation. At the time of presentation, these patients often require emergency tracheostomy.[2–4]

PHYSICAL EXAMINATION OF THE THYROID

After inspecting the neck, palpate the trachea for midline position. Place a thumb along each side of the trachea and compare the space between the trachea and the sternocleidomastoid muscle on each side. An unequal space may indicate displacement of the trachea from midline and presence of a mass. Tracheal deviation may be noted on chest radiography.

Palpation of the thyroid requires a gentle touch. Palpate the thyroid for size, shape, configuration, consistency, tenderness, and the presence of nodules. This part of the examination may be done with the examiner standing either in front of or behind the patient. To palpate the thyroid using a frontal approach, ask the patient to sit. Give the patient a cup of water to facilitate swallowing. Instruct the patient to hold a sip of water in the mouth until the examiner's hands are positioned correctly. Using the pads of the first two fingers, palpate the left lobe with the right hand and the right lobe with the left hand. To increase access to the lobe, gently move the skin medially over the sternocleidomastoid muscle and reach under its anterior borders with fingers just below the cricoid cartilage. Ask the patient to swallow while the isthmus is palpated, then to swallow again as the right and left lobes are palpated. The thyroid should move beneath the examiner's fingers on swallowing.

To examine the thyroid from behind, seat the patient on a chair with the neck at a comfortable level. Position two fingers of each hand on each side of the trachea just below the cricoid cartilage. Have the patient swallow as the examiner feels for movement of the isthmus. To palpate the main body of the right lobe, gently displace the trachea to the right, and ask the patient to swallow as the right lobe is palpated. Reverse to palpate the left lobe.[1]

In the case of thyroid gland enlargement, auscultate for vascular sounds. In a hypermetabolic state (Graves' disease), a bruit will be heard.[1, 6]

Fiberoptic or indirect laryngoscopy may be used to evaluate vocal cord movement. Tumor involvement of the recurrent laryngeal nerve may result in unilateral vocal cord palsy. All patients should undergo laryngoscopy prior to thyroid surgery. Unilateral palsy of the recurrent laryngeal nerve may be asymptomatic.[2, 4, 6]

DIAGNOSTIC EVALUATION

Knowledge of the natural history of the four types of thyroid cancer and the factors that influence prognosis enables the clinician to optimally evaluate and manage patients who have a thyroid nodule.

Thyroid function studies (TSH and thyroxine [T_4]) are of little value in differentiation between benign and malignant thyroid disease because thyroid nodules are usually hypofunctioning and therefore rarely alter the overall production of thyroid hormone. These studies are useful for determining hyperthyroidism or hypothyroidism; a suppressed TSH should alert the physician to the possibility of a toxic nodule(s).[2]

Although benign thyroid conditions may cause an increase in thyroglobulin secretion, papillary and follicular cancers are known to secrete thyroglobulin. Therefore, after ablative therapy, thyroglobulin values may be used to monitor for recurrent disease. Approximately 10% of patients have circulating endogenous antibodies that interfere with the measurement of thyroglobulin; these antibodies may be detected by serum antithyroid antibody screening.[2, 4]

MTC originates in the C cells of the thyroid. These cells produce carcinoembryonic antigen (CEA) and calcitonin, both of which can be measured in blood as specific, sensitive tumor markers of the disease. If MTC is suspected by the patient's presentation or family history, serum catecholamine levels should be evaluated to screen for pheochromocytoma as part of multiple endocrine neoplasia type II.[2, 4, 7]

The only definitive method of determining malignancy is pathologic examination of tissue. Fine-needle aspiration (FNA) biopsy is preferred because it is the most cost-effective and accurate method currently available. Accuracy depends on the cytopathologist's technique, but it is usually close to 90%. Occasionally, when insufficient material is available for cytologic analysis, lobectomy may be necessary. By cytologic evaluation, however, a benign follicular adenoma cannot be distinguished from a follicular cancer because the aspirate does not provide sufficient material for assessing vascular or capsular invasion.[2, 4, 9, 10]

IMAGING STUDIES

Until recently, thyroid scans were used to help determine the malignant potential of a thyroid nodule. Malignant thyroid neoplasms appear as "cold" areas on a thyroid scan, whereas hyperfunctioning nodules (almost always benign) appear as "hot" spots. As the accuracy of FNA biopsy has improved, imaging is no longer recommended for evaluation of malignant potential.[3, 4, 6] Following FNA, a cervical ultrasound is performed to accurately stage the extent of local-regional tumor spread.

ULTRASONOGRAPHY

Ultrasound is a useful tool when a thyroid nodule or lymph nodes are difficult to palpate, for ultrasound-guided FNA biopsy of suspicious lymph nodes; to characterize thyroid nodules (calcifications or cysts); and to establish the number of thyroid nodules or to measure thyroid nodule size before suppressive therapy is initiated. Ultrasound is critical for accurate preoperative evaluation of lymphatic spread or local tumor extension. The usefulness of ultrasound is dependent to some extent on the experience of the operator.[3, 4]

RADIOGRAPHY

A chest radiograph is obtained to rule out lung metastasis. It may also show tracheal deviation caused by a thyroid mass or paratracheal lymphadenopathy. Computed tomography (CT) scans and magnetic resonance imaging (MRI) are useful tools for evaluating large tumor volume, recurrent disease, or suspected invasion of surrounding soft tissues.[2, 4]

TREATMENT

THYROID SUPPRESSION

Thyroid nodules may decrease in size following the administration of exogenous thyroid hormone. Levothyroxine sodium is prescribed, in a dosage based on body weight, to reduce endogenous TSH secretion while maintaining the euthyroid (normal functional) state. Approximately 30% of benign nodules may decrease in size (in contrast to malignant ones, which do not), so that thyroid suppression may be used if a patient refuses surgical intervention. Any nodule (except a hemorrhagic cyst or adenoma) that grows despite thyroid suppression usually requires surgical resection. If the nodule shrinks by 50% or more, suppression should be continued and thyroid function studies monitored. Thyroid suppression may be complicated by osteoporosis or cardiac arrhythmias, particularly in elderly patients.[2, 4, 6]

SURGERY

Surgical intervention remains the most effective technique for treating thyroid cancers. Total thyroidectomy versus subtotal thyroidectomy is a subject of debate among clinicians. In general, subtotal thyroidectomy (lobectomy) is recommended for tumors that are smaller than 1 cm with no evidence of extrathyroidal extension and a favorable histologic profile. Total thyroidectomy is recommended for follicular or medullary cancer, papillary cancers larger than 1 cm, patients older than 50 years, and in those patients with extrathyroidal extension of the tumor. Total thyroidectomy is recommended also for patients with familial MTC, who often have bilateral, multifocal disease, and for patients with presumed sporadic disease, who have a 20% to 30% incidence of multifocal disease. In addition, because of the frequent finding of lymph node metastasis in the central neck compartment, central neck dissection is advocated for all patients with palpable primary medullary thyroid cancers, even in the absence of clinically detectable lymph node metastasis. The lists that follow give further indications for surgical resection.[10]

Factors that prompt a decision for surgical intervention after benign FNA has indicated no malignancy are large goiter causing obstructive symptoms, repetitive findings of blood-filled cysts, history of irradiation, and a family history of papillary or medullary thyroid cancer.

Specific indications for surgical intervention in the case of thyroid abnormalities are as follows:

- Finding or suspicion of thyroid cancer on FNA, especially if the patient has a history of irradiation
- Nondiagnostic FNA in a patient older than 60 years of age
- Thyroid mass with suggestion of malignant disease (hard fixed mass, vocal cord paralysis, regional tissue invasion)
- Proof of metastasis by cervical lymph node biopsy.
- Hyperfunctioning nodule in a young patient
- Unrelieved fear of thyroid cancer in a patient with a nodule despite benign-appearing FNA.

Potential complications of thyroid surgery include transient or permanent hypocalcemia if the parathyroid glands are removed or damaged and vocal cord paralysis (and change in voice) if the recurrent laryngeal nerve is removed or damaged.[4]

ADJUVANT TREATMENT

Well-differentiated papillary and follicular cancers concentrate iodine, making radioactive iodine effective for treating residual or metastatic disease. If the thyroid scan with iodine 131 (^{131}I) reveals thyroid bed uptake, patients are treated with a therapeutic dose of ^{131}I, usually in the range of 29 to 100 mCi. Thyroid hormone is withheld for 4 weeks preceding the thyroid scan. A repeat thyroid scan is performed 1 year following initial ablative therapy. If there is iodine uptake, the patient may be treated again with 100 to 200 mCi ^{131}I. Patients rarely require further I^{131} therapy in the absence of extracervical metastatic disease. Thyroglobulin levels are monitored to detect recurrent or metastatic disease after ablative therapy.[2–4, 6]

MEDULLARY THYROID CANCER

Adjuvant external beam radiation therapy should be considered for patients at high risk of local or regional tumor recurrence after surgery.[7] Indications of high risk are positive surgical margins, extension of the tumor into muscle or extranodal soft tissue, and extensive mediastinal tumor that requires median sternotomy.[7]

ANAPLASTIC TUMOR

Anaplastic (undifferentiated) thyroid cancer is rarely amenable to surgical resection. The patient should be referred quickly for chemotherapy.[2, 4] Attention to airway management may be life-saving.

AFTER-TREATMENT SURVEILLANCE

Patients who have undergone total thyroidectomy are given levothyroxine sodium, with the dosage geared to body weight. Once the dosage is in the desired range, TSH and T_4 levels are measured routinely to monitor TSH suppression (desired range for suppression, <0.5 µU/mL). TSH should be kept suppressed to eliminate the growth potential of residual microscopic tumor tissue.[2–4, 6]

Routine follow-up should be geared to the patient and the illness. In general, for patients with differentiated thyroid cancers, follow-up should include routine physical examination, measurement of thyroglobulin level, chest radiography to check for pulmonary metastasis, and ultrasound examination of the neck to check for local recurrence. Given the favorable natural history of this disease, it is important not to incur costly or unnecessary follow-up procedures.[2, 4]

Patients with MTC should have a yearly physical examination. Measurements of CEA and calcitonin levels are specific and sensitive tests of recurrence. If the values are elevated persistently, radiologic evaluation for recurrent or metastatic disease should be considered. Attempts should be made to locate the disease by CT, sonography, or radionucleotide imaging. If disease is found, the patient is referred for surgical intervention; systemic therapy is occasionally used to treat distant metastasis.[2, 4, 7] Figure 6–1 presents a treatment algorithm for patients with suspected thyroid cancer.

THE PARATHYROID GLANDS

The parathyroid glands are so named because of their proximity to the thyroid gland, but they have a distinctly separate function: they help to regulate the body's calcium metabolism. Four parathyroids are usual, but a person may have three or occasionally five. Because of their close anatomic relation to the thyroid gland, parathyroid tissue may be removed at the time the thyroid gland is surgically resected. Parathyroid cancer, which is exceedingly rare, must be distinguished from other hypercalcemic states because of the severity of disease and treatment approach.[2, 4, 6]

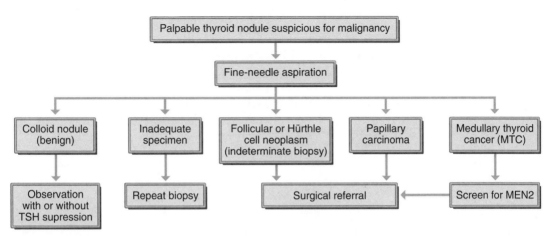

Figure 6–1. Decision algorithm for patients with thyroid cancer. (Adapted from Tyler DS, Winchester DJ, Carraway NP, et al: Indeterminate fine-needle aspiration biopsy of the thyroid: Identification of subgroup at high risk for invasive cancer. Surgery 1994;16:1054.)

EPIDEMIOLOGY AND RISK FACTORS

The cause of parathyroid adenomas is unknown, although persons who have a history of exposure of the head and neck to irradiation are postulated to be at increased risk.[2, 4] Parathyroid adenomas may be associated with the inherited syndromes MEN-I or MEN-2.[10]

HISTOLOGY AND PATHOLOGY

Primary hyperparathyroidism may develop from one of three possible conditions: adenoma (84%), hyperplasia (15%), or cancer (<1%). The three conditions may be identified by the following signs and symptoms:

Adenoma is most common; however, patients rarely present with a palpable mass. Double adenomas may occur, but most patients have single gland enlargement.

Hyperplasia usually follows a familial pattern and is of greatest clinical significance in patients with MEN I. Glands may be in ectopic locations, and supernumerary or fifth glands may occur (often within the thymus).

Cancer usually appears as a neck mass in a patient with the recent development of a very high serum calcium level. Local recurrence within the neck and distant metastases commonly occur.

Parathyroid adenoma is the most common cause of primary hyperparathyroidism. Parathyroid hyperplasia usually indicates multiple gland involvement and may be part of a MEN syndrome. Principal histologic features that distinguish cancer from adenoma include a trabecular pattern, mitotic figures, thick fibrous bands, and capsular and blood vessel invasion. Distant metastasis may develop to lung, bone, or liver.[2, 4]

PRESENTING HISTORY

The diagnosis of parathyroid cancer may be suspected at the time of the patient's initial examination. It usually involves severe hypercalcemia (14 mg/dl calcium or higher), a palpable neck mass, and bone and renal disease. Patients may also have symptoms related to increased urinary excretion of calcium (urinary calculi and nephrocalcinosis).[2, 4] One distinguishing feature of parathyroid cancer is the high rate of recurrence. Even though the patient may normalize serum calcium levels after surgical resection, recurrent hypercalcemia (indicative of tumor recurrence) may develop.[2, 4]

DIAGNOSTIC WORKUP

Laboratory studies include serial measures of serum calcium levels and intact PTH. Urinary calcium excretion should be measured to exclude familial hypocalciuric hypercalcemia (FHH). Localization studies (ultrasound, sestamibi scan, MRI) are usually reserved for reoperative cases.[2]

DIFFERENTIAL DIAGNOSIS

Primary hyperparathyroidism should be distinguished from the hypercalcemia of malignancy, which may be caused by bony metastasis from lung or breast. However, 50% to 80% of patients with hypercalcemia of malignancy present with no bony metastasis. Squamous cell cancers of any organ, renal cell cancer, transitional cell cancer of the bladder, and ovarian cancer may produce PTH-related peptide (PTH-RP) that can be measured. Its elevation helps to differentiate hypercalcemia of malignancy from primary hyperparathyroidism (in which case intact PTH is elevated, not PTH-RP).[2, 4, 6]

TREATMENT AND REFERRAL

The preferred treatment for parathyroid cancer is surgical resection. Before resection is considered, the patient is likely to need preoperative management of hypercalcemia, including hydration and administration of diuretics, most often furosemide.

Although parathyroid cancers grow slowly, most patients die from the metabolic complications of hypercalcemia. Therefore, an aggressive surgical approach is indicated to eliminate all PTH-secreting malignant tissue. Surgical resection should include en bloc resection, to include thyroid lobectomy and excision of tracheoesophageal tissue, regional lymph nodes, and the thymus.[4]

Medical therapy to treat recurrent disease should include hydration, diuresis, and possibly systemic therapy with multiagent chemotherapy. Recent medical treatments have focused on use of newer phosphonate derivatives such as pamidronic acid.[2, 4, 6]

THE ADRENAL GLANDS

The adrenal glands are located superior and medial to the upper pole of each kidney. The glands produce a large number of hormones, primarily in the adrenal cortex.[1, 6]

Cancers of the adrenal cortex constitute only 0.05% to 0.2% of all cancers. Women seem to develop functioning adrenocortical cancers more commonly than men, whereas the nonfunctioning adrenal tumors are more common in men. Patients with functioning adrenal tumors present with clinical features consistent with several syndromes of hormone hypersecretion. Nonfunctioning tumors often are discovered when they metastasize or when the primary tumor becomes large enough to produce abdominal symptoms. Differentiating between benign and malignant adrenocortical neoplasms is not always possible; the only reliable criterion is the presence of nodal or distant metastases.[2]

Pheochromocytomas are rare, usually benign tumors that arise in the chromaffin cells of the adrenal medulla. They secrete catecholamines which cause clinical symptoms, including tachycardia, palpitations, headache, anxiety attacks, and sustained hypertension. They may also produce other hormones such as ACTH; patients may present with concomitant Cushing's syndrome. Bilateral pheochromocytomas are components of MEN-2A and MEN-2B, as mentioned previously.[10, 11] Pheochromocytomas also occur in 25% of patients with von Hippel-Lindau disease and in occasional patients with neurofibromatosis or

Recklinghausen's disease.[10] The possible presence of pheochromocytoma should be evaluated preoperatively, because the tumor can cause hypertensive crisis and mortality during general anesthesia. As with adrenocortical cancers, it may be difficult to characterize its malignant potential. The only absolute criteria of malignancy are the presence of secondary tumors at sites where chromaffin cells are not normally present, and the presence of visceral metastases.[2]

Use of CT scans to evaluate clinical problems has resulted in the occasional serendipitous finding of a mass in the adrenal gland. Because they are discovered incidentally while the patient is undergoing evaluation, these tumors have been referred to as incidentalomas or incidental adrenalomas.[11, 12]

Three questions may help the clinician evaluate the patient who presents with a radiologically documented adrenal mass or suspicious clinical findings, or both: Is this a functioning or nonfunctioning tumor? Is this a benign or malignant tumor? Is this a primary or metastatic tumor? The evaluation is described in Table 6–1.[2, 11–13]

Surgery is the treatment of choice for adrenal tumors. Metastatic adrenocorti-

Table 6–1. Evaluation of Radiologically Documented Adrenal Mass and/or Suspicious Clinical Findings

FUNCTIONING OR NONFUNCTIONING ADRENAL TUMOR?

EVALUATION	FUNCTIONING	NEOPLASM
24-hr urine for vanillyl mandelic acid, metanephrine, catecholamines	If elevated, rule out pheomochromocytoma	
Physical examination	+ Virilization, + feminization, change in menses (indicating a functioning cortical adenoma or carcinoma)	Normal
Hypertension (HTN)	+ HTN (may occur with pheochromocytoma or aldosteronoma)	
Low serum potassium	Rule out hyperaldosteronism	
Family history	+ MEN, rule out pheochromocytoma	

BENIGN OR MALIGNANT ADRENAL TUMOR?

EVALUATION	MALIGNANT	BENIGN
Review/obtain CT or MRI	>6 cm or change from previous status or <6 cm and symptoms of nodal or distant metastasis	<6 cm
Physical examination	Weight gain, + feminization, + virilization	Normal

PRIMARY OR METASTATIC ADRENAL TUMOR?

EVALUATION	PRIMARY	METASTATIC
Careful history, imaging studies to evaluate for malignancy	Metastatic spread to lung, liver, or bone	Metastasis from lung, breast, kidney; melanoma or lymphoma

Table 6-2. Pancreatic Endocrine Cancers

TUMOR	PRIMARY PEPTIDE/ HORMONE	CLINICAL SYNDROME	PRESENTING/DEFINING SIGNS AND SYMPTOMS	RADIOLOGY	METASTATIC PATTERN
Nonfunctioning Islet Cell Carcinoma	None	None	Weight loss Abdominal pain Jaundice Rash (rare)	Hypervascular mass on CT scan	Liver Bone
Pancreatic Polypeptidoma	Pancreatic polypeptide	None	Weight loss Abdominal pain Jaundice ↑ Serum peptide level	Hypervascular mass on CT scan	Liver Bone
Insulinoma	Insulin	May be part of MEN I	Fasting hypoglycemia Altered consciousness Visual disturbances Weakness Sweating Weight gain ↓ Fasting glucose ↑ Serum insulin ↑ C-peptide	Tumor localization by endoscopic and intraoperative ultrasound	Liver
Gastrinoma	Gastrin	Zollinger-Ellison syndrome (gastrinoma, peptic ulcer, gastric hypersecretion) MEN I	Diarrhea (especially with ulcer) Ulcer in unusual location Recurrent/persistent ulcer ↑ Fasting serum gastrin Gastric hyperacidity	Localization by CT, MRI, or angiogram—90% in "gastric triangle"	Liver Lymph nodes Lung Bone
Glucagonoma	Glucagon	Glucagonoma syndrome	Weight loss Mild diabetes Dermatitis (migratory necrolytic erythema) Atrophic glossitis Angular stomatitis Normocytic, normochromic anemia Venous thrombosis Mental status changes ↑ Serum glucagon ↑ CEA	Hypervascular mass on CT	Liver Lung

Data from references 1, 6, 16, and 18.

cal cancer is treated with cytotoxic chemotherapy or mitotane. Chemoemboliza-
tion has been used in some circumstances.[5, 6]

PANCREATIC ENDOCRINE CANCER

Pancreatic endocrine tumors arise from the endocrine or islet cells of the
pancreas and are often referred to as islet cell cancers. They are an uncommon
malignancy. Pancreatic endocrine tumors are distinguished from pancreatic
exocrine tumors by their generally more indolent biologic behavior, higher
rate of surgical resectability, better response to chemotherapy, and better prognosis.[2, 14, 15]

Islet cell cancer may be classified as *functional* if it is associated with a clinical
syndrome related to ectopic hormone or peptide release or as *nonfunctional* if
it is not associated with a clinical syndrome.[13] Although one hormone or peptide
may predominate, multiple elevated peptide levels are not unusual for these
tumors. Currently available laboratory techniques can be used to measure gas-
trin, glucagon, vasoactive intestinal polypeptide, pancreatic polypeptide, neuro-
tensin, somatostatin, and insulin. Table 6–2 summarizes the clinical findings of
the more commonly seen pancreatic endocrine cancers.

The treatment of choice is surgery; many patients with these tumors can be
cured by surgical resection. Given the indolent nature of the disease, hepatic
metastasis is not an absolute contraindication to surgery. Chemotherapy is given
for metastatic disease, and radiation therapy may be effective for local control
and palliation.[2, 14–18]

REFERENCES

1. Siedel HM, Ball JW, Dains JE, Benedict GW (eds): Mosby's Guide to Physical Examination, 3rd
   ed. St. Louis, CV Mosby, 1994:219.
2. Norton JA, Levin B, Jensen RT: Cancer of the endocrine system. In DeVita VT, Hellman S,
   Rosenberg SA (eds): Cancer: Principles and Practice of Oncology, 4th ed. Philadelphia, JB
   Lippincott, 1993:1333.
3. Gagel RD, Goepfert H, Callender DL: Changing concepts in the pathogenesis and management of
   thyroid cancer. CA Cancer J Clin 1996; 46:261.
4. Horsley JS, Fratkin MJ: Cancer of the thyroid and parathyroid glands. In Murphy GP, Lawrence
   W, Lenhard RE (eds): American Cancer Society Textbook of Clinical Oncology, 2nd ed. Atlanta,
   American Cancer Society 1995:342–354.
5. Parker SL, Tong T, Bolden S, Wingo PA: Cancer statistics, 1997. CA Cancer J Clin 1997;47:5–27.
6. Burch WM: Endocrinology, 3rd ed. Baltimore, Williams & Wilkins, 1994.
7. Evans DB, Burgess AM, Mott, et al: Medullary Thyroid Cancer. Unpublished manuscript.
8. Wells SA: Recent advances in the treatment of thyroid cancer. CA Cancer J Clin 1996;46:258.
9. Tyler DS, Winchester DJ, Carraway NP, et al: Indeterminate fine-needle aspiration biopsy of the
   thyroid: Identification of subgroup at high risk for invasive cancer. Surgery 1994; 16:1054.
10. Antonelli A, Miccoli P, Derzhitski VE, et al: Epidemiologic and clinical evaluation of thyroid
    cancer in children from the Gomel region. World J Surg 1996;20:867.
11. Linos DA, Stylopoulus, Reptis SA: Adenoma: A call for more aggressive management. World J
    Surg 1996;20:788.
12. Cook DM, Loriaux L: The incidental adrenal mass. Am J Med 1996;101:88.
13. Evans DB, Lee JE, Merrell RC: Adrenal medullary disease in multiple endocrine neoplasia type
    2: Appropriate management. Endocrinol Metab Clin North Am 1994;23:167–176.
14. Delcore R, Friesen SR: Gastrointestinal neuroendocrine tumors. J Am Coll Surg 1994;178:187.
15. Lo CY, VanHeerden JA, Thompson GB, et al: Islet cell cancer of pancreas. World J Surg
    1996;20:878.
16. Evans DB, Skibber JM, Lee JE, et al: Nonfunctioning islet cell cancer of the pancreas. Surgery
    1993;114:1175.
17. Choksi UA, Sellin RV, Hickey RC, et al: An unusual skin rash associated with a pancreatic
    polypeptide-producing tumor. Ann Intern Med 1988;108:64.
18. Vassilopoulon-Sellin R, Ajani J: Islet cell tumors of the pancreas. Endocrin Metabol Clin North
    Am 1994;23(1):53–62.

Chapter 7

Pancreatic Cancer

Pamela A. Stanford, MN, RN, OCN, and
Douglas B. Evans, MD

The pancreas, located deep in the middle of the upper abdomen, is surrounded by the stomach, the small intestine, the liver, and the spleen. Shaped like a pear, the pancreas is divided into three sections: from the patient's perspective, these are the wider right end (head), the middle (body), and the narrow left end (tail). The pancreas performs both endocrine and exocrine functions. Endocrine functions include production and release of the hormones insulin and glucagon.

The pancreas' exocrine function is carried out in the acinar cells. These cells produce digestive juices that contain inactive enzymes for the digestion of proteins, fats, and carbohydrates. The collecting ducts empty the digestive juice into the pancreatic duct, which runs the length of the pancreas. The pancreatic duct joins the common bile duct (which runs through the pancreas) to form the ampulla of Vater, which enters the second portion of the duodenum. Once introduced into the duodenum, the digestive enzymes are activated. If the release of these enzymes is blocked for any reason, the body does not absorb food completely, and diarrhea and weight loss result (Fig. 7–1).[1]

Adenocarcinoma of the pancreas most often arises in the ductal cells. Because of its location deep in the abdomen and lack of early defining signs and symptoms, the disease may already have progressed beyond the curative stage at the time of diagnosis. For this reason, adenocarcinoma of the pancreas has been described as a "silent cancer."[2–4]

EPIDEMIOLOGY AND RISK FACTORS

The mortality rate for pancreatic adenocarcinoma almost equals the incidence rate, with very few patients surviving 5 years. Adenocarcinoma of the pancreas

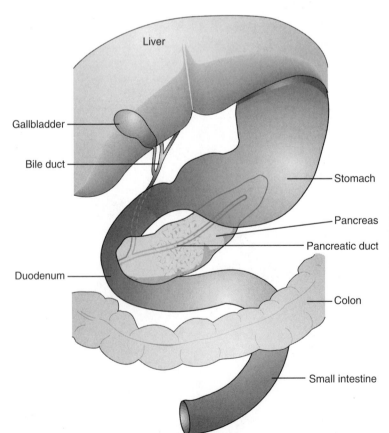

Figure 7–1. The pancreas and surrounding organs and viscera. (Adapted from Siedel HM, Ball JW, Dains JE, Benedict GW (eds): Mosby's Guide to Physical Examination, 3rd ed. St. Louis, CV Mosby, 1994.)

is the fifth leading cause of adult cancer deaths. In 1998, there will be an estimated 29,000 new cases of pancreatic carcinoma and an estimated 28,900 deaths. The disease occurs more frequently in black Americans than in white Americans.[2, 5]

Adenocarcinoma of the pancreas has been described as a cancer of the industrialized world. Increased risk is thought to be related to smoking, high-fat diets, ingestion of meats, and exposure to chemicals and metal working. One study conducted in Veteran's Administration hospitals showed the rate of pancreatic carcinoma to be twice as high in heavy smokers. Studies have failed to show a cause-and-effect relation between diabetes and pancreatic carcinoma although the data do indicate a fourfold increased risk. The onset of diabetes months before the diagnosis of pancreatic carcinoma has been recognized by clinicians for years.[2–4, 6]

GENETICS

The role of heredity in pancreatic cancer has not been clearly defined. There have been case reports of familial clustering. Studies have confirmed increased risk in persons who have a close relative with pancreatic malignancy.[3, 4]

The emerging role of oncogenes and growth factors in carcinogenesis is being researched. Point mutations in the K-*ras* oncogene (oncogenes are genes that are found to be mutated in many tumors) have been demonstrated in 75% to 90% of human pancreatic carcinomas. Increased expression of transforming growth factor-α, epidermal growth factor (EGF), and the EGF receptor—proteins often associated with tumor growth—has been demonstrated in most pancreatic cancer cell lines. These findings point to tumor growth mechanisms that are not responsive to normal cellular growth controls. One goal of ongoing research is to define cellular growth characteristics such as oncogene expression, growth factor expression, ploidy status (chromosome status), and other factors in relation to clinical outcome to identify patient groups who may benefit from more aggressive treatment.[6, 7]

HISTOLOGY AND PATHOLOGY

Most pancreatic carcinomas arise in the ductal epithelium even though less than 15% of the pancreas is composed of ductal tissue. Most (80%) are mucin-producing adenocarcinomas. Other tumors arising in the pancreas include acinar cell carcinoma, cystadenocarcinoma, adenosquamous carcinoma, carcinoid, sarcoma, and lymphoma.

Two thirds of adenocarcinomas arise in the head of the pancreas. Cancers that arise in the head of the pancreas should be distinguished from tumors that arise in the common bile duct, the ampulla of Vater, or the duodenum. Survival rates for all three are better than for pancreatic adenocarcinoma.

A characteristic pathologic feature of pancreatic adenocarcinoma is the development of early subclinical metastasis. In addition, 40% of patients present with locally advanced disease at diagnosis including regional lymph node involvement and direct extension to adjacent organs. The natural history of pancreatic adenocarcinoma is characterized by widespread metastasis to intra-abdominal organs (liver, peritoneal implants) and to extra-abdominal organs (lung).[3, 4, 6]

PRESENTING HISTORY AND PHYSICAL EXAMINATION

The classic triad of weight loss, jaundice, and abdominal pain is diagnostic for pancreatic carcinoma. Because of its location deep in the abdomen, pancreatic carcinoma has no early warning signs or symptoms (Table 7–1).[4, 6, 8] Patients may present with vague, nonspecific symptoms such as fatigue, anorexia, changes in bowel habits, and steatorrhea. Diabetes mellitus may occur concomitantly or precede the diagnosis by months.[3, 4] Psychiatric symptoms, usually depression, may also precede the diagnosis by months.[8–10] Migratory thrombophlebitis (Trousseau's sign) may be a presenting symptom.[3, 4]

Weight loss, a nonspecific symptom, usually is gradual and progressive. Some patients who have engaged in an active weight loss program for fitness report that their weight loss was more pronounced and rapid than anticipated. Some degree of weight loss may be attributed to subclinical malabsorption rather than inadequate calorie intake. Malabsorption is manifested by stools that are greasy, floating, frothy, and malodorous with increased frequency, indicating steatorrhea.

Jaundice is a common presenting symptom.[3, 11] Painless jaundice may also be a presenting symptom of periampullary or primary bile duct carcinomas. Because tumors that are strategically located in the pancreatic head are more likely to block the bile duct, jaundice may signify a localized, relatively small tumor that might be treated surgically. For this reason, any unexplained jaundice should be evaluated carefully. The initial presentation of jaundice may be icteric sclera or "yellow eyes." More than one patient has presented for evaluation because they were told by family, hairdressers, or work associates that they had "yellow eyes." Jaundice is often accompanied by itching, which at times may be intense.[3, 4, 6, 11]

Abdominal pain is another common presenting symptom of pancreatic carcinoma. Patients may present with vague and ill-defined pain that is worse at night and aggravated by lying flat. This vague presentation may contribute to a delay in diagnosis. Other patients may present with pain secondary to pancreatitis, a complication of pancreatic cancer. Severe pain is more often associated with carcinoma of the body or tail of the pancreas and may indicate tumor involvement of the retroperitoneum and splanchnic nerves, a possible sign of advanced disease. Patients whose tumor involves the celiac plexus may complain of a "gnawing" pain radiating to the back.[3, 4, 10, 11]

Diabetes may be diagnosed months before pancreatic carcinoma, or it may appear suddenly, indicating pancreatic endocrine insufficiency. Diabetes may be a sign of pancreatic carcinoma or a treatment sequela (after surgical resection). Not all patients who undergo pancreatectomy become diabetic, be-

---

Table 7–1. Moosa's High Index of Suspicion for Pancreatic Carcinoma in Patients Older Than 40 Years of Age

Obstructive jaundice
Recent unexplained weight loss (>10% body weight)
Recent unexplained upper abdominal or upper back pain
Recent vague unexplained dyspepsia with normal gastrointestinal evaluation
Sudden onset of diabetes mellitus without predisposition (obesity or family history)
Sudden onset of unexplained steatorrhea
Attack of idiopathic pancreatitis
History of heavy smoking (if so, the level of suspicion should be doubled)

Adapted from Beazeley RM, Cohn I: Tumors of the pancreas, gallbladder and extrahepatic bile ducts. In Murphy GP, Lawrence W, Lendhard RE (eds): American Cancer Society Textbook of Clinical Oncology, 2nd ed. Atlanta, American Cancer Society, 1995.

cause the pancreas may function normally even though a portion has been removed.[3, 4, 6]

Patients with pancreatic carcinoma are at higher risk for depression than those with other types of abdominal cancers. One study reported depression in 67% of patients with pancreatic carcinoma, compared with fewer than 10% of patients with colon carcinoma. A reactive depression may be anticipated in some patients because the delay in diagnosis of these cancers often leads to advanced disease, a finding that is emotionally distressing to the patient.[9, 10]

Because of their deep abdominal location, pancreatic tumors usually are not palpable unless the disease is progressive. However, approximately 33% of patients present with a distended, palpable gallbladder (the Courvoisier sign).[1, 3]

One uncommon physical finding in patients with pancreatic carcinoma is an enlarged spleen. Tumors of the distal pancreas spread by local extension to the anatomically nearby spleen. Patients may present with splenic vein occlusion and secondary splenomegaly demonstrated on computed tomography (CT) scans. Local tumor invasion may also cause gastric outlet or duodenal obstruction, or both, which may cause persistent nausea and vomiting. Ascites is associated with hepatic or peritoneal metastatic spread (carcinomatosis). Another physical finding suggestive of metastatic disease is a palpable left supraclavicular lymph node (Virchow's node).[1, 3, 4] The left supraclavicular region should be carefully palpated in all patients with suspected gastrointestinal malignancy.

DIFFERENTIAL DIAGNOSIS AND DIAGNOSTIC EVALUATION

As noted above, it is important to evaluate obstructive jaundice to differentiate between malignant and nonmalignant processes and to accurately stage (radiographically) malignant tumors of the pancreas or extrahepatic biliary tree (Table 7–2).

LABORATORY EVALUATION

Examination of laboratory values is helpful. In the absence of extrahepatic biliary obstruction, hepatitis serologies reveal chronic or active hepatitis. Levels of total bilirubin and alkaline phosphatase are increased in patients with mechanical biliary obstruction and continue to rise if biliary decompression is not performed. In the absence of a tumor mass on CT, biliary obstruction may be

Table 7–2. Common Nonmalignant Causes of Jaundice

Acute hepatitis
Cirrhosis
Acute pancreatitis
Stricture of the common bile duct (scarring secondary to chronic pancreatitis)
Gallstone pancreatitis (retained stone in duct)
Certain medications
Transfusion hemolysis
Hemolysis from chemicals or infection
Gilbert syndrome (benign hereditary hyperbilirubinemia)

Adapted from DeGowain RL: Diagnostic Examination, 6th ed. New York, McGraw-Hill, 1994.

secondary to choledocholithiasis. To differentiate neoplasm from choledocholithiasis, cholangiography is commonly performed as described below.[3, 4, 11]

ULTRASOUND OF THE ABDOMEN

Ultrasound of the abdomen can be used to visualize the liver and the intrahepatic and extrahepatic bile ducts. Ultrasound may reveal dilated bile ducts, gallstones, small tumors in the ampulla of Vater or head of the pancreas, or ascites. Advantages of ultrasound are that it is relatively inexpensive and readily available. Limitations of ultrasound include dependence on operator skill and the fact that evaluation is hampered by large patient size and by stomach and bowel gas.[3, 4, 6]

ENDOSCOPIC RETROGRADE CHOLANGIOPANCREATOGRAPHY

In symptomatic patients (pruritis, cholangitis), the first priority in managing obstructive jaundice that may be related to a malignant process is to relieve biliary obstruction. Endoscopic retrograde cholangiopancreatography (ERCP) is the procedure by which the endoscopist is able to cannulate the blocked duct and place an endobiliary stent, allowing drainage of bile into the duodenum. ERCP may be used to detect bile duct calculi, identify periampullary tumors, and obtain tissue for diagnosis by endoscopic brushing or biopsy. A pancreatogram may reveal small tumors in the head of the pancreas that compress the pancreatic ducts. The "double duct sign" refers to a cholangiogram demonstrating destruction of both the pancreatic and bile ducts. ERCP findings that suggest malignancy include abnormal tapering or stricture of the bile duct and suggestion of external compression of the duct by tumor.[3, 4, 6, 11]

Occasionally, it may not be possible to cannulate the ampulla endoscopically. In that case, a percutaneous transhepatic catheter (PTC) may be placed to relieve biliary obstruction. Usually with the percutaneous approach, the catheter enters the right hepatic lobe in the right subcostal region. A bag may be attached to the catheter to help drain bile. Potential problems with this approach include leakage at the exit site and at the connectors to the bile bag, creation of a portal for infection, and fluid and electrolyte imbalance if external drainage is used for a prolonged period of time.[11]

At some medical centers, an endoscope equipped with an ultrasound probe may be used to visualize a pancreatic tumor. A small needle at the end of the endoscopic ultrasound probe may be used to obtain a tissue sample.

COMPUTED TOMOGRAPHY SCAN

To radiologically document a suspected pancreatic tumor, CT scan is most commonly used. Radiologists prefer that the CT scan be obtained before endobiliary stenting because the stent can cause a "scatter" effect on the film. At M.D. Anderson Cancer Center, a particular approach is used in scanning the pancreatic region for suspected tumor. Three-millimeter-thick images (as opposed to the standard 10-mm-thick images) are taken of the pancreatic region while an intravenous contrast agent is injected simultaneously. The potential benefit of this high-resolution or "thin-cut" CT scan is to help clearly define the pancreatic and hepatic anatomy, define tumor size and location, define the extent of tumor involvement, define the tumor's relation to the major blood vessels (celiac axis, superior mesenteric vessels) in the abdomen, and detect evidence of hepatic metastasis. Such information is helpful because determination of surgical resectability is based on specific CT criteria. Once the pancreatic tumor is confirmed by CT scan, the decision algorithms shown in Figure 7–2 may help the clinician decide on the proper treatment approach.[12–16]

FINE-NEEDLE ASPIRATION

Percutaneous fine-needle aspiration (FNA) under CT guidance is the preferred method for obtaining tissue for definitive diagnosis.[13–15] The risks of this procedure include pain, pancreatitis, local inflammation, and false-negative results. The rate of false-negative findings is about 3% to 5%, although it varies significantly among institutions depending on the experience of individual radiologists. Some anecdotal reports have suggested that percutaneous FNA may result in peritoneal spread of tumor cells. However, data from 60 patients at the M.D. Anderson Cancer Center failed to substantiate those reports.[13] As noted earlier, an endoscopic ultrasound probe may be used to obtain a biopsy specimen.

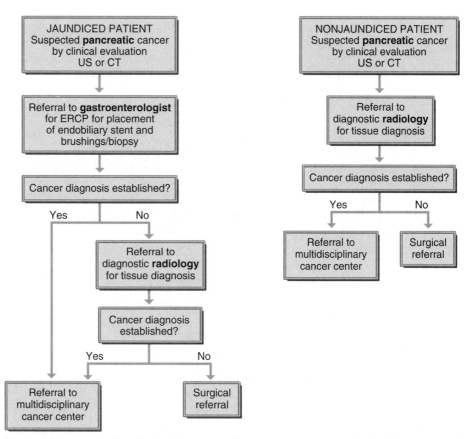

Figure 7–2. Treatment algorithm for the patient with pancreatic cancer. (US, ultrasound; CT, computed tomography; ERCP, endoscopic retrograde cholangiopancreatography.)

LAPAROSCOPY

The role of laparoscopy in diagnostic evaluation is to obtain tissue for definitive diagnosis and to determine the extent of disease. Laparoscopy may help to determine the presence of hepatic and peritoneal metastases too small to be imaged by standard radiologic studies. Laparoscopy may also be indicated to determine the resectability of pancreatic tail tumors and the extent of organ invasion. Laparoscopic evaluation may be a requirement for initiation of some research studies. Exploratory laparotomy, however, is rarely indicated for diagnosis of adenocarcinoma of the pancreas.[3, 4, 6, 13]

OTHER RADIOLOGIC STUDIES

On diagnostic workup, a chest radiograph is routinely obtained to rule out the presence of metastatic disease.[13] Angiography may be indicated to evaluate the tumor's relationship to major abdominal vessels and to outline the hepatic artery anatomy before surgical resection is considered.[3, 4, 6, 13]

TREATMENT AND REFERRAL

When evaluating a patient for referral for treatment options, several factors must be considered. Some of these factors are comorbid disease, performance status, nutritional status, accessibility of treatment facilities, and the patient's health beliefs and desire for medical treatment options. As for other solid tumors, treatment options include surgery, chemotherapy, and radiation therapy.

RESECTABLE TUMORS

Surgery offers the only curative approach for treatment of carcinoma of the pancreas.[3, 4, 6, 13] Specific CT criteria are used to determine surgical resectability (Table 7–3).[13, 15–17]

Studies have demonstrated that the addition of chemotherapy and radiation therapy to surgery improves outcome in the treatment of pancreatic carcinoma. Therefore, patients with potentially resectable tumors and a definitive tissue diagnosis should be offered chemoradiation before or after surgery. The standard chemotherapy regimen is based on 5-fluorouracil (5-FU), to which leucovorin or

Table 7–3. Computed Tomographic Criteria for Resectability of Pancreatic Tumors

Absence of extrapancreatic metastatic disease
No evidence of tumor extension to the celiac axis or superior mesenteric artery
Patent superior mesenteric-portal vein confluence

Data from Evans DB, Abbruzzese JL, Lee JE, et al: Preoperative chemoradiation for adenocarcinoma of the pancreas: The M.D. Anderson experience. Semin Oncol 1995;11:132; Evans DB, Rich TA, Byrd DR: Preoperative chemoradiation and pancreaticoduodenectomy for adenocarcinoma of the pancreas. Arch Surg 1992;27:1335; Staley CA, Lee JE, Cleary KR, et al: Preoperative chemoradiation, pancreaticoduodenectomy, and intraoperative radiation therapy for adenocarcinoma of the head of the pancreas. Am J Surg 1996;171:118; and Rich TA, Evans DB, Curley SA, Ajani JA: Adjuvant radiotherapy and chemotherapy for biliary and pancreatic cancer. Ann Oncol 1994;5:75.

mitomycin C may be added. Patients with biopsy-proven adenocarcinoma and localized disease are offered preoperative hyperfractionated chemoradiation. Radiation is given over a period of 10 days, with weekends off. Chemotherapy (5-FU) is also given during this time as a slow infusion via ambulatory pump on an outpatient basis. Currently under study is the use of chemotherapy agents such as paclitaxel (Taxol) or gemcitabine (Gemzar) that have known activity in solid tumors.[13-17] A current clinical trial at M.D. Anderson Cancer Center involves gemcitabine as a radiosensitizing chemotherapy agent in combination with hyperfractionated radiation therapy as a preoperative treatment. After completion of preoperative chemoradiation, patients are given a rest period of 3 to 4 weeks, followed by a restaging workup that includes a physical examination, laboratory studies, a chest radiograph, and a repeat thin-cut CT scan of the abdomen.[13, 15-17]

Patients who meet the specific CT criteria for resection are then taken to the operating room for surgical resection of the tumor.[13, 14, 16, 17] Patients with tumors in the body or tail of the pancreas may undergo partial pancreatectomy with possible splenectomy. Total pancreatectomy is rarely indicated. Most resectable adenocarcinomas of the pancreas occur in the head of the pancreas.[3, 4, 6]

In a pancreaticoduodenectomy, part of the pancreas is removed along with the contained tumor, the distal stomach, the gallbladder, the common bile duct, and the duodenum (Fig. 7–3). Three separate anastomoses are then made: choledochojejunostomy (between the bile duct and jejunum); pancreaticojejunostomy (between the pancreas remnant and jejunum), and gastrojejunostomy (between the gastric pouch and jejunum).[6, 18]

At the time of surgery, before construction of the anastomoses, the patient may be given a dose of intraoperative radiation therapy to optimize local tumor control.[13, 19] Intraoperative radiation therapy, however, is available only at some specialty medical centers. After completion of the surgical procedure, two abdominal drains are placed. These two abdominal drains are removed prior to hospital discharge. A gastrostomy tube is placed to relieve gastric distention, and is removed 4 to 6 weeks after surgery, and a jejunostomy feeding tube is placed and is left in for 4 to 8 weeks after surgery for supplemental nutrition (Fig. 7–4). The average length of hospital stay is 10 to 14 days. After pancreaticoduodenectomy, patients should be given a histamine$_2$ blocker for life to prevent marginal gastrointestinal ulceration, a potential complication of this surgical procedure.[18]

LOCALLY ADVANCED (UNRESECTABLE) TUMORS

If the listed CT criteria (see Table 7–3) are not met, it should be determined whether the tumor is locally advanced (i.e., has spread locally to adjacent organs) or metastatic. If it is locally advanced, chemoradiation may be considered. This principle of treatment is based on the synergistic effect of chemotherapy and radiation therapy for local control of tumor growth. Standard chemotherapy regimens are based on 5-FU. Chemotherapy may be given as a slow infusion via ambulatory pump at the same time as radiation therapy on an outpatient basis. Side effects include nausea and vomiting, fatigue, malaise, anorexia, and crampy diarrhea. Once this course of chemoradiation is completed, the patient is monitored by physical examination, routine laboratory studies, and radiologic evaluation.[13, 14, 19-21] Currently under clinical study at M.D. Anderson Cancer Center is gemcitabine, a new chemotherapy agent approved by the U.S. Food and Drug Administration in 1996 for treatment of metastatic pancreatic carcinoma, in

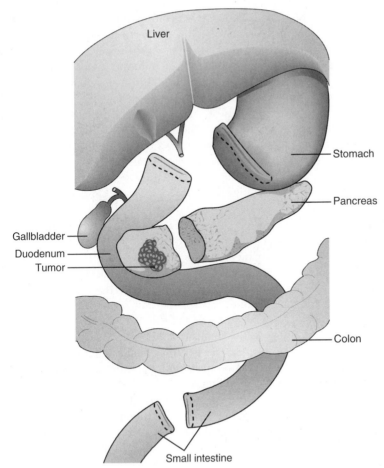

Figure 7-3. Pancreaticoduodenectomy. (Adapted from Davidson BS, Lee JE, Pisters PWT, Ames FC, Evans DB: Teaching complex surgery: A standardized approach to pancreaticoduodenectomy. Surgical Rounds 1995:450; and Wanebo HJ, Vereridis MP: Pancreatic carcinoma in perspective: A continuing challenge. Cancer 1996;78(Suppl 3):580.)

combination with radiation therapy. The aim is to determine whether the combination therapy provides more effective local tumor control.[22] At present, however, chemoradiation is palliative rather than curative, with several reports describing significant relief of pain and improved quality of life. Progression of disease or metastatic spread is an indication for referral for systemic therapy.[3, 4, 6, 20–22]

The role of surgery in locally advanced or metastatic disease is palliative and may include management of obstructive or motility problems. A biliary bypass or relief of gastric outlet obstruction can result in improved quality of life.[3, 6, 11]

METASTATIC DISEASE

Standard approaches to systemic therapy (chemotherapy) have included 5-FU, streptomycin, doxorubicin, and the nitrosoureas. Studies have not conclusively demonstrated a survival advantage, for the use of chemotherapy. The recently developed nucleoside analog gemcitabine has been associated with an increase in survival duration and a clinical benefit. This agent currently represents the

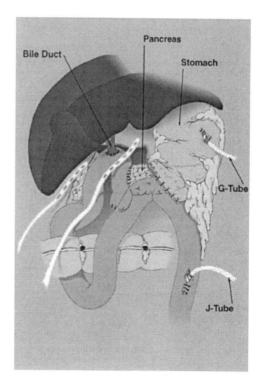

Figure 7–4. Placement of abdominal drains after pancreaticoduodenectomy. The gastrostomy tube (G-tube) relieves gastric distention, and the jejunostomy feeding tube (J-tube) allows supplemental nutrition. (Adapted from Davidson BS, Lee JE, Pisters PWT, Ames FC, Evans DB: Teaching complex surgery: A standardized approach to pancreaticoduodenectomy. Surgical Rounds 1995:450.)

first line systemic therapy for patients with metastatic or recurrent pancreatic cancer. Improvement in quality of life has been reported.[20, 22]

Other systemic approaches may include hormonal agents. One agent currently used is tamoxifen, which is also used in breast cancer.[6, 20, 21] A study conducted in a Canadian hospital demonstrated a prolonged survival benefit for patients with unresected or metastatic adenocarcinoma of the pancreas who took tamoxifen (20 mg twice daily). This potential benefit was most prominent in postmenopausal women.[24]

Failure of currently available agents to significantly impact the survival of patients with pancreatic carcinoma suggests that novel therapeutic approaches may be needed for this disease. Currently under clinical investigation are antiangiogenesis agents that may help inhibit tumors from forming the new blood vessels they need to survive.[21]

MANAGEMENT ISSUES

PANCREATIC INSUFFICIENCY

Obstruction of the pancreatic duct can lead to a decreased secretion of pancreatic enzymes, resulting in malabsorption and steatorrhea. These enzymes must be replaced with pancreatic enzyme supplements, and it may even be necessary to provide supplemental feeding for patients undergoing treatment to ensure adequate intake of nutrients and calories. After pancreaticoduodenectomy, jejunostomy tube feedings are given for approximately 4 to 8 weeks to ensure intake of sufficient calories and protein to promote healing.

ANOREXIA

Clinicians should assess patients for factors contributing to anorexia, such as poorly controlled pain, reduced gastric motility, and narcotic-induced constipation, and institute symptom management as appropriate. Patients who present with anorexia or malabsorption may benefit from nutritional counseling on how to choose foods that maximize protein and calorie intake and how to limit fats and sweets (which may contribute to rapid gastric emptying). Small, frequent meals may be more acceptable to patients who complain of early satiety. Liquid nutritional supplements may be encouraged to boost protein and calorie intake.

PAIN

Patients with pain related to pancreatic carcinoma also may experience fatigue, malaise, and nausea. This combination of symptoms taken together with the patient's emotional reaction to the illness may result in "suffering" that challenges management.[8, 9]

For many patients, pain can be managed adequately with oral narcotic analgesics. The World Health Organization analgesic ladder[23] should be followed (see Chapter 22). Use of nonsteroidal anti-inflammatory drugs should be limited, however, because their long-term use can contribute to marginal gastrointestinal ulceration. If NSAIDs are used, gastric acidity should be decreased with histamine receptor antagonists or proton-pump inhibitors. Side effects of narcotic administration (constipation, decreased gastrointestinal motility) can contribute to other existing symptoms such as nausea and vomiting and may contribute to obstipation. For patients taking narcotic analgesics, a bowel management program should be instituted to prevent constipation.[11, 23]

If oral narcotic analgesics do not satisfactorily control pain or if they produce unacceptable side effects, percutaneous chemical splanchnicectomy can be useful. This involves injecting a neurotoxic substance (alcohol or phenol) into the celiac nerve plexus. Substantial pain relief may be obtained for months with this procedure.[6, 11, 12, 23] This technique is discussed more completely in Chapter 22.

DIABETES

Diabetes mellitus may result from surgical treatment. However, not all patients who undergo pancreatic surgery become diabetic. The pancreas has a large functional hormone reserve and may function normally even after a portion of the organ has been removed. Diabetes varies with the individual patient; some patients are able to control blood glucose levels by taking oral hypoglycemic agents, and others require insulin therapy to manage hyperglycemia.[3, 6]

FATIGUE

Clinicians should assess patients who complain of fatigue for contributing factors such as unrelieved pain or inadequate hydration and apply appropriate symptom management. Unrelieved pain may contribute to insomnia and daytime sleepiness. For most patients, emphasis should be placed on maintaining a balance between rest and activity tailored to the individual. Patients who undergo surgical resection should be advised that with time they will feel less tired.[10, 23]

DEPRESSION

In about half of patients who have cancer-related symptoms of depression, the symptoms gradually disappear, with the help of supportive family and friends. Clinicians may aid this process by providing clear medical and treatment information to both patient and family. Providing information in terms the patient and family can comprehend is often viewed as the most supportive way in which the health care team can intervene. Also, the health care team can outline a clear treatment plan that offers a sense of hope. Clinicians should carefully assess patients for distressing symptoms that may contribute to depression, such as unrelieved pain or nausea, and institute symptom management as appropriate. Some patients may require a hypnotic or low-dose antidepressant to permit normal sleep or a daytime sedative (e.g., benzodiazepine) to reduce anxiety during crisis periods and help them adapt.[8, 9, 23]

POSTTREATMENT SURVEILLANCE

After definitive treatment, the patient should be seen on a regular basis, usually every 3 to 4 months, for a physical examination, laboratory studies, a chest radiograph, and radiologic evaluation to check for disease progression or spread. Evidence of spread of disease is an indication for referral or for consideration of further systemic therapy.

REFERENCES

1. Siedel HM, Ball JW, Dains JE, Benedict GW (eds): Mosby's Guide to Physical Examination, 3rd ed. St. Louis, CV Mosby, 1994.
2. Landis SH, Murray T, Bolden S, Wingo PA: Cancer statistics, 1998. CA Cancer J Clin 1998;8:6–29.
3. Brennan MF, Kinsella TJ, Casper ES: Cancer of the pancreas. In DeVita VT, Hellman S, Rosenberg SA (eds): Cancer: Principles and Practice. Philadelphia, JB Lippincott, 1993:849.
4. Beazeley RM, Cohn I: Tumors of the pancreas, gallbladder and extrahepatic bile ducts. In Murphy GP, Lawrence W, Lendhard RE (eds): American Cancer Society Textbook of Clinical Oncology, 2nd ed. Atlanta, American Cancer Society, 1995.
5. Parker SL, Tony T, Bolden S, Wingo PA: Cancer statistics 1996. CA Cancer J Clin 1996;45:5.
6. Wanebo HJ, Vereridis MP: Pancreatic carcinoma in perspective: A continuing challenge. Cancer 1996;78(3 suppl):580.
7. Byrd DR, Mansfield PF, Evans DB: Pancreatic cancer: Biology and changing clinical management. Cancer Bulletin 1992;292–300.
8. Kelsen DP, Portenoy RK, Thaler HT, et al: Pain and depression in patients with newly diagnosed pancreatic cancer. J Clin Oncol 1995;3:748.
9. Passik SD, Breitbart WS: Depression in patients with pancreatic carcinoma: Diagnostic and treatment issues. Cancer 1996;78(3 suppl):615.
10. Caraceni A, Portenoy RK: Pain management in patients with pancreatic carcinoma. Cancer 1996;78(3 suppl):639.
11. Lilliemoe K, Pitt HA: Palliation: Surgical and otherwise. Cancer 1996;78(3 suppl):605.
12. Fuhrman GM, Charnsangavej C, Abbruzzese JF, et al: Thin section contrast-enhanced computed tomography accurately predicts the resectability of malignant pancreatic neoplasms. Am J Surg 1994;167:104.

13. Evans DB, Abbruzzese JL, Lee JE, et al: Preoperative chemoradiation for adenocarcinoma of the pancreas: The M.D. Anderson experience. Semin Oncol 1995;11:132.
14. Hoffman JP, O'Dwyer P, Agarwal P, Slaazar H, Neelofur A: Preoperative chemoradiotherapy for localized pancreatic carcinoma: A perspective. Cancer 1996; 78(3 suppl):592.
15. Evans DB, Rich TA, Byrd DR, et al: Preoperative chemoradiation and pancreaticoduodenectomy for adenocarcinoma of the pancreas. Arch Surg 1992;27:1335.
16. Staley CA, Lee JE, Cleary KR, et al: Preoperative chemoradiation, pancreaticoduodenectomy, and intraoperative radiation therapy for adenocarcinoma of the head of the pancreas. Am J Surg 1996;171:118.
17. Rich TA, Evans DB, Curley SA, Ajani JA: Adjuvant radiotherapy and chemotherapy for biliary and pancreatic cancer. Ann Oncol 1994;5:75.
18. Davidson BS, Lee JE, Pisters PWT, Ames FC, Evans DB: Teaching complex surgery: A standardized approach to pancreaticoduodenectomy. Surgical Rounds 1995;450–457.
19. Evans DB, Termuhlen PM, Byrd DR, Ames FC, Ochran TB, Rich TA: Intraoperative radiation therapy following pancreaticoduodenectomy. Ann Surg 1993;218:54.
20. Clark JW, Glicksman AS, Wanebo HJ: Systemic and adjuvant therapy for patients with pancreatic carcinoma. Cancer 1996;78(3 suppl):688.
21. Ahlgren JD: Chemotherapy for pancreatic carcinoma. Cancer 1996;78(3 suppl):654.
22. Moore M: Activity of gemcitabine in patients with advanced pancreatic carcinoma: A review. Cancer 1996;78(3 suppl):633.
23. Clinical Practice Guidelines: Management of Cancer Pain. AHCPR Publication No. 94-0592. Silver Springs, MD, Publications Clearinghouse, 1994.
24. Wong A, Chan A: Survival benefit of tamoxifen therapy in adenocarcinoma of pancreas: A case-control study. Cancer 1993;71:2200.
25. DeGowain RL: Diagnostic Examination, 6th ed. New York, McGraw-Hill, 1994.

Chapter 8

Cancers of the Upper Gastrointestinal Tract

Patricia Spencer-Cisek, MS, RN, CS, ANP, OCN,
and Bernard Levin, MD

Cancers of the upper gastrointestinal tract develop insidiously and cause only vague presenting symptoms. In the United States, where screening for such cancers is not routine, the vague symptoms and a tendency for patients to treat themselves result in late-stage diagnoses and poor long-term survival rates. The astute clinician recognizes high-risk patients and monitors for symptoms that may be worthy of evaluation. This chapter covers cancers of the esophagus and stomach.

ESOPHAGEAL CANCER

EPIDEMIOLOGY

Cancer of the esophagus is not a high-incidence cancer in the United States, where 12,300 new cases and 11,900 deaths were predicted for 1998.[1] In contrast to China and other countries where cancer of the esophagus is more common, the incidence and mortality rates in the United States are not high enough to sustain widespread screening of asymptomatic persons. This results in predominantly late-stage diagnosis, and fewer than 10% of patients in the United States diagnosed with late-stage disease survive for 5 years.

The epidemiology of esophageal cancer follows a pattern similar to that of many other cancers, with the peak age at onset falling between 50 and 70 years. Men are affected more often than women, and black men have the highest incidence in the United States.

ETIOLOGY

Large variations in the incidence of esophageal cancer around the world point to environmental and nutritional risk factors. Incidence rates are significantly higher in China, Japan, Finland, and Iran than they are in the United States. It is therefore important to determine country of origin when assessing a patient's risk for this cancer. Persons who emigrated to the United States in their teenage years or later may have a risk similar to that of people in their country of origin. Dietary habits, including exposure to nitrosamines, selenium deficiency, and vitamin deficiency, appear to play an important role in these intercountry variations.

In assessing risk, it is also important to ask about previous injury to the esophagus with a caustic substance such as lye. Stricture resulting from such injuries has been linked to an increased risk of esophageal cancer. Tobacco use and excessive alcohol consumption can be considered independent risk factors for the development of squamous cell carcinoma of the esophagus. Furthermore, the two can act synergistically, increasing risk to an even greater extent.

A history of achalasia is also significant and may increase the risk of squamous cell carcinoma of the esophagus by up to 10%.[2] In achalasia, the smooth muscle of the gastrointestinal tract fails to relax because of degeneration of ganglion cells in the organ wall. A common location for this occurrence is in the distal esophagus on swallowing. Achalasia can lead to dilatation of the esophagus above the area of constriction and decrease in or absence of peristalsis in the area. The exact cause of achalasia is unclear, but stress and anxiety appear to exacerbate the condition.

Persons with a history of Barrett's esophagus, a syndrome in which the gastric columnar epithelium extends more than 3 cm into the distal esophagus, have a higher incidence of adenocarcinoma of the esophagus. This group demands close follow-up, because studies report a 30% higher risk of esophageal cancer than that of the normal population.[2] The presence of a hiatal hernia with chronic reflux also has been implicated in the development of adenocarcinoma in the area of the distal esophagus and gastroesophageal junction.[3]

The only evidence for a genetic basis of cancer of the esophagus identified thus far is an increased incidence among persons with tylosis palmaris et plantaris. Among those with this rare inherited autosomal dominant syndrome, esophageal cancer rates of more than 37% have been reported. Persons with a diagnosis of Plummer-Vinson syndrome (characterized by dysphagia, splenomegaly, anemia, and atrophy of the mouth, pharynx, and upper esophagus) also have an increased risk of esophageal cancer that is probably related to nutritional deficiencies. Table 8–1 summarizes the risk factors associated with cancer of the esophagus.[3]

PRESENTING HISTORY AND PHYSICAL EXAMINATION

The exact location of the tumor plays a key role in the presentation and extent of symptoms. The distribution of esophageal cancers is as follows: 25% occur in the cervical esophagus, 50% in the upper thoracic esophagus, and 25% in the lower thoracic esophagus.[4] The proximity of the esophagus to other organs and the extensive lymphatic network in this area facilitate the rapid spread of esophageal tumors. Cervical tumors most frequently invade the carotid artery, pleural space, laryngeal nerve, trachea, and larynx. Upper thoracic lesions spread to the left main stem bronchus, thoracic duct, aortic arch, and pleura. Tumors that develop in the lower esophagus invade the pericardium, pleura, descending aorta, and diaphragm.[5]

The symptoms of esophageal cancer are often vague, and physical findings may occur only after the disease is extensive. Complaints of heartburn and indigestion should be evaluated, and self-medication should be assessed. Most patients complain of progressive dysphagia, which may begin with solids and progress ultimately to liquids. A detailed history of eating patterns and the nature of the dysphagia should be obtained. When did it first begin? Was it sporadic? What foods were affected? How has the pattern changed or progressed? A patient may experience symptoms for many months but not seek attention until the problem becomes significant. Odynophagia (painful swallowing) is also a common complaint.

Table 8–1. Risk Factors for Cancer of the Esophagus

Nutrition and environmental factors
Resident of Japan, Finland, Iran, or northern China
Heavy alcohol and/or tobacco use
Poor nutrition (vitamin deficiency, selenium deficiency)
Nitrosamine exposure
Chronic irritation related to reflux, hiatal hernia, diverticuli
Achalasia
Barrett's esophagus
History of ingestion of caustic substance (e.g., lye)
Tylosis palmaris et plantaris

As the disease progresses, weight loss, regurgitation, and aspiration may result. The pattern and extent of weight loss should be assessed; decreases of 10% to 20% from baseline may occur. Questions to evaluate the potential for aspiration are important. Coughing or choking while eating or drinking may indicate a tracheoesophageal fistula, which must be closely monitored because it can lead to aspiration pneumonia.

The person who presents with complaints of dysphagia and weight loss requires a thorough evaluation. A complete physical examination should be performed. In the early stages of esophageal cancer there may be no significant physical findings, but as the disease progresses systemic signs become apparent.

On inspection, there may be significant wasting and cachexia when weight loss is substantial. Mucous membranes and skin turgor should be assessed for signs of dehydration. Pale mucous membranes, rapid pulse, and other signs of anemia may be present. A complete survey of all lymph node chains should be performed. The left supraclavicular node is a common site for nodal spread. The voice and the patient's history should be assessed for evidence of hoarseness, which may indicate laryngeal nerve involvement. Cardiac and respiratory evaluation may reveal signs of anemia, and adventitious breath sounds may indicate aspiration pneumonitis. Hepatomegaly noted on abdominal examination may indicate liver metastasis. A neurologic examination also should be performed to rule out a neurologic cause for the dysphagia. Significant findings include tremor, rigidity, and cranial nerve disruption.[6] Presenting signs and symptoms are summarized in Table 8–2.

DIAGNOSTIC EVALUATION

Persons who present with dysphagia, odynophagia, or other complaints associated with esophageal cancer should be evaluated radiologically and with endoscopy. The provider should initially order a double-contrast (air-contrast) barium swallow. When a lesion is present in the esophageal lumen, the mucosal pattern typically is irregular and ragged with luminal narrowing.[2] A chest roentgenogram is helpful for assessing metastatic disease but has limited use in evaluating the primary tumor. Once the diagnosis is established, a computed tomography scan of the abdomen and chest should be obtained to assess for local invasion, regional node involvement, and metastatic disease. Table 8–3 details the components of the workup.[3, 4]

Referral to a gastroenterologist for evaluation with upper endoscopy is vital to

Table 8–2. Presenting Signs and Symptoms of Esophageal Cancer

Vague pressure, fullness, indigestion, substernal discomfort
Dysphagia (present in 90% of cases; begins with solids and progresses to total)
Odynophagia (painful swallowing; present in 50% of patients)
Weight loss (10%–20% of usual weight is common)
Anorexia
Anemia
Dehydration
Aspiration related to tracheoesophageal fistula formation
Wasting and cachexia°
Nodal involvement (left supraclavicular common)°
Hepatomegaly°
Hoarseness (laryngeal nerve involvement)°

°Present with advanced disease only.

Table 8–3. Recommended Workup for Suspected Cancer of the Esophagus

TEST	PURPOSE
Radiologic evaluations	
Barium swallow (double contrast)	Determine location, length, circumference of tumor
Chest radiograph	Evaluate metastatic disease to lung
Computed tomography scan of abdomen (chest if high lesion)	Evaluate invasion of surrounding tissue, metastatic disease
Laboratory tests	
Complete blood cell count	Check for anemia
Chemistry profile	Check liver function
Electrocardiography	Obtain preoperative information and aid treatment planning
Evaluation by gastroenterologist	
Upper endoscopy with biopsy and cytology brushings	Help in diagnosis and staging
Endoscopic ultrasonography	Assess depth of invasion
Bronchoscopy (by pulmonologist)	Evaluate tracheobronchial tree involvement for high lesions

the diagnosis and in some areas of the country is the primary step in evaluating symptoms. Biopsies and cytology brushings have an accuracy rate of 90% for the diagnosis of esophageal cancer.[2] Endoscopic ultrasonography is proving very useful in the evaluation of these cancers. When it is available, this technique provides a valuable tool for visualizing the tumor and evaluating depth of invasion and the presence of local adenopathy.

DIFFERENTIAL DIAGNOSIS

A history of dysphagia always indicates an esophageal problem and should be evaluated. The causes fall into two categories: motility disorders resulting from muscular or neurologic disease and obstructions caused from inside or extrinsically. See Figure 8–1 for an algorithmic approach to the patient with dysphagia.

Among persons who report heartburn, those with atypical presentations should be evaluated further. Heartburn is a very common complaint in the primary care setting: 30% of adults experience heartburn caused by gastroesophageal reflux disease at least once a month. In a person younger than 45 years of age, who has no recent weight loss or evidence of bleeding and describes the classic burning substernal pain that radiates upward and is relieved by antacids, a history alone may be sufficient. If any other factors are present or the symptoms do not dissipate, a thorough examination for signs of an esophageal tumor should be undertaken.[6]

HISTOLOGY

The histologic type and patient profile for persons diagnosed with esophageal cancer have changed over the past several decades in the United States. In the 1970s, squamous cell carcinoma was by far the most common histologic type and was associated with smoking, use of alcohol, and the development of head and neck cancer. The incidence of distal esophageal and proximal gastric-area tumors has been increasing since the 1980s. Not only has the location changed,

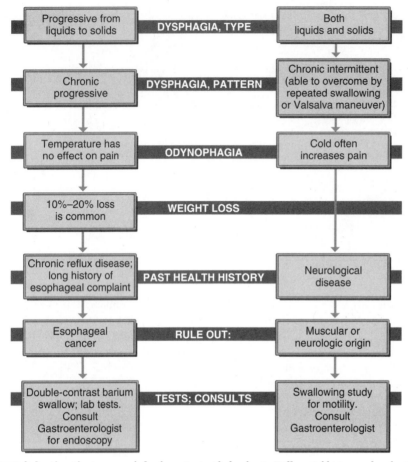

Figure 8–1. Algorithmic approach for the patient with dysphagia: Differential history and evaluation.

but the histologic type is evolving: the incidence of adenocarcinoma of the distal esophagus and gastroesophageal junction is increasing at a rate of 4% to 10% per year. In several studies of esophageal cancer, the incidence of adenocarcinoma has been reported to be as high as 60%. The exact cause of this trend remains speculative, but the cancers seem to be occurring predominantly in white men. Among this group, it has been reported that 40% of patients have a history of hiatal hernia.[3]

TREATMENT OVERVIEW

The amount of esophagus involved with tumor has been correlated with outcome in several studies. In a Japanese study of squamous cell carcinomas, among patients diagnosed with esophageal involvement of 5 cm or less in length, 65% had localized tumors and 35% had metastatic disease. Among patients with more than 5 cm involvement, however, 25% had localized tumors and 75% had metastatic disease.[7] These findings emphasize the need for early diagnosis if one hopes to have an impact on the outcome of this disease. Many authorities believe that subclinical metastases are a common occurrence at the time of diagnosis and account for the low long-term survival rates. Esophageal cancers typically metastasize to the lung, liver, bone, brain, adrenals, and kidney.

Table 8–4. TNM Staging for Esophageal Cancer

Primary tumor (T)
TX	Minimum requirements to assess the primary tumor cannot be seen
T0	No evidence of primary tumor
Tis	Preinvasive carcinoma (carcinoma in situ)
T1	Tumor invades into but not beyond the submucosa
T2	Tumor invades into but not beyond the muscularis propria
T3	Tumor invades into the adventitia
T4	Tumor invades contiguous structures

Regional lymph nodes (N)
Cervical esophagus (cervical and supraclavicular lymph nodes)
NX	Lymph nodes cannot be assessed
N0	No demonstrable metastasis to regional lymph nodes
N1	Regional lymph nodes contain metastatic tumor

Thoracic esophagus (nodes in the thorax, not those of the cervical, supraclavicular, or abdominal areas)
N0	No nodal involvement
N1	Nodal involvement

Distant metastasis (M)
MX	Distant metastasis cannot be assessed
M0	No evidence of distant metastasis
M1	Distant metastasis present

From Roth JA, Putnam JB Jr, Lichter AS, Forastiere AA: Cancer of the esophagus. In Devita VT, Hellman S, Rosenberg SA (eds): Cancer: Principles and Practice of Oncology, 4th ed. Philadelphia, JB Lippincott, 1993:781–782.

The tumor-nodes-metastasis (TNM) classification system is used to stage cancers of the esophagus. The tumor is evaluated and ranked according to depth of invasion. A stage I esophageal cancer is a small tumor that invades the lamina propria or submucosa but has no nodal or distant involvement. Tables 8–4 and 8–5 present the complete TNM staging system.

Nutritional status is important in determining the outcome of surgery, and surgical procedures may be delayed to allow for nutritional supplementation. The primary care provider can assume a proactive role in implementing nutritional support measures during the diagnosis phase. A percutaneous gastrostomy or jejunostomy tube may be required for adequate supplementation.

Surgical resection is the preferred intervention for persons with early-stage disease. Patients with stage I or II disease without penetration into other organs, with no evidence of metastatic disease, and with no coexisting conditions that would compromise recovery are candidates for curative resection. Among those with T1 or T2 disease without nodal involvement at the time of resection, 5-year survival rates of about 80% have been reported. However, fewer than 20% of candidates are able to have definitive surgery.[8] Table 8–6 outlines the typical surgical procedures performed.

Table 8–5. Stage Grouping for Esophageal Cancer

Stage I	T1	N0	M0
Stage II	T2	N0	M0
	T1	N1	M0
	T2	N1	M0
Stage III	T3	N0	M0
	T3	N1	M0
	T4	N1	M0
Stage IV	Any T	Any N	M1

From Roth JA, Putnam JB Jr, Lichter AS, Forastiere AA: Cancer of the esophagus. In Devita VT, Hellman S, Rosenberg SA (eds): Cancer: Principles and Practice of Oncology, 4th ed. Philadelphia, JB Lippincott, 1993:781–782.

Table 8–6. Surgical Procedures for Cancers of the Upper Gastrointestinal Tract

PROCEDURE	DESCRIPTION
Esophageal	
Ivor-Lewis esophagectomy	Right thoracotomy and laparotomy. Stomach is pulled up with intrathoracic anastomosis. Used for tumor in upper to middle third of esophagus.
Radical en bloc esophagectomy	Laparotomy with resection of thoracic esophagus, mediastinal lymph nodes, stomach, spleen, and celiac and thoracic nodes. Colon is used to replace esophagus by bowel interposition with intrathoracic anastomoses. Used for tumors in lower esophagus and cardia.
Total thoracic esophagectomy	Thoracotomy, laparotomy, and neck exploration with resection of head of left clavicle. Cervical (retrosternal) anastomosis using stomach.
Transhiatal esophagectomy	Neck exploration to mobilize and remove esophagus. Laparotomy with cervical anastomosis using stomach. Used for tumors at any level. Preferred for cervical or thoracic inlet locations.
Gastric	
Total gastrectomy	Used for lesions in midsection. Stomach removed en bloc with mesentery and nodes. Esophagus anastomosed with jejunum. Laparotomy with or without thoracotomy.
Subtotal gastrectomy	En bloc removal of large part of stomach with greater and lesser omentum, with or without spleen and with or without distal pancreas.
Billroth I	Anastomosis—gastroduodenostomy (stomach to duodenum).
Billroth II	Anastomosis—gastrojejunostomy (stomach to jejunum; close duodenum).

Modified from Spencer-Cisek PA: Upper gastrointestinal cancer. In Liebman MC, Camp-Sorrell D (eds): Multimodal Therapy in Oncology Nursing. St. Louis, CV Mosby, 1996:174–175.

Monitoring of patients who undergo resection should anticipate potential gastroesophageal reflux, esophagitis, early satiety, and dysphagia. Continued nutritional supplementation and a gradual loosening of dietary restrictions after surgery are dictated by surgeon preference and patient tolerance. Reappearance of symptoms after initial improvement may be indicative of recurrence.

Radiation therapy alone is seldom recommended except for palliation of symptoms in the setting of metastatic disease. Squamous cell tumors respond more readily than adenocarcinomas to radiation therapy. In patients with squamous cell carcinoma who are not candidates for surgery, radiation therapy may significantly improve symptoms of dysphagia and quality of life. Squamous cell tumors may respond rapidly, and the development of a tracheoesophageal fistula may be precipitated by tumor reduction. Patients should be closely observed for signs of aspiration during this period.

Multimodality therapy and radiation therapy have been used increasingly in both the preoperative and postoperative settings. In early cancers of the cervical esophagus, radiation therapy may allow preservation of the larynx. In advanced disease, palliative radiotherapy to areas of bone or brain metastasis may be very helpful in controlling symptoms. Complications of radiation therapy that may be encountered include stricture formation, esophageal fistula, radiation pneumonitis, and local skin reactions.[4]

Chemotherapy is used in all stages of esophageal cancer and in the past decade has assumed a greater role, especially in combination with other therapy. In clinical trials, combination chemotherapy regimens are used both preoperatively and postoperatively. New regimens are also being evaluated for palliation of symptoms in the setting of advanced disease. Combinations with a demonstrated effect include cisplatin-based regimens for squamous cell carcinomas and fluorouracil-based regimens for adenocarcinomas. New investigative therapies are continually being tried against this disease.

The primary care provider may be called on to support and monitor the patient between courses of chemotherapy. The oncologist should advise the primary care provider of the drugs being used and their common side effects, and together they should establish guidelines for reporting of symptoms and test results. Common side effects of chemotherapy include alopecia, nausea and vomiting, mucositis, and cytopenias. Patients receiving combined-modality therapy may have worse side effects that can lead to dehydration or complications of infection.

POSTTREATMENT SURVEILLANCE

In the United States, most patients with esophageal cancer have advanced disease at the time of diagnosis or, despite available therapy, have recurrence within a short period. Patients who have undergone therapy for esophageal cancer may develop complications related to the therapy and advancing disease. They should be monitored closely by an oncologist for signs of metastatic disease. The follow-up plan must take into account the therapy received and the expected long-term outcome. A standard schedule of radiologic evaluation, physical examinations, and laboratory tests should be established by the oncology team.

Indications of progressive disease may include recurrence of initial presenting symptoms, hoarseness, hepatomegaly, new onset of bone pain, signs of aspiration related to fistula development, and confusion and other signs of brain metastasis. In patients with advanced disease, the primary care provider may play a key role in providing palliative treatment and monitoring for disease progression and symptom management. Pain control, nutritional support, hydration, and supportive-care issues are key for this population. Dysphagia related to stricture development may be relieved through dilation of the area by a gastroenterologist. Laser therapy, either alone or in combination with a photosensitizing agent, may be used in some settings for tumor ablation. Thanks to improved technology, a stent can often be used to allow the patient with a fistula to resume oral intake. The patient and the family should be involved in decision making to determine the extent of intervention and comfort measures as the disease progresses.

GASTRIC CANCER

As with esophageal carcinoma, the incidence and outcome of gastric carcinoma differ dramatically depending on geographic location. Adenocarcinoma of the stomach is the second most common cancer throughout the world, although it is not as common in the United States. Two subtypes of adenocarcinoma of the stomach are recognized: the *intestinal type*, which is the dominant subtype in areas where gastric cancer is epidemic, and the *diffuse type*, which is dominant in areas where gastric cancer is endemic.[9]

EPIDEMIOLOGY

The intestinal type of gastric carcinoma is the most common cancer in several countries, including Japan. In the United States, 22,600 new cases and 13,700 deaths from gastric carcinoma were predicted for 1998.[1] The incidence of gastric cancer has decreased significantly over the past 30 years in the United States. Many other countries are beginning to see a decline as well.

In the United States, the average age at onset for the intestinal type of gastric cancer is 50 to 70 years, and men are affected more often than women. The epidemiology of diffuse gastric cancer follows a different pattern. Its incidence is increasing, the age at diagnosis tends to be younger, and women are affected at the same rate as men.

ETIOLOGY

As demonstrated by the geographic distribution of gastric cancer, nutrition and environmental exposures play a large role in the development of this disease. The countries of the Far East, Europe, the former Soviet Union, and Central and South America have the highest rates of gastric cancer. One theory holds that gastritis induced by environmental factors progresses to chronic atrophic gastritis and intestinal metaplasia with exposure to salts and nitrosamines.[9]

Persons with a history of pernicious anemia have a higher-than-average incidence of gastric cancer, although the exact cause is unclear. As in esophageal cancer, the combination of heavy tobacco and heavy alcohol use has been implicated in the development of gastric cancer. Occupational history can be significant for crop workers, miners of coal or iron, and workers exposed to coke gas.

Changes in the acidity of the stomach appear to increase the incidence of gastric cancer: the incidence is higher among those with documented hypochlorhydria or achlorhydria. An increased incidence is also reported among persons treated previously with a gastrectomy and Billroth II anastomosis for peptic ulcer disease. Substantial evidence exists for an increased risk due to *Helicobacter pylori* infection.[10] Table 8–7 presents a concise listing of risk factors.[9, 10]

A familial predisposition for the diffuse type of gastric cancer has been identified. In persons younger than 40 years of age, more than 90% of gastric cancers are of the diffuse type.[9] Some investigators, however, believe that the major influence is environment and that familial tendency decreases over generations in a lower-risk area.

Table 8–7. Risk Factors for Cancer of the Stomach

Nutrition and environmental factors
Resident of the Far East, Europe, countries of the former Soviet Union, Central and South America, and Iceland
Poor nutrition (vitamin A deficiency, vitamin C deficiency, diets low in fresh vegetables and fruit)
Nitrosamine exposure
Food preparation that includes salting and smoking
Chronic atrophic gastritis
Intestinal metaplasia of gastric mucosa
Helicobacter pylori infection
Pernicious anemia
Past history of gastric resection for benign peptic ulcer disease
Heavy alcohol and tobacco use
Occupational exposure (coal miners, iron workers, crop workers, workers exposed to coke gas)

PRESENTING HISTORY AND PHYSICAL EXAMINATION

Like the symptoms of cancer of the esophagus, those associated with gastric cancer are vague and nonspecific. They include complaints of weight loss, epigastric pain, early satiety, belching, nausea, vomiting, and anorexia. These symptoms should be evaluated thoroughly by the clinician if they last for 2 weeks or longer.

A thorough history, including country of origin, age at emigration, dietary patterns, and onset and character of symptoms, should be obtained. About 10% of persons with gastric cancer present with classic symptoms of peptic ulcer disease. In the absence of other risk factors, it is reasonable to treat according to standard therapy for that disorder. If the symptoms do not improve with short-term therapy, further investigation is warranted.

A thorough physical examination should be performed, although significant findings do not appear until the disease is advanced. Signs of chronic disease (e.g., weight loss, complaints of weakness, anemia) may be present. A complete nodal assessment may reveal a positive left supraclavicular node, left axillary adenopathy, and a positive umbilical node. Abdominal examination may reveal hepatomegaly and ascites. Findings on rectal examination may include a rectal shelf. In young women with suspected gastric cancer, a pelvic examination should be performed to assess for ovarian masses as well. Table 8–8 summarizes the typical findings.

WORKUP

Initial diagnosis and staging is performed through the use of an upper gastrointestinal series combined with endoscopic evaluation and routine laboratory tests. On radiologic evaluation, gastric cancers characteristically appear as lesions with elevated, irregular margins and rugal folds that do not radiate from the ulcer.[2]

During endoscopy, in addition to the multiple biopsies and cytologic brushings, endoscopic ultrasonography is also being used to evaluate depth of invasion. Computed tomography scans may be helpful in identifying metastatic disease and surgical candidates. The most complete staging cannot be performed until the time of surgery, and many centers are promoting the use of staging laparoscopy to determine the most appropriate therapy. Table 8–9 presents a summary of the recommended workup for gastric cancer.[9,11]

Table 8–8. Presenting Signs and Symptoms of Gastric Cancer

Vague epigastric discomfort, indigestion
Occasional vomiting, belching, postprandial fullness
Classic symptoms of peptic ulcer disease (5%–10% of patients)
Nonspecific symptoms of chronic disease: anemia, weight loss, weakness (10% of patients)
Advanced disease
　Fecal occult blood test positive
　Left supraclavicular adenopathy (Virchow node)
　Left axillary adenopathy (Irish node)
　Hepatomegaly, jaundice
　Ascites
　Acanthosis nigricans
　Umbilical node (Sister Mary Joseph node)
　Ovarian metastases (Krukenberg tumor)
　Rectal shelf (Blumer)

Table 8-9. Recommended Workup for Suspected Gastric Cancer

TEST	PURPOSE
Radiologic evaluation	
Upper gastrointestinal series (double contrast recommended)	To find small lesions
Computed tomographic scan	Staging
Evaluation by gastroenterologist	
Endoscopy with biopsy and cytology brushings	Diagnosis and staging
Endoscopic ultrasonography	Diagnosis and staging
Laboratory tests	
Complete blood cell count	Detect abnormalities (one third of patients are anemic)
Electrolytes	Detect abnormalities
Liver function tests	Prognostic for length of survival in advanced disease
Carcinoembryonic antigen	Detect abnormalities (may be elevated in one third to one half of patients)

HISTOLOGY

Adenocarcinoma is the most common type of gastric cancer, accounting for about 90% of cases. Primary lymphomas, leiomyosarcomas, and other rare histologic types comprise the remaining cases. Most adenocarcinomas occur in the distal stomach. Proximal lesions have the worst prognosis.[11]

DIFFERENTIAL DIAGNOSIS

People from areas of the world with a high incidence of gastric cancer maintain that risk after emigrating to the United States. This should be kept in mind when gastric symptoms are evaluated in immigrant populations. Because true signs of gastric cancer are not present until advanced stages, anyone who presents with persistent upper gastrointestinal tract complaints should be examined thoroughly by the clinician. The differential diagnosis includes gastric (peptic) ulcer, polyps, leiomyoma, and pseudolymphoma, all of which require biopsy for definitive diagnosis.

TREATMENT

Staging of gastric cancers is completed at the time of resection with the use of the TNM system. A description of TNM staging for gastric cancer can be found in Table 8–10. The tumor is classified according to depth of invasion. The lymph nodes are classified on the basis of proximity to the primary tumor, with N1 indicating one or more involved nodes within 3 cm of the primary tumor and N2 indicating more distant nodal spread.

Surgical resection is the primary modality for curative treatment of gastric cancers. In Japan, where the high incidence of this cancer supports widespread screening, many cases are diagnosed very early, and the 5-year survival rate has been reported to be high as 90%.[9] In the United States, most patients present with incurable disease. The goals of surgery in such patients are removal of the

Table 8–10. AJCC Staging of Gastric Cancer, 1988

Primary tumor (T)

TX	Primary tumor cannot be assessed
T0	No evidence of primary tumor
Tis	Carcinoma in situ
T1	Tumor invades lamina propria or submucosa
T2	Tumor invades muscularis propria
T3	Tumor invades adventitia
T4	Tumor invades adjacent structures

Regional lymph nodes (N)

NX	Regional lymph node(s) cannot be assessed
N0	No regional lymph node metastasis
N1	Metastasis in perigastric lymph node(s) within 3 cm of edge of primary tumor
N2	Metastasis in perigastric lymph node(s) more than 3 cm from edge of primary tumor, or in lymph nodes along left gastric, common hepatic, splenic, or celiac arteries

Distant metastasis (M)

MX	Presence of distant metastasis cannot be assessed
M0	No distant metastasis
M1	Distant metastasis

Stage grouping

Stage 0	Tis	N0	M0
Stage IA	T1	N0	M0
Stage IB	T1	N1	M0
	T2	N0	M0
Stage II	T1	N2	M0
	T2	N1	M0
	T3	N0	M0
Stage IIIA	T2	N2	M0
	T3	N1	M0
	T4	N0	M0
Stage IIIB	T3	N2	M0
	T4	N1	M0
Stage IV	T4	N2	M0
	Any T	Any N	M1

From Alexander HR, Kelsen DP, Tepper JE: Cancer of the stomach. In Devita VT, Hellman S, Rosenberg SA (eds): Cancer: Principles and Practice of Oncology, 4th ed. Philadelphia, JB Lippincott, 1993:828.

primary tumor and palliation of symptoms with the least surgical morbidity and mortality.

The primary care provider can play an important role in preparing the patient for surgical intervention. Stabilization of fluid and electrolyte status, correction of anemia, and nutritional intervention assist in attaining a successful operative outcome. The most common surgical interventions are outlined in Table 8–6.

Radiation therapy has not been effective in the primary treatment of gastric cancer. It has, however, been used successfully in combination with surgery and chemotherapy, or both, especially for those with locally advanced disease. Short-term effects of radiation therapy on the stomach include abdominal cramping, diarrhea, anorexia, nausea, vomiting, and weight loss. In Japan, intraoperative radiation therapy has met with success and is frequently used.

In patients who present with advanced disease, single-agent fluorouracil or combination chemotherapy may be used as the front-line therapy. Various combinations of chemotherapeutic agents have been tried, with the most successful being the combination of etoposide, doxorubicin, and cisplatin and that of fluorouracil, leucovorin, and etoposide.

The primary care provider may be called on to support and monitor the patient between courses of chemotherapy. The oncologist should advise the primary care provider of the drugs being used and their common side effects, and together they should establish guidelines for reporting of symptoms and test results. Common effects of chemotherapy include alopecia, nausea and vomiting, mucositis, and cytopenias. Patients receiving combined-modality therapy may have more intense side effects, which can lead to dehydration or complications of infection.

Current studies combine chemotherapy and radiation therapy with surgery in an attempt to improve the survival rates associated with this disease. With combination therapy comes the potential for worse side effects. Patients receiving combined-modality therapy may require additional monitoring and supportive intervention to complete their courses of therapy.

POSTTREATMENT SURVEILLANCE

Patients who have undergone potentially curative therapy for gastric carcinoma should be monitored closely by an oncologist for signs of recurrent disease. Follow-up evaluation should include radiologic monitoring of the most common sites of metastasis, routine laboratory tests to assess liver function and the presence of anemia, and measurement of carcinoembryonic antigen if it was increased at the time of diagnosis.

Routine management of any patient undergoing a gastric resection requires attention to several sequelae. Administration of vitamin B_{12} on a monthly basis is required to compensate for decreased absorption and to prevent anemia. Some patients experience dumping syndrome, which is urgency of the bowels approximately 30 minutes after meals. Complaints of palpitations and weakness during these episodes are common. Interventions to decrease this effect include eating frequent, small meals; separating intake of solids and liquids; and increasing fat and protein while decreasing carbohydrate intake. Medications to increase transit time may be used in severe cases.

Routine assessment for these sequelae and appropriate interventions may be the role of the primary care provider. Once the disease has spread, the main focus is comfort and symptom management, which can also be directed by the primary care provider.

REFERENCES

1. Landis SH, Murray T, Bolden S, et al: Cancer statistics, 1998. CA Cancer J Clin 1998;48:6–31.
2. Peacock JL, Keller JW, Asbury RF: Alimentary cancer. In Rubin P, McDonald S, Qazi R (eds): Clinical Oncology: A Multidisciplinary Approach for Physicians and Students, 7th ed. New York, WB Saunders, 1993:557–596.
3. Roth JA, Putnam JB Jr, Lichter AS, et al: Cancer of the esophagus. In Devita VT, Hellman S, Rosenberg SA (eds): Cancer: Principles and Practice of Oncology, 4th ed. Philadelphia, JB Lippincott, 1993:776–817.
4. Frogge MH: Gastrointestinal cancer: Esophagus, stomach, liver and pancreas. In Groenwald SL, Frogge MH, Goodman M, Yarbro C (eds): Cancer Nursing Principles and Practice, 3rd ed. Boston, Jones & Bartlett, 1993:1004–1043.
5. Leichman L, Israel V: Neoplasms of the esophagus. In Calabresi P, Schein PS (eds): Medical Oncology: Basic Principles and Clinical Management of Cancer, 2nd ed. New York, McGraw-Hill, 1993:649–667.
6. Uphold CR, Graham MV: Clinical Guidelines in Adult Health. Gainesville, FL, Barmarrae Books, 1993:377–381.
7. Takagi I, Karasawa K: Growth of squamous cell esophageal carcinoma observed by serial esophagographies. J Surg Oncol 1982;8:1897.
8. John MJ, Flam MS: Esophagus. In John MJ, Flam MS, Legha S, Phillips T (eds): Chemoradiation: An Integrated Approach to Cancer Treatment. Philadelphia, Lea & Febiger, 1993:285–301.

9. Bruckner HW, Kondo T, Kondo K: Neoplasms of the stomach. In Holland JF, Frei E III, Bast RC Jr, et al (eds): Cancer Medicine, 4th ed. Baltimore, Williams & Wilkins, 1997:1879–1922.
10. Neugut AI, Hoyek M, Howe G: Epidemiology of gastric cancer. Semin Oncol 1996;23:281–291.
11. Schein PS, Haller DG: Gastric cancer. In Calabresi P, Schein PS (eds): Medical Oncology: Basic Principles and Clinical Management of Cancer, 2nd ed. New York, McGraw-Hill, 1993:671–690.

Chapter **9**

Colorectal Cancer

Patricia Ewert-Flannagan, MSN, RN, BA, OCN, CNS, and Bernard Levin, MD

Colorectal cancers remain a significant problem in the United States and other westernized countries. Mortality rates for colorectal cancer have dropped by 4% to 5% in the past 5 years. An infant born in the United States in 1997 has a 5% chance of developing colorectal cancer in his or her lifetime.[1]

EPIDEMIOLOGY

Cancer of the large intestine is one of the most common cancers in the United States. It occurs equally in men and women. About three fourths of new cases occur in the colon and the rest in the rectum. The incidence of colon cancer in the United States is about 30 per 100,000 people, and that of rectal cancer is about 18.2 per 100,000. Because they are anatomically contiguous, they are often lumped together as "colorectal cancers."[2] However, in some instances it is difficult to distinguish whether the tumor originates in the colon or rectum.[3]

Colorectal cancer is second only to lung cancer among the internal malignancies. Yet, incidence rates have fallen substantially in recent years.[2] In fact, the American Joint Committee on Cancer in 1993 reported a marginal but steady increase in survival.[4] The projected 5-year survival rate for colorectal cancer is currently 60%, with survival being determined by the stage and grade of tumor. Survival among blacks is generally poorer than among whites.

In whites, mortality is declining for both men and women. Reports in the literature predict a further decline in female mortality as a result of coincidental screening for cervical cancer with Papanicolaou (Pap) smears and pelvic examinations that should include a rectal examination.[5]

Although cancer of the large intestine can occur at any age, its incidence increases with age. Incidence begins to rise after the age of 40 years and peaks after age 60. The mean age at diagnosis is 63 years for men and 62 years for women. Rare subgroups of patients seem to develop colon cancer much earlier (20 to 30 years of age) as a result of an inherited predisposition.[6]

In countries with a high incidence of colorectal cancer, colorectal cancers tend to cluster in the sigmoid area and in the cecum and ascending colon. Recently, an increased occurrence of colorectal cancer in the proximal versus distal portion of the large bowel has been noted.[1] This may be a result of wider use of flexible sigmoidoscopy, which allows biopsy and/or polypectomy. Because colorectal tumors are so easy to access, colorectal carcinoma is among the most studied and best understood of the human cancers.

ETIOLOGY

Colon carcinogenesis results from a complex interaction of confounding environmental, dietary, and genetic factors. The incidence of colorectal cancer has been increasing worldwide for the past several decades, not only in high-incidence Western countries but also in countries such as Japan, where the rate historically has been low. This may be a result in part to the "globalization" of diets.[1, 2] On the other hand, the mortality rate has leveled off and has even declined in some high-incidence countries. One explanation for the gap between rising incidence and falling mortality may be that earlier, more accurate diagnosis and improved surgical techniques have offset continued exposure to environmental and dietary carcinogens and the increased longevity of populations.[3]

ENVIRONMENTAL AND DIETARY RISK FACTORS

Diet is generally accepted as a major risk factor for colorectal cancer. The incidence of colorectal cancer is higher in the northeastern United States than in the western and southern parts of the country. In the past, high incidence rates also have been correlated with factors such as higher income, higher education, and urban living. However, since dietary habits are now similar across socioeconomic classes and regions, regional variations in incidence rates within the United States cannot be attributed solely to differences in socioeconomic class or dietary habits. Sun exposure and vitamin D status may be responsible in part for such variations.[6]

In general the rate of colorectal cancer is high in the Western world. This is attributed to a diet high in animal fat and low in fiber and fresh fruits and vegetables. Tobacco exposure and lack of physical activity may also be contributing factors. Two religious groups in the United States, the Seventh-Day Adventists and the Mormons, have a cancer mortality rate below that of the general population; the lower rate is thought to be related to diet. Both groups limit their intake of meat, appear to eat more vegetables, and restrict the use of tobacco, alcohol, and caffeine-containing products.[7, 8]

Although it is unclear how dietary substances act within the gastrointestinal tract to initiate a carcinogenic process, certain foods, such as fats, are known to promote abnormal cellular changes in the bowel mucosa. There are several possible explanations for this. When large amounts of dietary fat are present, more fecal bile acid comes into contact with the gastrointestinal mucosa.[9, 10] In turn, metabolites of fecal bile acid and sterol conversion products present in the gastrointestinal mucosa may become carcinogenic or enhance or promote other cancer-causing agents that are present. Fat also slows the transit of food through the gastrointestinal tract, thus increasing the time that bile acids and other carcinogenic substances may stay in direct contact with the bowel lining. Low-fiber and high-fat foods are thought to work synergistically to increase the risk of colorectal cancer. Consuming large amounts of alcohol has been shown to increase the risk for rectal cancer.[9]

MIGRATION AND DIETARY FACTORS

A person's geographic migration history and its effects on dietary habits influence the risk of colorectal cancer. For example, immigrants to the United States from Japan, which traditionally has had a low rate of colorectal cancer, have a much higher rate after they immigrate.[10, 11] However, it cannot be simply assumed that the increased occurrence results from a high-fat, low-fiber diet acquired as a result of immigration. There could be other environmental factors such as physical activity.

Extensive studies of dietary habits in black and white Africans by Burstein suggest that refined carbohydrates and low-fiber diets may increase the risk of colon cancer.[7, 8] The hypothesis suggested by Burkitt is that the slow transit of food through the gut of patients with low-fiber diets exposes the mucosa to exogenous carcinogens for longer periods. However, this explanation does not always hold because, in some normal persons, certain types of fiber can slow down fecal transit time. Moreover, fiber may directly bind carcinogens and increase the levels of fatty acids, mucosal nutrients that help cells to differentiate.

Fiber also decreases ammonia in the colonic lumen, which modifies the acid-base balance of the colon, thereby creating an opportunity for feces to become mutagenic.[12] More recent studies have questioned this hypothesis by noting that dietary fiber is not just a simple chemical entity but rather a diverse group of compounds that originate in plants and are resistant to human digestive enzymes.[8-14]

GENETIC RISK FACTORS

The genes responsible for malignant transformation are divided into three groups: oncogenes, tumor suppressor genes, and mismatch-repair genes. All three types may be involved in colorectal carcinogenesis. *Oncogenes* are proto-oncogenes that when activated in humans may cause tumors; only one allele needs to be activated to produce a tumor. The oncogenes most commonly involved in colon cancer development are the *ras*, *myc*, and *src* genes.[15] *Tumor suppressor genes* normally produce proteins that keep tumor cells from replicating. When the expression of such genes is disrupted, tumor cells can reproduce uncontrollably. However, both alleles of a tumor suppressor gene must be defective to cause a tumor (the *p53* gene is an exception in that only one allele needs to be lost). The APC (adenomatous polyposis coli) tumor suppressor gene is mutated or deleted in familial polyposis. *Mismatch-repair genes* produce proteins that recognize and correct errors in replicating DNA. Mismatch-repair gene mutations have been found in 80% of hereditary nonpolyposis colorectal cancers (HNPCC) and 13% of sporadic colorectal cancers. Besides these specific gene alterations, other genetic factors also appear to be important in colorectal neoplasia.[16-18] One suggestion is that colorectal cancer may be caused by the accumulation of mutations in oncogenes and tumor suppressor genes, since more than 90% of colorectal cancers have two or more genetic defects (Fig. 9–1).[19-21]

It is now accepted that colorectal cancer is not often an inherited disease;

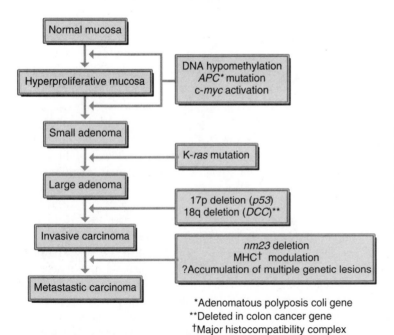

Figure 9–1. Schematic diagram interrelating the types of genetic alterations found in colorectal tumors. (From Burt LW, DiSario JA, Cannon-Albright L: Genetics of colon cancer: Impact of inheritance on colon cancer risk. Annu Rev Med 1995;46:371–379.)

*Adenomatous polyposis coli gene
**Deleted in colon cancer gene
†Major histocompatibility complex

only about 5% to 7% of colorectal cancers are considered to be hereditary. The major known hereditary polyposis syndromes are familial adenomatous polyposis (FAP); Gardner syndrome, which includes desmoid tumors, osteomas, fibromas, and colorectal adenomas; Peutz-Jeghers syndrome; and familial juvenile polyposis.[22, 23] FAP is transmitted in autosomal dominant fashion and is characterized by pancolonic adenomatous polyps. If not treated by colectomy, patients with FAP develop cancer before the age of 45 years.[24-26]

HNPCC also is transmitted in an autosomal dominant fashion. The term "nonpolyposis" is misleading, however, because polyps are present, although not in the numbers seen in FAP. There are two types of HNPCC. Lynch I syndrome is specific to the colon and causes an early onset of colorectal cancer (average age at diagnosis, 45 years); the resulting tumor is often located proximally and is accompanied by synchronous and metachronous tumors. Lynch II syndrome includes extracolonic adenocarcinomas such as those of the endometrium, stomach, ovary, urinary tract, small bowel, and bile duct.[16-18, 22-27]

The inherited syndromes account for about 7% of all colon cancers (FAP and Gardner syndrome, 1%; HNPCC, 6%).[24-26] This leaves another 93% of colon cancers that were once viewed as "sporadic" but are now confirmed to have a hereditary component in approximately 15% to 20% of cases. Persons with a first-degree relative with colon cancer have a risk of colon cancer threefold higher than that of the general population. There is also an increased risk for adenomas in first-degree relatives of individuals with colorectal cancer and an increased risk for colorectal cancers in first-degree relatives with adenomas.[27, 28]

Inflammatory bowel disease predisposes to colorectal cancer. Persons who have ulcerative colitis develop colorectal cancer at higher rates than the general population. Risk factors for subsequent cancer development include total involvement of the colon and long-standing colitis. Risk increases significantly if the colitis lasts longer than 7 to 10 years and increases about 20% with each following decade of life.[29-31]

Crohn disease (Crohn colitis) of the colon slightly increases the risk for colon cancer but not as much as ulcerative colitis. The risk for people with Crohn disease is higher than for the general public but less than for people with chronic ulcerative colitis. Crohn disease may progress to dysplasia and then to colorectal cancer. Diverticulosis and cancer may be found together, but there is no evidence that diverticula are important in the development of cancer.[31]

BACTERIA

As already discussed, fecal bacteria may act on bile salts to produce metabolites that act as carcinogens or cocarcinogens. Burkitt proposed that distal bowel carcinoma is more common than proximal disease because of the increased concentration of bacteria in the distal bowel.[11] Futhermore, secondary bile acids are increased in people with cancer. Secondary bile salts may be chemical carcinogens, as has been shown in experimental studies.[11]

PRIOR NONCANCER SURGERY OR IRRADIATION

Prior surgery or irradiation for a noncancerous condition may influence the risk of colorectal cancer. In some studies, elderly women had an increased incidence of right-sided colon cancer 10 years after cholecystectomy. However, any connection between colorectal cancer and prior surgery is controversial.[13, 14] Patients who undergo ureterosigmoidostomy have a higher incidence of large bowel cancer than those who do not; this appears to be caused by a higher concentration of cancer-causing or cancer-promoting compounds in the mixed secretions of urine and fecal matter. Although it is not clearly understood, an association also has been made between colorectal cancer and prior pelvic irradiation.[32]

PREVIOUS MALIGNANT DISEASE

People previously treated for colorectal adenocarcinoma are three times more likely to have a second large bowel tumor, at the same time as the primary or later, than people of the same age without colorectal cancer.[33, 34] Clustering of breast, ovarian, and colon cancers has been seen in the same patient (Table 9–1).[35]

MISCELLANEOUS HYPOTHETICAL RISK FACTORS

Nulliparity is being examined as a risk factor. The incidence of colorectal cancer is decreased in women who have had two or three children. Exposure to estrogens may be an important component of this decrease.[36] Exposure to asbestos may also be a risk factor.[33]

CLINICAL DETECTION

With the increasing use of screening technology, more colorectal cancers are found in asymptomatic patients (Fig. 9–2 and Tables 9–2 through 9–5). However, most patients with diagnosed colorectal cancers present with symptoms. The symptoms depend on the size and location of the tumor. In patients with a colorectal cancer, the patient's history and a physical examination should reveal the following: large tumor size, occult bleeding, and anemia leading to fatigue and/or heart failure for right-sided cancers; small tumor size and bowel obstruction for left-sided tumors. The obstructive symptoms in left-sided tumors can

Table 9–1. Risk Factors for Colorectal Cancer

Average risk	Hamartomatous polyposis syndromes
Age 50 years and older	Peutz-Jeghers syndrome
Asymptomatic	Juvenile polyposis
Increased risk	Family history
Inflammatory bowel disease	Colorectal cancer
Chronic ulcerative colitis	Colorectal adenomas
Crohn disease, long-standing	Hereditary nonpolyposis colorectal cancer
Familial adenomatous polyposis (including	Personal history
Gardner and Turcot syndromes)	Colorectal adenomas
	Breast, ovarian, or uterine cancers

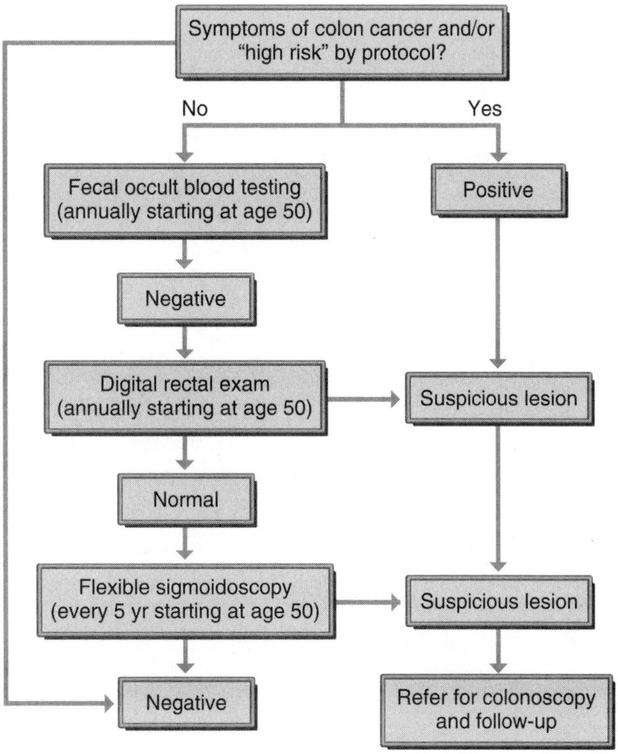

Figure 9-2. Colorectal cancer screening. The age at which regular colonoscopic examinations begin depends on risk assessment. This algorithm is part of the Colorectal Cancer Screening Protocol used at the University of Texas M.D. Anderson Cancer Center's Cancer Screening Clinic.

manifest as abdominal cramps or a change in bowel habits (see Table 9–2). The spread of tumor to the regional lymph nodes generally correlates with the depth of invasion by the primary tumor and with tumor grade. Cancers of the rectum tend to spread to hypogastric lymph nodes along the pelvic side walls, to mesorectal lymph nodes along the pelvic side wall, and to mesorectal lymph nodes along the superior hemorrhoid artery. The spread of tumor through the blood to the liver usually occurs through the portal vein. Colorectal tumors rarely spread to bone or brain.

Table 9-2. Anatomic Areas of Large Intestine and Correlating Colorectal Symptoms

SITE	SYMPTOMS
Right colon	Microcytic anemia
	Occult blood in stool
	Palpable mass in right lower quadrant
Left colon	Hematochezia
	Obstructive symptoms
	Small-caliber (pencil-size) stools
	Crampy, vague abdominal pain
	Change in bowel habits
Rectum	Rectal bleeding
	Change in bowel habits
	Pain
	Change in stool caliber
	Tenesmus

Adapted from Faintuch JS, Levin B: Clinical aspects of malignant tumors of the large intestine and anal canal, including therapies. In Kirsner JB, Shorter RG (eds): Disease of the Colon, Rectum, and Anal Canal. Baltimore, Williams & Wilkins, 1988:395–414.

Table 9-3. Colorectal Cancer Diagnostic Workup Procedures

Laboratory studies
  CBC with differential and platelet count
  Liver enzymes (SGOT, SGPT, alkaline dehydrogenase, and lactate dehydrogenase)
  Electrolytes
  PT and PTT
  BUN and creatinine
  CEA
Staging workup procedures°
  Colonoscopy and/or double-contrast barium enema (used to identify synchronous carcinomas
    and adenomas)
  Chest-radiograph
  CT scan (in staging rectal cancer, it is helpful to evaluate local spread to adjacent organs, pelvic
    bones, or liver)
  MRI (for staging rectal cancer)
  Endoluminal ultrasonography (useful for finding local spread into rectal wall and occasionally for
    detecting perirectal nodes)
  Biopsy of lesion
  Cystoscopy (for low sigmoid or rectal lesions)
  HIV testing (anal cancers are associated with acquired immunodeficiency disease syndrome)

CBC, complete blood count; PT, prothrombin time; PTT, partial thromboplastin time; CEA, carcinoembryonic antigen; SGOT, serum glutamic-oxaloacetic transaminase; SGPT, serum glutamate pyruvate transaminase; BUN, blood urea nitrogen.
  °The colon and rectum are evaluated by available clinical diagnostic procedures as to spread and extension but require surgical and pathologic evaluation in the AJCC staging.
  Adapted from Rubin P (ed): Clinical Oncology: A Multidisciplinary Approach for Physicians and Students, 7th ed. Philadelphia, WB Saunders, 1993:576–589.

Table 9-4. AJCC/UICC Staging Classification of Colorectal Cancer

Primary tumor (T)
  TX   Primary tumor cannot be assessed
  T0   No evidence of tumor in resected specimen
  Tis   Carcinoma in situ (intraepithelial or invasion of the lamina propria)
  T1   Tumor invades the submucosa
  T2   Tumor invades the muscularis propria
  T3–4   Depends on whether serosa is present
          If serosa is present:
              T3 invades through muscularis propria into subserosa, serosa (but not through),
              and pericolic fat within the leaves of the mesentery
              T4 invades through serosa into free peritoneal cavity or through serosa into a
              contiguous organ
          If no serosa (distal two thirds of rectum, posterior left or right colon):
              T3 invades through muscularis propria
              T4 invades other organs (vagina, prostate, ureter, kidney)
Regional lymph nodes (N)
  NX   Nodes cannot be assessed (e.g., local excision only)
  N0   No regional lymph node metastases
  N1   Metastases to 1 to 3 pericolic or perirectal lymph nodes
  N2   Metastases to >4 pericolic or perirectal lymph nodes
  N3   Metastases to any lymph node along the course of a named vascular trunk and/or
          metastasis to apical node(s) (when marked by surgeon)
Distant metastasis (M)
  MX   Presence of distant metastases cannot be assessed
  M0   No distant metastasis
  M1   Distant metastasis

Modified from American Joint Committee on Cancer, Manual for Staging of Cancer, 3rd ed. Philadelphia, JB Lippincott, 1988; and Union International Contre le Cancer, TMN Classification of Malignant Tumors, 4th ed. Geneva, UICC, 1987.

Table 9–5. Comparison of AJCC/UICC Stage Grouping and Dukes Stage Grouping Used in the Past

AJCC/UICC				DUKES
Stage 0	Tis	N0	M0	
Stage I	T1	N0	M0	A
	T2	N0	M0	
Stage II	T3	N0	M0	B
	T4	N0	M0	
Stage III	Any T	N1	M0	C
	Any T	N2	M0	
	Any T	N3	M0	
Stage IV	Any T	Any N	M1	

Modified from American Joint Committee on Cancer, Manual for Staging of Cancer, 3rd ed. Philadelphia: JB Lippincott, 1988; and Union International Contre le Cancer, TMN Classification of Malignant Tumors, 4th ed. Geneva: UICC, 1987.

HISTOPATHOLOGY

ADENOMATOUS POLYPS

Adenomas usually precede or accompany colorectal cancers. Neoplastic polyps in the large bowel may be tubular or villous; the former type is four times more common and usually is smaller. In general, larger polyps (more than 2 cm in diameter) are more likely to be malignant. About one in four patients with one tubular polyp has others. Tubular adenomas occur more often in the colon; villous tumors, more often in the rectum.[37, 38] Villous adenomas are 8 to 10 times more likely to become malignant than are tubular polyps. The adenoma-carcinoma sequence is now well accepted. The fact that a cancer usually occurs where adenomas are found is strong circumstantial evidence in support of this theory (Table 9–6).[39, 40] Controversy is being resolved in several other areas: (1) prognostic significance of high tumor grade and lymphatic invasion[40, 41]; (2) prognostic significance of invasion into the head, neck, or stalk of the polyp; and (3) extent of the surgery necessary when adenomas show poor prognostic factors or invasive cancer at varying levels.[40]

Adenocarcinomas may be classified as either polypoid or annular constricting lesions. Polypoid tumors can appear throughout the colon but usually occur on the right side. They usually are large and only occasionally constrict the bowel lumen. Within the rectum, the adenocarcinomas include sessile or polypoid

Table 9–6. Polyps as a Significant Prognostic Factor in Colorectal Cancer

POLYP TYPE	LEVEL OF INVASION	EXTENT OF INVASION	INDICATION
Pedunculated/sessile	0	None	Endoscopic/surgical removal
Pedunculated	1	Head	Endoscopic/surgical removal
Pedunculated	2	Neck	Endoscopic/surgical removal
Pedunculated	3	Stalk	Endoscopic/surgical removal
Pedunculated/sessile	4	Submucosa	Bowel resection

From Cooper HS, Deppisch LM, Gourley WK, et al: Endoscopically removed malignant colorectal polyps: Clinicopathologic correlations. Gastroenterology 1995;109:1801–1807.

lesions that can ulcerate and extend into adjacent organs. Annular lesions often appear in the left colon but sometimes in the sigmoid or rectum. They appear as nodular infiltrating lesions that may ulcerate.[38–43]

Adenocarcinoma is the major histologic type of colorectal tumor, accounting for 94% of all cases. Adenocarcinomas include mucinous tumors; signet ring tumors (which metastasize early and can extend along the bowel without greatly disturbing the mucosa, but make the large intestine extremely rigid); and scirrhous carcinoma (a leathery tumor). The remaining 6% of colorectal tumors include squamous cell, carcinoid, basaloid, and small cell carcinomas; adenocanthoma; basal cell epithelioma; and the colorectal sarcomas including lymphoma, leiomyosarcoma, rhabdomyosarcoma, liposarcoma, and melanoma.[38, 39] The prognosis for these rare malignancies is poor. They extend into adjoining organs or spread by way of the lymphatics to regional lymph nodes and through the bloodstream to distant sites.[38]

The progression of a colorectal neoplasm and the patient's survival depend on the tumor's histologic type, grade, and local and distant metastasis. The earlier the malignancy is found, the greater the chance of survival. Primary cancer of the large bowel grows slowly. However, once the tumor spreads, its doubling rate increases, from 1.6 years for a primary tumor to 9 months for a metastatic one.[42]

In most patients, by the time colorectal cancer is diagnosed the primary tumor has at least penetrated through the bowel wall, and in 20% to 25% of cases it has distantly metastasized. As one example, patients with FAP should have a total colectomy before the age of 20 to 21 years.[42, 43] At presentation, 8% of colorectal cancers are stage A, 39% are stage B, 28% are stage C, and 25% are stage D. After curative surgery, 20% of stage A, B, or C colorectal cancers recur locally or regionally with or without distant metastases, 30% recur locally or regionally with distant metastases, and 11% recur with distant metastases alone. The liver is the prime target for metastasis in 65% of cases, lung in 25%, and bone or brain in 10%. Most recurrences (70%) appear within 2 years and almost all (90%) occur within 5 years.[43] For an overview of treatment and referral criteria, see Table 9–7.[44]

MANAGEMENT

As previously discussed, the initial management of most patients with colorectal cancer usually includes surgical resection of the primary tumor. The goal of surgery is to remove the involved segment of bowel and its lymphatic drainage. The extent of surgery is determined by the blood supply and location of the regional lymph nodes. Surgery is not always possible if (1) the surgery will compromise the supply of blood to portions of the colon, (2) lymph nodes are extensively involved, (3) the lesion is large and bulky, and/or (4) the tumor has spread locally to the pelvis. Most stage I and II colonic tumors are treated with surgery alone.[45]

Chemotherapy is used for stage II through IV colorectal cancers. When the lesion carries a poor prognosis (e.g., local invasion into other organs, poorly differentiated histology, venous or lymphatic invasion), the patient is given adjuvant chemotherapy. Patients with stage II rectal cancer receive preoperative or postoperative combined adjuvant therapy (radiation and chemotherapy). The reasoning is that after surgery all macroscopic lesions with lymph node metastases have a high rate of recurrence due to undetected micrometastases. Adjuvant therapy is aimed at killing microscopic metastases. Research indicates that the

Table 9–7. Overview of Treatment and Referral Criteria

Colon

Stage 0 (superficial lesions and limited to mucosa without invasion of lamina propria)

Local excision or polypectomy leaving clean margins or colon resection for larger lesions that cannot be locally removed

Stage I   Surgery (wide segmental resection of primary and regional nodes in mesentery and primary anastomosis)

Stage II   Surgery same as for stage I and placement on carefully controlled clinical trials using systemic or regional chemotherapy, radiation therapy, or biologic therapy

Stage III   Surgery as above and postoperative chemotherapy (available to the postsurgical patient who qualifies for clinical trials evaluating various postsurgical chemotherapy, radiation, or biologic therapy; these trials may be for one type of treatment or a combination of two or more)

Stage IV Surgery (resection if feasible and/or anastomosis or bypass of obstruction caused by primary lesion if possible)

Surgical resection of isolated metastases (liver, lung, ovaries)

Palliative therapy (either radiation or chemotherapy)

Clinical trials for new drugs and biologic therapy under investigation

Recurrent (treatment options aimed at extending patient's quality of life)

Resection of liver metastases, isolated pulmonary metastases, or ovarian metastases

Palliative therapies as previously mentioned

Biologic therapy clinical trials

Phase I and II chemotherapy clinical trials

Rectum

Stage 0 (lesions limited to mucosa without invasion)

Surgery (local excision or polypectomy)

Surgery for large lesions through the anal canal or through the coccygeal area that cannot be locally removed

Electrofulguration (a type of high-frequency electrocautery)

Endocavitary irradiation or local external radiation therapy

Stage I   Abdominoperineal resection (APR) for lesions if a low anterior resection cannot be performed

Local transanal or other resection with or without preoperative chemotherapy (fluorouracil [5-FU]) plus radiation therapy

Endocavitary radiation therapy in selected patients with tumors <3 cm

Electrofulguration in a very restricted population of patients

Local transanal or other resection in selected patients with or without external beam irradiation and preoperative 5-FU treatment

Stage II   Surgical resection and LAR with colorectal or coloanal reanastomosis

Postsurgical radiation therapy and/or concurrent chemotherapy (if possible)

Wide resection with APR with adjuvant chemotherapy and postsurgical radiation therapy

Presurgical radiation therapy and/or chemotherapy followed by surgery attempting to preserve sphincter function and then postsurgical chemotherapy

Intraoperative radiation therapy

Stage III   Same as for stage II

Palliative chemoradiation

Stage IV Surgical resection/anastomosis or bypass of obstructing lesions in selected cases or resection for palliation

Surgical removal of metastatic isolated lesions in liver, lung, or ovaries

Palliative chemoradiation

Investigative protocols for new drugs and biologic therapy

Modified from Accessed National Cancer Institute—Physicians Desk Query, Nov. 15, 1996. Treatment of Colon Cancer. Internet http://wwwicic.nci...cer-Physician.html.

combination of fluorouracil (5-FU) plus levamisole or 5-FU plus leucovorin is effective adjuvant therapy for stage II or III colorectal cancers.[46]

Chemotherapy for advanced disease has produced disappointing results. Responses are often short-lived (6 months), and survival rates have not been much improved. Various combinations of 5-FU plus leucovorin, fluorodeoxyuridine (FUDR), the nitrosoureas, mitomycin C, and, more recently, CPT-11, have been used. Liver metastases have been treated by infusing 5-FU or FUDR into the common hepatic artery; this method is associated with significant hepatotoxicity, and the effect on overall survival has been marginal (Tables 9–8 and 9–9).[47]

Table 9–8. Posttreatment Monitoring and Surveillance For Colon Cancer*

Interim history and physical examination including DRE every 3 mo for 2 yr, then every 6 mo
   to 5 yr
CBC + chemistries every 3 mo for 2 yr, then every 6 mo to 5 yr
If CEA elevated at diagnosis or within 1 wk of colectomy, repeat CEA every 6 mo for 2 yr, then
   annually for 5 yr
Chest radiograph
   every 12 mo to 5 yr of treatment if stage B2 or C, or
   every 6 mo for 5 yr of treatment if liver or abdominal metastases resected, or
   every 3 mo for 5 yr of treatment if lung metastases resected
Abdominal CT every 6 mo to 5 yr, then annually for 3 yr if liver or abdominal metastases resected,
   or
   every 6 mo to 5 yr, then annually for 3 yr if rectal tumor resected
Chest CT every 6 mo to 5 yr if lung metastases resected
Colonoscopy in 1 yr if negative for multiple synchronous polyps; repeat in 1 yr if negative, then
   repeat every 3 yr

*Implementation of these guidelines, after aggressive surgical intervention, depends on individual clinical circumstances. These guidelines are rated Category 2—"somewhat controversial"—by the NCCN expert panels.
   From National Comprehensive Cancer Network: Colorectal Cancer Practice Guidelines, Oncology 1996; 11(suppl):140–175.
   The NCCN guidelines are a statement of consensus of its authors regarding their views of currently accepted approaches to treatment. Any clinician seeking to apply or consult any NCCN guideline is expected to use independent medical judgment in the context of individual clinical circumstances to determine any patient's care or treatment. The National Comprehensive Cancer Network makes no warranties of any kind whatsoever regarding their content, use, or application and disclaims any responsibility for their application or use in any way.
   The colon and rectal guidelines are works in progress that will be refined as often as new significant data become available.
   All NCCN guidelines are copyrighted by the National Comprehensive Cancer Network. All rights reserved. These guidelines may not be reproduced without the express written permission of the NCCN.

The patterns of failure in adjuvant therapy for rectal cancer differ from those for colon cancer. Rectal cancer recurs both locally and distantly. The combination of postoperative radiation therapy with 5-FU chemotherapy has been shown to reduce cancer-related deaths in stage II and III rectal cancers.[48] The combination of continuous 5-FU with pelvic radiation therapy postoperatively in patients with high-risk rectal cancer has enhanced survival.[48]

Table 9–9. Posttreatment Monitoring and Surveillance for Rectal Cancer*

Physical examination including DRE every 3 mo for 2 yr, then every 6 mo for 5 yr
CBC + blood chemistries every 3 mo for 2 yr, then every 6 mo for 5 yr
If CEA elevated at diagnosis or within 1 wk of colectomy,
   repeat CEA every 6 mo for 2 yr, then annually for 5 yr
Chest radiograph every 12 mo to 5 yr if stage B2 or C, or
   every 6 mo to 5 yr if liver or abdominal metastases resected, or
   every 3 mo to 5 yr if lung metastases resected
Abdominal CT every 6 mo to 5 yr, then every 12 mo for 3 yr
   if liver or abdominal metastases resected, or
   every 6 mo to 5 yr, then every 12 mo for 3 yr if rectal tumor resected
Chest CT every 6 mo to 5 yr if lung metastases resected
Flexible sigmoidoscopy at 3 mo and 6 mo
Colonoscopy in 1 yr; repeat in 1 yr if negative for multiple synchronous polyps, then every 3 yr

*Implementation of these guidelines, after aggressive surgical intervention, depends on individual patient circumstances. These guidelines are rated Category 2—"somewhat controversial"—by the NCCN expert panels.
   From National Comprehensive Cancer Network: Colorectal Cancer Practice Guidelines, Oncology 1996;11(suppl):140–175.
   The NCCN guidelines are a statement of consensus of its authors regarding their views of currently accepted approaches to treatment. Any clinician seeking to apply or consult any NCCN guideline is expected to use independent medical judgment in the context of individual clinical circumstances to determine any patient's care or treatment. The National Comprehensive Cancer Network makes no warranties of any kind whatsoever regarding their content, use, or application and disclaims any responsibility for their application or use in any way.
   The colon and rectal guidelines are works in progress that will be refined as often as new significant data become available.
   All NCCN guidelines are copyrighted by the National Comprehensive Cancer Network. All rights reserved. These guidelines may not be reproduced without the express written permission of the NCCN.

The future direction for colorectal cancer treatment may include metalloproteinase inhibitors, synthetic peptides that decrease tumor cell adhesion, growth factor inhibitors, and antibodies, vaccines, or immunotoxins directed against tumor cell antigens (see Tables 9–8 and 9–9).

CANCER PREVENTION AND EARLY DETECTION

Several screening tools are available to the health care provider for the prevention and early detection of colorectal cancers (Table 9–10). These tools include (1) digital rectal examination, (2) the fecal occult blood test, and (3) flexible sigmoidoscopy. Colonoscopy or a barium enema may be chosen instead. Each has its strengths and weaknesses, and each should be applied only after considering a patient's risk profile, the procedure's potential for causing morbidity, and the availability of the procedure in the screening setting. Because colorectal cancer has been linked to genetic mutations, screening guidelines have also been established for patients, from low risk to highest risk.[49]

CHEMOPREVENTION

Laboratory studies have shown that carcinogenesis can be blocked by administration of substances that interfere with the development of a tumor. These findings have led to the concept of chemoprevention of colorectal cancer through the use of anticarcinogenic agents. Current clinical trials are focusing on several agents, including nonsteroidal anti-inflammatory drugs, calcium, ascorbic acid, vitamin E, wheat bran, and other components of fiber.[32–35, 37–42] Selenium, a trace element and possible chemopreventive agent, has been found to inhibit carcinogenesis by deactivating carcinogens and protecting cells from the formation of free radicals.[7–10, 50–54] Another suggested prevention tactic is to limit or reduce fat intake and increase the intake of fresh fruits and vegetables. Many potential chemopreventive agents are found in fruits and vegetables, including limonene (citrus fruits) and dithiolthiones (in garlic and onions).[55]

Table 9–10. Screening Guidelines for Colorectal Cancer Patients by Risk

Average risk°	Annual DRE starting at age 50 yr
	Annual FOBT (if negative, F/S every 5 yr)
High risk†	Annual DRE and FOBT starting at age 40
	F/S every 5 yr
Higher risk‡	Annual DRE and FOBT starting at diagnosis
	Colonoscopy 6 mo to 1 yr after diagnosis (depending on findings)
	Colonoscopy every 3 yr if follow-up colonoscopy normal
Highest risk§	Identification and counseling of patient and family
	Consultation with and surveillance by a specialist
	Prophylactic colectomy if necessary

FOBT, Fecal occult blood test; F/S, flexible sigmoidoscopy.
°Patients who are asymptomatic.
†Patients with prior breast, ovarian, or endometrial cancer or family history of colorectal cancer.
‡Patients with adenomatous polyps and prior colorectal cancer.
§Patients with chronic inflammatory bowel disease, FAP, or HNPCC.
Data from Nixon DW: Diet and chemoprevention of colon polyps and colorectal cancer. Semin Surg Oncol 1995;11:411–415.

CONCLUSION

Colorectal cancer is the third most common cancer in the United States and the second leading cause of cancer deaths for both men and women. A hierarchy of risk can be developed for each patient by taking a personal and family history. Primary prevention measures include a diet lower in fats and higher in fiber, including fresh fruits and vegetables. Detection depends on screening for adenomas and early colorectal cancer and performing a colonoscopic polypectomy when adenomas are found during a screening flexible sigmoidoscopic examination. Specific screening programs should be based on a patient's risk assessment. Patients with long-standing inflammatory bowel disease and those with known or suspected hereditary colon cancer syndromes should be referred to a specialist for long-term care and surveillance. The overall 5-year survival rate for colorectal cancer is approximately 50%. However, more than 80% of patients whose disease is localized at presentation survive, compared with fewer than 5% of those with disseminated disease. Therefore, it is essential that the general public be informed about this disease and the importance of preventive measures

REFERENCES

1. Groenwald SL, Hansen-Frogge M, Goodman M, et al (eds): Cancer Nursing Principles and Practice, 3rd ed. Boston, Jones & Bartlett, 1995:1044–1064.
2. Cancer Facts & Figures. Atlanta, American Cancer Society, 1997:11-13.
3. Faintuch JS, Levin B: Clinical aspects of malignant tumors of the large intestine and anal canal, including therapies. In Kirsner JB, Shorter RG (eds): Disease of the Colon, Rectum, and Anal Canal. Baltimore, Williams & Wilkins, 1988:395–414.
4. Collins FS: Colon cancer screening. Response Science 1994;264:13–14.
5. Kwale G, Heuch I: Is the incidence of colorectal cancer related to reproduction? A prospective study of 63,000 women. Int J Cancer 1991;47:390–395.
6. Beart RW: Colorectal cancer. In Holleb AI, Fink DJ, Murphy GP (eds): Clinical Oncology. Atlanta, American Cancer Society, 1991:213–219.
7. Burstein MJ: Dietary factors related to colorectal neoplasms. Surg Clin North Am 1993;73:13–29.
8. Wynder EL, Reddy BS, Weisburger JH: Environmental dietary factors in colorectal cancer: Some resolved issues. Cancer 1992;70(5 suppl):1222–1228.
9. Young GP, Rozen P, Levin B (eds): Prevention and Early Detection of Colorectal Cancer. Philadelphia, WB Saunders, 1996:24–34.
10. Shike M: Body weight and colon cancer. Am J Clin Nutr 1996; 63(3 suppl):4425–4445.
11. Levin B: Nutrition and colorectal cancer. Cancer 1992;70(6 suppl):1723–1726.
12. Burkitt DP: Epidemiology of cancer of the colon and rectum. Dis Colon Rectum 1993;36:1071–1082.
13. Levin R, Tenner S, Fromm H: Prevention and early detection of colorectal cancer. Am Fam Physician 1992;45:663–668.
14. McFarlane MJ, Welch KE: Gallstones, cholecystectomy, and colorectal cancer. Am J Gastroenterol 1993;88:1994–1999.
15. Woolfson K: Tumor markers in cancer of the colon and rectum. Dis Colon Rectum 1991;34:506–511.
16. Tobi M, Luo FC, Ronai Z: Detection of K-*ras* mutation in colonic effluent samples from patients without evidence of colorectal carcinoma. J Natl Cancer Inst 1994;86:955–956.
17. Giardiello FM, Krush AJ, Peterson GM, et al: Phenotypic variability of familial adenomatous polyposis in 11 unrelated families with identical APC gene mutation. Gastroenterology 1994;106:1542–1547.
18. Fearon ER: Molecular genetics studies of the adenoma-carcinoma sequence. Adv Intern Med 1994;39:123–147.
19. Scates DK, Spigelman AD, Nugent KP, et al: DNA adducts, detected by ^{32}P post labelling, in DNA treated in vitro with bile from patients with familial adenomatous polyposis and from unaffected controls. Adv Intern Med 1993;14:1107–1110.
20. Hamilton SR, Liu B, Parsons RE, et al: The molecular basis of Turcot's syndrome. N Engl J Med 1995;332:839–847.
21. Dunlop MG: Colorectal cancer genetics. Semin Cancer Biol 1992;3:131–140.
22. Jagelman DG: Choice of operation and familial adenomatous polyposis. World J Surg 1990;15:47–49.

23. Fitzsimmons ML: Hereditary colorectal cancers. Semin Oncol Nurs 1992;8:252–257.

24. Burt LW, DiSario JA, Cannon-Albright L: Genetics of colon cancer: Impact of inheritance on colon cancer risk. Annu Rev Med 1995;46:371–379.

25. Rustgi AK: Molecular genetics and colorectal cancer. Gastroenterology 1993;104:1223–1225.

26. Dunlap MG: Colorectal cancer genetics. Semin Cancer Biol 1992;3:131–140.

27. Winawer SJ, Zauber AG, Gerdes H, et al: Risk of colorectal cancer in the families of patients with adenomatous polyps: National Polyp Study Workgroup. N Engl J Med 1996;334:82–87.

28. Bazzoli F, Fossi S, Sottibi S, et al: The risk of adenomatous polyps in asymptomatic first-degree relatives of persons with colon cancer. Gastroenterology 1995;109:783–788.

29. Bansal P, Sonnenberg A: Risk factors of colorectal cancer in inflammatory bowel disease. Am J Gastroenterol 1996;9:44–48.

30. Bachwich DR, Lichtenstein GR, Traber PG: Cancer in inflammatory bowel disease. Med Clin North Am 1994;78:1399–1412.

31. Choi PM, Zelig MP: Similarity of colorectal cancer in Crohn's disease and ulcerative colitis: Implications for carcinogenesis and prevention. Gut 1994;35:950–955.

32. Singh S, Sheppard MC, Langman MJ: Sex differences in the incidence of colorectal cancer: An exploration of oestrogen and progesterone receptors. Gut 1993;34:611–615.

33. Kimura T, Iwayak H, Hizesta A, et al: Colorectal cancer after irradiation for cervical cancer: Case reports. Cancer Res 1995;15:557–558.

34. Ahsan H, Neugut AI, Bruce SN: Association of malignant brain tumors and cancers of other sites. J Clin Oncol 1995;13:2931–2935.

35. Rubin P (ed): Clinical Oncology: A Multidisciplinary Approach for Physicians and Students, 7th ed. Philadelphia, WB Saunders, 1993:576–589.

36. Ekbom A, Yuen J, Adami HO, et al: Cholecystectomy and colorectal cancer. Gastroenterology 1993;105:142–147.

37. Sugarbaker PH: Follow-up of colorectal cancer (review). Tumori 1995;81(3 suppl):126–134.

38. Schroen RE, Weissfeld JL, Kuller LH: Are women with breast, endometrial, or ovarian cancer at increased risk for colorectal cancer? Am J Gastroenterol 1994;89:835–842.

39. Colon and rectum. In American Joint Committee on Cancer: Manual for Staging of Cancer, 4th ed. Philadelphia, JB Lippincott, 1992:75–82.

40. Teixeira CR, Tanaka S, Harwina K, et al: The clinical significance of the histologic subclassifications of colorectal carcinoma. Oncology 1993;50:495–499.

41. Levi F, Ramdinbison L, La Vechia C: Incidence of colorectal cancer following adenomatous polyps of the large intestine. Int J Cancer 1993;55:415–418.

42. Simons BD, Morrison AS, Lev R, et al: Relationship of polyps to cancer of the large intestine. J Natl Cancer Inst 1992;84:962–966.

43. Alabaster O: Colorectal cancer: Epidemiology, risk, and prevention. In Ahlgren JD, Macdonald JS (eds): Gastrointestinal Oncology. Philadelphia, JB Lippincott, 1992:243–259.

44. NCI PDQ. Treatment of colon cancer. 1997:1–20. Available at: http://wwwicic.nci...cer-Physician.html. Accessed National Cancer Institute—Physicians Desk Query, Nov. 15, 1996.

45. Hafstrom L, Engraeas B, Holmberg SB, et al: Treatment of liver metastases from colorectal cancer with hepatic artery occlusion, intraportal 5FU infusion, and oral allopurinol: A randomized clinical trial. Cancer 1994;74:749–756.

46. American Gastroenterological Association: Colorectal cancer screening and surveillance: Clinical guidelines and rationale. Gastroenterology 1997;112:596–642.

47. National Comprehensive Cancer Network: Colorectal cancer practice guidelines. Oncology 1996;11(suppl):140–175.

48. Buroker TR, O'Connell MJ, Wieand HS, et al: Randomized comparison of two schedules of fluorouracil with leucovorin in the treatment of advanced colorectal cancer. J Clin Oncol 1994;12:14–20.

49. Kampman E, Giovannucci E, Van't Veer P, et al: Calcium, vitamins, dairy foods, and the occurrence of colorectal adenomas among men and women in two prospective studies. Am J Epidemiol 1994;139:16–29.

50. Greenwald P, Kelloff GJ, Boone CW, et al: Genetic and cellular changes in colorectal cancer: Proposed targets of chemopreventive agents. Cancer Epidemiol Biomarkers Prev 1995;4:691–702.

51. Nelson RL, Davis FG, Sutter E, et al: Serum selenium and colonic neoplastic risk. Dis Colon Rectum 1995;38:1306–1310.

52. Corman ML: Carcinoma of the colon. In Corman ML (ed): Colon and Rectal Surgery. Philadelphia, JB Lippincott, 1989:248–259.

53. Williams ST, Beart RW: Staging of colorectal cancer. Semin Surg Oncol 1992;8:89–93.

54. Kleibeuker JH, Cats A, Van de Meer R, et al: Calcium supplementation as prophylaxis against colon cancer? Dig Dis 1994;12:85–97.

55. Nixon DW: Diet and chemoprevention of colon polyps and colorectal cancer. Semin Surg Oncol 1995;11:411–415.

Chapter 10

Genitourinary Cancers

Shellie M. Scott, PA-C, and
Louis L. Pisters, MD

Genitourinary cancers are among the most commonly diagnosed cancers and are responsible for a large proportion of cancer deaths (Table 10–1). The median age of incidence for prostate, renal cell, and bladder cancers is more than 50 years. With an increasing population age in this country, the incidence of genitourinary carcinomas is most likely to increase. The diagnosis of these cancers is made by a urologist, but there is an important place for primary care providers in their early detection, evaluation, and management. Surgery is the primary treatment; however, other reliable treatment options do exist. This chapter discusses current information and strategies for prostate, renal cell, and bladder cancers. Testicular cancer is discussed in a separate chapter.

PROSTATE CANCER

EPIDEMIOLOGY

Prostate carcinoma is the most frequently diagnosed cancer (other than skin cancer) and the second most common cause of cancer-related death in U.S. men. The number of newly diagnosed prostate cancers continues to rise annually.[1] Some of this increase is probably a result of increased screening, improved screening techniques, and a larger elderly population. The incidence of prostate cancer increases with each decade of life after age 50, and it rarely is diagnosed in men younger than 50 years of age. The average age at diagnosis is 70 years.[2] The incidence of clinically significant prostate cancer is very different among populations worldwide, but according to autopsy data there is little difference in the incidence of latent microscopic prostate cancer among different populations.[1] In the United States, black men have a greater incidence of prostate cancer and a higher cancer-related mortality rate than do white men.

ETIOLOGY

Environmental influences appear to be important in prostate cancer. The Japanese have a very low incidence of prostate cancer, possibly because of their low-fat diets. High-fat diets may increase androgen bioavailability, which may stimulate prostate cancer.[1]

Although the cause of prostate cancer is unknown and no specific prostate cancer gene has been identified, there are data demonstrating a Mendelian pattern of inheritance of cancer risk within some families. There is a 2.1% to

Table 10–1. 1994 Incidence and Mortality Rates for Genitourinary Cancers

CANCER	NEW CASES	PERCENTAGE OF ALL CANCERS	CANCER DEATHS
Prostate	200,000	32	38,000
Bladder	51,200	2	10,600
Renal	27,600	2	11,300

Data from Kassabian VS, Graham SD: Urologic and male genital cancers. In Murphy GP, Lawrence W, Lenhard RE (eds): American Cancer Society Textbook of Clinical Oncology, 2nd ed. Atlanta, American Cancer Society, 1995.

2.8% greater risk of prostate cancer among men who have a first-degree relative with prostate cancer than in men with no family history of the disease.[1]

When the primary risk factors of age, race, and inheritance are considered, it is obvious that there are no means of avoiding them. Therefore, prevention efforts must focus on secondary means, those of screening and early detection. Screening for prostate cancer is controversial in part because of the likelihood of detecting clinically insignificant prostate cancer. Prostate cancer has a long natural history, and the benefit of initiating early treatment for cancers found by screening has not been proven. Before widespread screening, which began in the early 1980s, most prostate cancers were advanced at diagnosis, with 25% to 30% of patients having distant metastases.[3] Today, about 58% of patients have clinically localized disease at diagnosis.[2] The best treatment modality for early-stage prostate cancer also is controversial, as is the cost-effectiveness of treatment at this stage. Currently, several investigators are looking at the impact of early detection on the natural history of the disease and on patient survival.

EVALUATION

HISTORY AND PHYSICAL EXAMINATION

Clinically, localized disease is notoriously asymptomatic, whereas patients with advanced prostate cancer may present with urinary-obstructive symptoms. Classic obstructive symptoms include urinary frequency, urgency, an intermittent urine stream, decreased force and caliber, nocturia, and dribbling. Patients with more advanced disease may present with nonspecific symptoms, such as fatigue, weight loss, loss of appetite, or symptoms related to metastatic lesions, such as bone pain.

Critics of digital rectal examination (DRE) cite variability among practitioners, subjectivity, and lack of sensitivity for early-stage disease as drawbacks to using DRE as a diagnostic tool. Findings for early-stage disease are quite subtle; they include mild asymmetry and slight changes in tissue consistency. Abnormal DRE findings have a relatively low positive predictive value (between 17% and 31%[4]). Abnormal DRE results have been found in more than 30% of patients with prostate cancer.[5]

LABORATORY STUDIES

Prostate-specific antigen (PSA), a protein produced by benign or malignant prostatic epithelial cells, can be measured in serum. PSA is an independent risk indicator and the most important marker for both diagnosis and monitoring of prostate cancer.[6] Although it is not specific for prostate cancer, the serum PSA concentration has a direct relation to prostate volume and patient age, and age-adjusted normal PSA values are often cited (Table 10–2). The positive predictive value of PSA is between 40% and 49%,[7] and it has been reported that between 25% and 30% of patients with a PSA value higher than 4 ng/mL have prostate cancer, regardless of the DRE findings.[8] The PSA value may also be elevated in patients with benign prostatic hypertrophy, prostatitis, prostatic infarction, and injuries such as those caused by biopsy or transurethral resection of the prostate (TURP). Up to 20% of patients with an elevated PSA value do not have

Table 10–2. Age-Adjusted Normal Values for Serum Prostate-Specific Antigen

AGE RANGE	NORMAL VALUE (ng/mL)
40 but <50 yr	2.5
50 but <60 yr	3.5
60 but <70 yr	5.0
70 but <80 yr	6.5

Data from Osterling JE, et al: Serum prostate-specific antigen in a community-based population of healthy men: Establishment of age-specific reference ranges. JAMA 1993;207:860. Copyright 1993, American Medical Association.

detectable prostate cancer.[9] By contrast, up to 30% of patients with clinically significant prostate cancer have a normal PSA value (i.e., less than 4 ng/mL), underscoring the need for annual DRE.[9] Most clinicians believe that optimal screening for prostate cancer includes both DRE and PSA determination annually and that patients with abnormal DRE or PSA results should undergo a transrectal ultrasound examination.[10]

IMAGING

Transrectal ultrasound is an excellent, noninvasive adjunct tool in the diagnosis and surveillance of adenocarcinoma of the prostate. It is used primarily in patients with abnormal DRE or PSA findings. Used alone, it has a moderate to low positive predictive value and only a 2.6% cancer detection rate.[7] It is also considered to be expensive as a screening modality (average cost, $125 to $175 per patient). Prostate tumors frequently demonstrate hypoechoic areas on transrectal ultrasound; therefore, ultrasound can improve the accuracy of biopsy when it is used for guidance to biopsy locations. Transrectal ultrasound remains an imperfect tool, however, because not all prostate cancers are hypoechoic.

BIOPSY

The diagnosis of prostate cancer is made by tissue sampling. Ideally, because most prostate cancers are multifocal, a minimum of six different locations are biopsied with ultrasound guidance. In addition, biopsy specimens are taken from any abnormal hypoechoic areas and from extracapsular tissue if there is suspicion of spread. If the biopsy results are positive for cancer, further workup depends on PSA value, grade of tumor, and signs and symptoms of the disease. If the biopsy results are negative, serial PSA tests, repeat DRE, and another biopsy may be performed depending on the clinician's degree of suspicion based on the initial PSA value and the rate of change of PSA over time.

Adenocarcinoma is by far the most common cell type. Tumor grading is based on cellular architecture; the Gleason system is normally used. The Gleason score is reported as a value between 2 and 10, which is the sum of the grades of the major and minor patterns within the tumor. Well-differentiated cells have a low score; poorly differentiated cells have a high score. Tumor grade is highly predictive of outcome, and high-grade tumors are suggestive of metastatic disease, especially if there is a high PSA value or DRE evidence of extracapsular extension.

MANAGEMENT

There remains much controversy concerning the treatment of both local and advanced adenocarcinoma of the prostate. Development of therapeutic recommendations involves balancing the goals of preserving the patient's quality of life and eradicating the disease. Criteria to consider in selecting therapy include tumor grade and stage, the patient's risk factors for complications from any particular therapy, the patient's predicted lifespan considering other health problems, and the patient's preference.

STAGING

Clinical stage is used with grade for predicting prognosis and choosing treatment. Clinical stage is based on DRE results, transrectal ultrasound findings, and, in selected patients, further imaging studies such as bone scans, computed tomography (CT) scans, and plain roentgenographic films. An increased level of serum prostatic acid phosphatase (PAP), as determined by the enzymatic (Roy) method, may indicate the presence of metastatic disease. The American Joint Committee on Cancer (AJCC) staging of prostate cancer is a widely accepted staging system (Table 10–3).

Common sites of spread for prostate cancer are the pelvic and retroperitoneal lymph nodes and bones. The disease metastasizes in various ways: through lymphatic and venous drainage, along nerve bundles, and by direct extension into neighboring tissues. If the PSA value, the PAP level, or the physical examination or ultrasound findings raise concern that metastatic disease may be present, a CT scan of the abdomen and pelvis to image pelvic lymphadenopathy

Table 10–3. American Joint Committee on Cancer Staging System for Prostate Cancer

Primary Tumor	pT (Pathological Stage)
T1	Clinically unapparent tumor, not palpable nor visible by imaging
T1a	≤5 % of tissue from TURP, incidental
T1b	>5% of tissue from TURP, incidental
T1c	From needle biopsy performed for elevated PSA only
T2	Palpable, confined within prostate
T2a	One (1) lobe of prostate
T2b	Both lobes
T3	Tumor extends outside prostate capsule
T3a	Unilateral or bilateral extension
T3b	Invades seminal vesicle(s)
T4	Tumor invades adjacent structures other than seminal vesicles
Regional Lymph Nodes (N)	
N0	No nodes
N1	Regional metastasis
Distant Metastasis (M)	
M0	No metastasis
M1	Distant metastasis

Adapted from Fleming ID, Cooper JS, Henson DE, et al (eds.): American Joint Committee on Cancer Staging Manual, 5th ed. Philadelphia, Lippincott Raven, 1997:219.

is appropriate. Disease metastatic to the pelvic lymph nodes can be confirmed using tissue obtained from either CT-guided fine-needle aspiration or bilateral pelvic lymph node dissection done laparoscopically or at the time of prostatectomy. A chest radiograph is not routinely needed in healthy patients with clinically localized disease but can be useful to exclude the presence of pulmonary metastases (which are rare but possible) in patients with advanced disease. Treatment may be recommended either on the basis of clinical staging, when tests are convincing, or after pelvic lymph node dissection and pathologic staging.

Criteria for ordering a bone scan vary among clinicians; they typically include a significantly increased PSA value (higher than 20 ng/mL), signs and symptoms of bone pain, a high-grade tumor, or an increased PAP value. If abnormal uptake is demonstrated on a bone scan, plain films may be used to further evaluate the areas in question. About 80% of prostate cancer metastatic bone lesions are osteoblastic.[11]

LOCAL DISEASE

For locally confined disease, therapeutic options include observation, surgery, hormone-ablative therapy, radiation therapy, and cryotherapy.

Observation

Observation (watchful waiting) means testing PSA and performing a DRE on a routine basis—either every 3, 6, or 12 months—until a progressive rise in PSA value is demonstrated or symptoms develop. Observation includes the option of delayed hormone-ablative therapy, radiation, or surgery, should the cancer progress with potential morbidity or mortality. Observation is a viable option for selected patients in whom the perceived risk of death from other causes exceeds the perceived risk of death from prostate cancer. It may be appropriate for older patients with low-stage, low-grade tumor, who may not experience tumor-related complications for up to 10 years after initial diagnosis because of the slow progression of the disease.[5]

Surgery

Radical prostatectomy—removal of the prostate gland, seminal vesicles, and ampulla of the vas—is the most definitive therapy for clinically localized prostate cancer. A retropubic prostatectomy involves an incision in the lower abdomen and can include a pelvic lymph node dissection. A perineal prostatectomy is performed through an incision between the rectum and the scrotum. The 15-year survival rate after radical prostatectomy for patients with clinically localized disease is approximately 93%.[5]

The major surgical risk in otherwise healthy persons is bleeding, which may require a blood transfusion (5% to 10% of patients).[5] The major long-term complications are urinary incontinence and impotence. Urinary incontinence occurs in 4% to 20% of men who have undergone a radical prostatectomy and is age influenced.[12] Improvement in urinary continence can continue up to 1 year postoperatively. It is rare for a patient to experience complete urinary incontinence after radical retropubic prostatectomy. Urinary incontinence can be treated by placement of an artificial urinary sphincter or by collagen injection therapy.

The cavernous nerves, which lie along the prostate, are important for normal erectile function and may be preserved to improve the chances of a return of normal erectile function after surgery. The selection criteria for a nerve-sparing radical retropubic prostatectomy are strict because tumor cells that are left behind could cause subsequent recurrence of disease. The treatment choices for postprostatectomy impotence currently include the use of an external vacuum appliance, the surgical placement of a prosthesis, and pharmacologic therapy by intracavernous injection or urethral suppository. The loss of erectile function has no physiologic relation to penile sensation or libido.

Hormone-Ablative Therapy

The first evidence of a therapeutic effect of hormone-ablative therapy was demonstrated by Dr. Charles Huggins. He won the Nobel Prize in 1966 for demonstrating that the elimination of testosterone by bilateral orchiectomy improved symptoms in patients with metastatic prostate cancer.[13] This is not a curative modality, and no clear survival advantage has been demonstrated for early as opposed to late hormone therapy. Hormone ablation may be accomplished either surgically, by bilateral scrotal orchiectomy, or chemically, by injection of a luteinizing hormone-releasing hormone (LH-RH) agonist, which blocks testosterone production by decreasing the release of luteinizing hormone from the pituitary gland. Complete hormone-ablative therapy would include an oral antiandrogen, which blocks the uptake or binding of androgens in target cells. The disadvantages of hormone-ablative therapy include vasomotor instability with resulting hot flashes, loss of libido, and impotence. Some antiandrogens have gastrointestinal side effects and carry a risk of liver toxicity.

Radiation Therapy

External beam radiation therapy for clinically localized disease can be used with curative intent either alone or in combination with other treatment modalities; it is also used for palliative treatment in more advanced disease. For primary treatment, about 7000 cGy are given to the pelvis in a 5-day-per-week regimen for a duration of 7 weeks. This dosage is associated with a low incidence of serious complications, about 1.8% in an M.D. Anderson Cancer Center series.[14] About 19% of patients treated with radiation therapy complain of mild transient complications, including gastrointestinal symptoms (diarrhea, hematochezia, rectal urgency) and genitourinary symptoms (frequency, urgency, hematuria, impotence, urinary incontinence).[15] Five-year survival rates are comparable to those achieved with radical surgery; however, 36% of patients with stage T1 or T2 disease have clinical or biochemical evidence of recurrence at 5 years.[16] Pretreatment PSA values may help predict the risk of relapse.

Until recently, brachytherapy had fallen out of favor because of difficulty with seed placement and seed migration, which resulted in uneven radiation delivery and a high percentage of treatment failures and treatment complications. Renewed interest in brachytherapy for low-stage (local) disease has come about because of the development of transrectal ultrasound technology, which can be used to guide seed placement, and the use of new isotopes.

Cryosurgery

One of the newest treatment options for adenocarcinoma of the prostate is cryosurgical ablation, or freezing, of the prostate gland by means of probes placed transperineally. The procedure is well tolerated and requires only a very short hospitalization, usually no more than 1 day. Although short-term data indicate that cryoablation is an excellent modality for tumor destruction, long-term results are unavailable. Long-term complications and side effects can be quite variable and include incontinence, impotence, pain, obstruction, and infection. Cryotherapy should be regarded as investigational until further data accumulate.

ADVANCED DISEASE

Survival data for stage T3 disease, even after therapy, are disappointing. The 5-, 10-, and 15-year survival rates for patients who have had external-beam radiation therapy at M.D. Anderson Cancer Center are 72%, 47%, and 17%, respectively.[11] Combination therapy, including radiation for local control and hormone-ablative therapy for systemic control, is advocated, but no long-term data are available.

Although optimal treatment for stage T4 and metastatic disease is controversial, total androgen ablation involving either orchiectomy or an LH-RH agonist with oral antiandrogens is a common first step. Up to 85% of patients respond to hormone ablation initially, and the median survival rate is 36 months.[5] Patients' serum testosterone levels can be checked to monitor the effectiveness of the androgen-ablative therapy or if compliance is an issue.

Chemotherapeutic protocols do exist; they employ medications such as ketoconazole, estramustine, and vinblastine. Treatment for symptoms of metastatic disease can include radiation therapy to bone metastatic sites, the use of intravenous strontium 89, and TURP for bladder obstruction. The use of chemotherapy, strontium 89, and other salvage agents is generally reserved for patients with progressive symptomatic disease after failure of hormone-ablative therapy, because all of these modalities have complications and are noncurative.

SURVEILLANCE

After either definitive treatment or watchful-waiting protocols, patients are monitored with a DRE and serum PSA test. Initially, these tests are repeated every 3 months, but as time progresses without changes the interval may be extended to every 6 months. A rising PSA value or abnormal DRE findings should initiate a repeated staging workup, which may include transrectal ultrasound, prostate biopsy, bone scan, and CT.

RENAL CELL CARCINOMA

EPIDEMIOLOGY

Renal cell carcinoma (RCC) accounts for 2% to 3% of all new adult cancers diagnosed each year[17] (see Table 10–1). The highest incidence of RCC is in people between the ages of 50 and 70 years, and the ratio of affected men to affected women is 2:1.[17] Five-year survival rates by stage are 80% for T1 disease, 70% to 78% for T2 disease, 30% to 50% for T3 disease, and 5% to 14% for T4 disease.[18] The 5-year survival rate for patients with nodal or visceral metastases rarely exceeds 5%.

ETIOLOGY

The cause of RCC is still unknown, and most patients diagnosed with RCC have no identifiable risk factor. Abnormalities of the kidney, including polycystic kidney disease, renal cystic disease, and von Hippel-Lindau syndrome, are associated with RCC. A correlation also has been demonstrated between RCC and environmental exposures. Persons working in the tanning industry, in petroleum refineries, or with asbestos exposure have an increased incidence of RCC; in addition, epidemiologic studies have implicated smoking as a weak risk factor for RCC. Genetic studies have demonstrated that a tumor supressor gene on chromosome 3 is responsible for some if not all cases of RCC.[17]

Approximately 74% of all adult kidney tumors are adenocarcinomas.[19] Within this classification, there are several cell types; the most common is clear cell, but there are granular and sarcomatoid (spindle) cell types as well. It is believed that RCC originates in the proximal renal tubule and spreads to the surrounding tissue by various means, including direct invasion and extension into the renal vein and lymphatics.[17]

Although the renal capsule and Gerota fascia are anatomic barriers to local extension and metastatic spread, approximately 30% of RCCs are diagnosed as metastatic at presentation.[20] The most common sites for metastatic disease are the lung, lymph nodes, liver, bone, adrenal gland, opposite kidney, brain, and subcutaneous tissue.[17]

No staging system is totally satisfactory for predicting outcome of patients with RCC. At the M.D. Anderson Cancer Center the AJCC staging system is used (Table 10–4). Factors suggesting a poor prognosis include perinephric fat extension, renal vein involvement, extension into regional lymph nodes, involvement of contiguous organs such as the adrenal gland, and distant metastatic disease. At this center the Fuhrman grading system is used; a high Fuhrman grade indicates a relatively poor prognosis.

EVALUATION

HISTORY AND PHYSICAL EXAMINATION

RCC may have a very subtle presentation, and almost 40% of all RCCs are found serendipitously by imaging studies.[21] The "classic triad" of flank pain, abdominal mass, and gross hematuria is seen in fewer than 15% of patients who

Table 10–4. American Joint Committee on Cancer Staging System for Kidney Cancer

Primary Tumor (T)
T1	Tumor ≤7 cm limited to kidney
T2	Tumor >7 cm limited to kidney
T3	Tumor extends into major veins or invades adrenal gland or perinephric tissues, but not beyond Gerota's fascia
T4	Tumor invades beyond Gerota's fascia

Regional Lymph Nodes (N)
N0	No nodal metastasis
N1	Single regional node
N2	More than one regional node with metastasis

Distant Metastasis (M)
M0	No distant metastasis
M1	Distant metastasis

Data from Fleming ID, Cooper JS, Henson DE, et al (eds.): American Joint Committee on Cancer Staging Manual, 5th ed. Philadelphia, Lippincott Raven, 1997:231.

present with RCC and is usually associated with advanced disease. Gross hematuria is the most common symptom; it is seen in 60% of patients with RCC.[20] Patients also commonly present with nonspecific symptoms such as weight loss, loss of appetite, fatigue, fever, night sweats, or flank pain.

It is essential to take a good medical history when investigating the cause of a renal mass, especially considering the various benign lesions that can be caused by trauma, stone disease, or abscess. For a renal mass, the differential diagnoses to consider include cyst, benign oncocytoma, hematoma, abscess, arteriovenous malformation, renal infarction, lymphoma, sarcoma, transitional cell carcinoma (TCC) of the collecting system, Wilms' tumor, and angiomyolipoma. A very small percentage of solid renal masses are angiomyolipomas; patients with these lesions commonly present with flank pain. For angiomyolipomas the CT usually is diagnostic because of the visibility of fat in the tumor.[17] Abscesses can cause fever, flank pain, pyuria, and leukocytosis; have a characteristic CT appearance; and are confirmed with urine culture and sensitivity. The most common pediatric urinary neoplasm is Wilms' tumor, which is seen in approximately 1 of every 100,000 children younger than 5 years of age and commonly appears as a palpable abdominal mass.

There is a paucity of physical findings in patients with RCC; fewer than a third have a palpable abdominal mass, the most common physical finding.[21] Occasionally, hypertension or hepatomegaly without icterus is found. Rarer still are palpable supraclavicular lymph nodes, which suggest metastatic disease. Occasionally, a varicocele that does not collapse when the patient is in a supine position may indicate a renal vein obstruction and lead to the diagnosis of RCC.

LABORATORY STUDIES

Laboratory studies in the workup for RCC include a complete blood count (CBC) and serum creatinine, alkaline phosphatase, serum calcium, and liver function studies. A serum creatinine value is basic to the evaluation of renal function. A normochromic, normocytic anemia may be seen in advanced disease. RCCs can produce a number of biologically active substances that result in a variety of metabolic abnormalities, loosely termed paraneoplastic syndromes, including erythrocytosis and hypercalcemia. Stauffer syndrome, a dysfunction of the liver seen in approximately 15% of patients with nonmetastatic RCC,[19] may be reversible with nephrectomy. An increased alkaline phosphatase level could reflect metastasis to bone and suggests the need for further evaluation by bone scan.

IMAGING

Most commonly, the diagnosis of RCC is made by imaging studies. The initial evaluation tool for a palpable abdominal mass is an abdominal ultrasound study, and staging is done with CT or magnetic resonance imaging. The workup for a patient who presents with hematuria includes an intravenous pyelogram (IVP) and cystoscopy. If a lesion is found on IVP, the most important question to answer is whether it is a cystic or solid lesion.

Ultrasound is the best imaging modality for differentiating cystic from solid renal masses; its accuracy in defining a simple cyst approaches 98%.[20] The criteria for a simple cyst include a lack of internal echoes; a smooth, well-defined wall with a smooth inner surface; a round or oval shape with good sound transmission; and an acoustic shadow arising from the edge of the lesion. If the criteria for a simple cyst are met and the patient is asymptomatic, no further workup, treatment, or follow-up is indicated.

As a general rule, any enhancing renal mass found on CT is an RCC unless proved otherwise.[19] Findings on CT that suggest a renal cell malignancy include an enhancing solid mass with or without the following: amputation of a portion of the collecting system, poor definition between the renal parenchyma and the lesion, invasion of perinephric fat or adjacent structures, presence of abnormal periaortic adenopathy, or evidence of distant metastatic disease. CT examination is the best means for deriving information concerning spread of the disease, and it provides information concerning renal vein involvement. It is thought by many to be the best single diagnostic study for RCC.[17]

The workup for RCC should include a chest radiograph, both as a screening tool for metastatic disease and as part of a preoperative evaluation if the patient is recommended for surgery. A bone scan is ordered only if the patient appears symptomatic or the alkaline phosphatase level is increased. Other possible preoperative studies include magnetic resonance imaging if there is a concern about vascular extension, particularly to the inferior vena cava. Today, angiography is used primarily in surgical planning for partial nephrectomy. Almost 95% of all RCCs demonstrate hypervascularity with angiography.[19] Occasionally, a renal scan is done to determine the function of the affected kidney or of the contralateral kidney.

Needle biopsy has a very limited role in the evaluation of RCC. It is used to differentiate between primary RCC and metastatic lesions in patients with other primary cancers of nonrenal origin. It is also used to diagnose lymphoma when lymphoma is suspected. Urine cytologic analysis, in which voided urine is examined for exfoliated cells, is used in the diagnosis of renal pelvic and ureteral tumors but is not part of the routine workup for RCC.

MANAGEMENT

LOCAL DISEASE

The standard treatment for local disease (stages T1 through T3) is surgery. The objective of radical nephrectomy is to remove all tumor with adequate surgical margins.[17] Various surgical incisions and surgical approaches are used, depending on regional anatomy, tumor location, and tumor size. Radical nephrectomy includes removal of the entire kidney along with the surrounding fat, adrenal gland, and regional lymph nodes. There is no consensus on whether a survival advantage is conferred by regional lymphadenectomy.[17]

Partial nephrectomy, which is the removal of the tumor and only a portion of the kidney surrounding the tumor, is appropriate only under special circumstances because it has not shown to reduce morbidity or cost or to provide survival advantage over radical nephrectomy. These special circumstances include situations in which renal function is or may become critically compromised, as in patients with bilateral renal tumors, renal insufficiency, a solitary kidney or abnormal contralateral kidney, or von Hippel-Landau syndrome.[19]

ADVANCED DISEASE

Results of treatment for advanced RCC have been very disappointing. In general, surgery does not improve survival and is rarely performed for palliation except in combination with experimental immunotherapy protocols.[22] New immunologic therapies have been developed because of the resistance to multiple chemotherapeutic agents often seen in RCC.[17] Termed "biologic response modifiers," various drugs such as the antiviral agents interferon-α and interleukin-2, which enhance T-cell proliferation and killer cell activity, have induced partial responses in patients with a small tumor burden.[17]

SURVEILLANCE

Patients with local disease should be monitored every 3 to 4 months for the first 2 years after surgery with a chest radiograph, CBC, serum creatinine determination, history update, and physical examination. Every 6 to 12 months, a CT examination should be performed to evaluate the renal bed and the opposite kidney, particularly for patients with stage T3 and higher disease. After 2 years without recurrence, patients may be monitored on an annual basis with renal ultrasound, chest radiography, CBC, serum creatinine determination, history update, and physical. Patients need lifelong follow-up because late recurrences (even 10 years after initial diagnosis) have been documented. Similarly, the recommended follow-up for patients with metastatic disease is every 3 months with a chest radiograph, CBC, serum creatinine determination, history update, and physical. Frequency of CT examination in patients with metastatic disease varies depending on the clinician; standard criteria have not been established.

BLADDER CANCER

EPIDEMIOLOGY

Bladder cancer is the most common cancer of the urinary tract (see Table 10–1). It is diagnosed 2.5 times more frequently in men than in women. The age of onset usually is between the ages of 60 and 70 years; the average age at diagnosis is 67 years.[23] There is a slightly greater incidence in whites than in blacks. Because more than 90% of bladder cancers are TCCs,[24] this discussion is limited to TCC.

ETIOLOGY

Although the cause of bladder cancer remains unproved, most investigators believe that cell transformation or the promotion of abnormal cell proliferation occurs, potentially by several mechanisms. The exact genetic events leading to cell transformation are not known, but many investigators believe that activation of an oncogene or inactivation of tumor suppressor genes occurs. Data linking abnormalities in chromosomes 9, 11, and 17 and mutation of the *p53* gene to bladder cancer have been reported by several investigators.[25]

Risk factors for bladder cancer include smoking, environmental exposure, and abuse of analgesics. The aromatic amines α- and β-naphthylamine, which are present in cigarette smoke, are believed to be initiators of cell transformation. A large percentage of patients with bladder cancer smoke or have smoked. There is also a relation between bladder cancer and occupational exposure for persons working in the textile, rubber, petroleum, leather, and printing industries, who may be exposed to certain aromatic amines. The incidence of bladder cancer is higher in patients with histories of analgesic abuse, but this exposure has a prolonged latency period (more than 25 years). The analgesic agent implicated in these studies is phenacetin.[23]

EVALUATION

HISTORY AND PHYSICAL EXAMINATION

Unlike other urinary tract and genitourinary carcinomas, bladder cancer has a classic symptom: gross, painless hematuria, which is seen in 80% to 90% of patients.[23] This hematuria may be intermittent or there may be only a single episode, so all patients who present with this complaint merit evaluation.

The history and physical examination are key to working through the differential diagnosis of gross hematuria. The list of possible diagnoses includes the following:

- Infectious causes, including bacterial cystitis
- Stone disease
- RCC, bladder cancer, and other neoplasms
- Trauma
- Coagulopathy (including drug-induced)
- Sickle cell disease
- Hemorrhagic cystitis: sequelae of radiation therapy or chemotherapeutic drugs (e.g., cyclophosphamide)
- Collagen vascular disease
- Glomerular nephritis

Irritative voiding symptoms, such as frequency, urgency, and dysuria, are the second most common presentation of bladder cancer. Patients may also present with a urinary tract infection, because the presence of infection does not rule out a tumor. Patients with metastatic disease may present with bone pain, ureteral obstruction from a retroperitoneal mass, flank pain, lower extremity edema, a palpable pelvic mass, and weight loss. Most patients present with no physical findings unless the tumor mass is quite large.

LABORATORY STUDIES

The workup for hematuria includes urinalysis, IVP, and cystoscopy. Cystoscopic examination provides the clinical information for the diagnosis of bladder cancer. Urine cytologic analysis may be used as an adjunct to cystoscopy, but it is more useful for monitoring the response to therapy. Flow cytometry detects cells with increased DNA.[25] An alkaline phosphatase determination is informative in patients suspected of having metastatic disease.

IMAGING

Patients with stage T1 and higher disease require CT of the abdomen and pelvis to rule out metastatic spread to pelvic or retroperitoneal nodes and to the liver. Fine-needle aspiration of questionable lymph nodes seen on CT is used to verify regional metastasis. Other studies in the workup for metastatic disease include chest radiography and a bone scan. An IVP or retrograde pyelogram is used to evaluate the kidneys, ureters, and bladder for the origin of the bleeding if the upper urinary tract is suspected; however, these are not reliable tests for ruling out bladder lesions.

BIOPSY

Cystoscopic examination should be performed in all patients with suspected bladder cancer.[23] Usually the first-look cystoscopic examination can be done in a urologist's office without anesthesia; however, if an abnormality is discovered, cystoscopy with anesthesia is required. Examination under anesthesia is essential for staging of the tumor. Transurethral resection of the bladder tumor and, in selected patients, random bladder biopsies are performed. If no muscle is present in the specimen, it is considered an inadequate specimen for diagnosis and staging. Prostatic urethral biopsies may also be performed in cases suggestive of invasive tumor or when the surgeon is considering an orthotopic reconstruction.

MANAGEMENT

Management of TCC is based primarily on stage. The staging system that is currently used is the AJCC system, which is based on depth of tumor invasion and metastatic involvement (Table 10–5). The goals for management include differentiating superficial from invasive tumor and determining which patients

Table 10–5. American Joint Committee on Cancer Staging System for Bladder Cancer

Primary Tumor (T)
Ta	Noninvasive papillary tumor
Tis	Carcinoma in situ
T1	Tumor invades subepithelial connective tissue
T2	Tumor invades muscle
T3	Tumor invades perivesical tissue
T4	Tumor invades any of the following: prostate, uterus, vagina, pelvic side wall, or abdominal wall

Regional Lymph Nodes (N)
N0	No regional lymph node metastasis
N1–3	Regional lymph nodes

Distant Metastasis (M)
M0	No distant metastasis
M1	Distant metastasis

Data from Fleming ID, Cooper JS, Henson DE, et al (eds.): American Joint Committee on Cancer Staging Manual, 5th ed. Philadelphia, Lippincott Raven, 1997:241.

will benefit from aggressive therapy. The potential for recurrence or progression depends on grade, stage, number of tumors, initial size of the tumor, and the previously established history of the patient's disease.[25]

In terms of prognosis, bladder cancers can be divided into two groups: superficial tumors, which include stages Ta, Tis, and T1 and are associated with a 5-year survival rate of almost 70%,[23] and invasive tumors, which include stages T2 through T4, require surgical treatment, and carry a much poorer prognosis. Approximately 70% of bladder cancers are superficial, low-grade tumors. The risk of developing invasive or metastatic tumors is about 3% for patients with stage Ta disease and almost 15% for patients with stages Tis or T1 disease.[23]

LOCAL DISEASE

For superficial bladder cancer, the concern in managing treatment is tumor recurrence; more than 50% of superficial bladder cancers recur in less than 12 months. The initial treatment is transurethral resection of the bladder tumor, with a follow-up cystoscopy in 3 months. As long as there is no evidence of recurrence, patients initially diagnosed with superficial tumors are traditionally monitored with cystoscopic examination every 3 months for the first 2 years, then every 4 months for 1 year, every 6 months for the next 2 years, and yearly thereafter.

If during the surveillance recurrent bladder cancer is discovered and remains low grade and low stage (Ta, Tis, or T1), intravesical chemotherapy or immunotherapy may be recommended. The therapeutic agents are introduced into the bladder through a catheter. The number of courses of treatment and their frequency and duration vary depending on the prescribed medication. Four agents currently are being used for intravesical therapy: thiotepa, mitomycin C, doxorubicin, and bacillus Calmette-Guérin (BCG).

Thiotepa is an alkylating agent that carries significant side effects. Between 15% and 20% of patients develop leukopenia because of the myelosuppressive activity of thiotepa. This drug has been noted to be less effective than other drugs on carcinoma in situ. Mitomycin C is an antitumor antibiotic and alkylating agent that inhibits DNA synthesis. Its known side effects include development of a rash, particularly on the hands and genital area where contact with the medication may occur, and various degrees of cystitis. Doxorubicin is an intercalating agent and antibiotic. It can produce severe cystitis with irritative voiding symptoms. Probably the most effective medication used in intravesical therapy is BCG, which is an attenuated mycobacterium. The mechanism for its activity is unknown but probably involves an immunologically mediated response. Side effects of BCG include irritative voiding symptoms, hematuria, and a flu-like syndrome; 7% of patients develop hemorrhagic cystitis, and almost 6% develop a persistent fever that requires antituberculosis therapy. Because of the risk of tuberculosis, this medication is not given if there has been a traumatic catheterization or severe hematuria. Granulomatous prostatitis as a result of BCG therapy is fairly common. Death from systemic tuberculosis has been reported in BCG-treated patients but is rare. The therapy is very well tolerated by most patients and remains the treatment of choice for carcinoma in situ.

ADVANCED DISEASE

The management of invasive bladder tumors begins with transurethral resection of the tumor. Laser surgery for this disease does not produce a specimen adequate for staging. Radical cystectomy is indicated in most patients with stages T2, T3, or T4a bladder cancer. The 5-year survival rates after radical cystectomy are about 75% for stage T2 disease, 44% for stage T3 disease, and 33% for stage T4a disease.[5] The rate of local recurrence is low, between 4% and 6%, in patients who undergo cystectomy.

In men, radical cystectomy consists of removal of the bladder, pelvic lymph nodes, seminal vesicles, prostate, and urethra if the prostatic urethral biopsy specimen is positive for TCC.[25] In women, the operative procedure is an anterior pelvic exenteration. This includes removal of the bladder, pelvic lymph nodes, uterus, cervix, anterior vaginal wall, ovaries, fallopian tubes, and urethra. The operative mortality with radical surgery is less than 2%,[23] and the incidence of serious complications is relatively low.[24] Operative complications can include wound infection, prolonged ileus, hemorrhage, rectal injury (in fewer than 2% of patients), bowel injury, and complications of ureteral anastomosis. Late complications can include stomal stenosis. This is managed either conservatively with dilatation of the stoma or surgically with a revision. Parastomal hernia and ureteroenteric anastomotic stricture are other possible late complications. Upper tract deterioration and nephrolithiasis have been documented.

Radical surgery includes a urinary diversion, of which there are three basic types. The gold standard in urinary diversion is the ileal conduit, which has no storage capability and requires an external appliance for storage. A good internal reservoir mimics the normal bladder—that is, it has low-pressure storage capability and a good storage capacity. The second type of diversion, the continent catheterizable reservoir, is a constructed pouch that requires catheterization at regular intervals through a small stoma on the abdominal wall. Variations of this type of reservoir include the Indiana, Florida, and Koch pouches. These vary in construction techniques and materials (which portion of the bowel), but the result and management are the same. The third choice is the orthotopic neobladder. These are bladders built from bowel and anastomosed to the urethra. Variations of the neobladder—including the Studer pouch, the Hauptman pouch, and the hemi-Koch neobladder—have different advantages and disadvantages, and the type that is recommended depends primarily on the surgeon's preference. The advantage of orthotopic neobladders is that the patient continues to urinate through the urethra as before surgery. However, these reconstructions do have several limitations. Except in experimental protocols, orthotopic neo-bladders are not an option for women because of the risk of urethral recurrences. Up to 20% of patients experience nocturnal enuresis because of the lack of normal external sphincter recruitment during bladder filling.[24] This problem can be managed quite well with timed voiding, the use of a condom catheter, and medical therapy. Patients learn to void with new techniques using abdominal pressure and pelvic floor relaxation. They learn to check for postvoid residual urine with a catheter to prevent overdistention of the neobladder. Metabolic abnormalities, including hyperchloremia, metabolic acidosis, and, rarely, B_{12} malabsorption, occasionally arise in patients with neobladders.

Partial cystectomy can be considered in a small number (approximately 5%) of patients, primarily those with a solitary infiltrating tumor and either T1 or T2 disease. The location of the tumor on the dome or posterior wall of the bladder is critical in obtaining an adequate surgical margin.[24] Recurrence rates after this treatment have been as high as 70% in some reports.[23]

Bladder-sparing treatment options that involve combination chemotherapy and radiation therapy are being studied in patients with T2 disease.[25] The recurrence rate after radiation therapy alone is between 50% and 70%, with a 5-year survival rate of 30%, for patients with all stages of bladder cancer.[23]

The primary therapeutic option for patients with metastatic disease is chemotherapy. Almost 15% of patients who present with bladder cancer have metastatic disease.[25] Multiagent chemotherapy regimens have higher response rates than single-agent regimens and are the mainstay in treatment. The MVAC chemotherapy regimen is a combination of methotrexate, vinblastine, doxorubicin (Adriamycin), and cisplatin. Complete response rates for combination chemotherapy range between 13% and 35%.[25] The 5-year survival rate after MVAC is as high as 32% in patients with nodal metastases and 17% in patients with distant metastases.[24] Fluorouracil (5-FU) and interferon-α plus platinum is a biologic therapy active against bladder cancer.[24] Combination chemotherapy has significant toxicity; primary side effects are myelosuppression, infectious complications, nephrotoxicity, and mucositis.

SURVEILLANCE

Follow-up for patients treated for invasive bladder cancer includes evaluation every 6 months for the first 2 years after surgical treatment. This includes a chest radiograph, liver function tests, and determinations of blood urea nitrogen and serum creatinine level. If a continent diversion was created, B_{12} levels and electrolytes should be checked to monitor for malabsorption and acidosis. A CT examination can be included in this 6-month evaluation, particularly for patients who had an invasive tumor, to rule out nodal disease, metastasis to the liver, or recurrence. An IVP can be performed every other year to image the upper tract, again as a surveillance modality.

REFERENCES

1. Brawley OW, Kramer BS: Epidemiology of prostate cancer. In Vogelzang NJ, Scardino PT, Shipley WA, et al (eds): Comprehensive Textbook of Genitourinary Oncology. Baltimore, Williams & Williams, 1996:565–572.

2. Kassabian VS, Graham SD: Urologic and male genital cancers. In Murphy GP, Lawrence W, Lenhard RE (eds): American Cancer Society Textbook of Clinical Oncology, 2nd ed. Atlanta, American Cancer Society, 1995:311–329.
3. Hudson MA: Screening for prostate cancer. In Ball TP, Novicki DE, Montano G, et al (eds): AUA Update Series, lesson 25, vol 15. Houston, American Urological Association, 1996:198–203.
4. Brawer MK: Screening for prostate cancer. In Vogelzang NJ, Scardino PT, Shipley WA, et al (eds): Comprehensive Textbook of Genitourinary Oncology. Baltimore, Williams & Williams, 1996:684–698.
5. Seigne JD, Grossman HB: Malignant tumors of the urogenital tract. In Rakel RA (ed): Conn's Current Therapy. Philadelphia, WB Saunders 1997:712–724.
6. Babaian RJ, Camps JL: The role of prostate specific antigen as part of the diagnostic triad and as a guide when to perform a biopsy. Cancer 1991;68:2060.
7. Osterling JE, Cupp MR: Prostate specific antigen, digital rectal examination and transrectal ultrasonography: Their role in diagnosing early prostate cancer. Mayo Clin Proc 1993;68:297.
8. Narayan P: Neoplasms of the prostate gland. In Tanagho EA, McAninch JW (eds): Smith's General Urology, 14th ed. Norwalk, CT, Appleton & Lange, 1995:392–433.
9. Pisters LL, Babaian RJ: Evaluating screening tools for prostate cancer. Hospital Medicine 1993;11:62.
10. Catalona WJ, Smith DS, Ratliff TL, et al: Measurement of prostate specific antigen in serum as a screening test for prostate cancer. N Engl J Med 1991;324:1156.
11. Delworth MG, Dinney CP: Genitourinary cancer. In Berger DH, Feig BW, Fuhrman GM (eds): The M.D. Anderson Surgical Oncology Handbook. Boston, Little, Brown, 1995:308–325.
12. Rukstalis DB: Recent advances in the surgical management of localized prostate cancer. In Dawson WA, Vogelzang NJ (eds): Prostate Cancer. New York, Wiley-Liss, 1994:151–164.
13. Huggins C, Hodges CV: Studies of prostatic cancer: 1. Effect of castration, estrogen and androgen injections on serum phosphatases in metastatic carcinoma of the prostate. Cancer Res 1941;293.
14. Zagars GK, von Eschenbach AC, Johnson DE, et al: The role of radiation therapy in stages A2 and B adenocarcinoma of the prostate. Int J Radiat Oncol Biol Phys 1988;14:701.
15. Greskovich FJ, Zagars GK, Sherman NE, et al: Complications following external beam radiation therapy for prostate cancer: An analysis of patients treated with and without pelvic lymphadenectomy. J Urol 1991;146:798.
16. Zagars GK: Prostate specific antigen as an outcome variable for T1 and T2 prostate cancer treated by radiation therapy. J Urol 1994;152:1786.
17. deKernion JB, Belldegrun A: Renal tumors. In Walsh PC, Retik AB, Stamey TA, et al (eds): Campbell's Urology, 6th ed, vol 2. Philadelphia, WB Saunders, 1992:1053–1093.
18. McDougal WS, Garrnick MB: Clinical signs and symptoms of cinoma. In Vogelzang NJ, Scardino PT, Shipley WA, et al (eds): Comprehensive Textbook of Genitourinary Oncology. Baltimore, Williams & Williams, 1996:154–159.
19. Kumar A, Pontes JE: Tumors of the kidney and ureter. In McKenna RJ, Murphy GP: Cancer Surgery. Philadelphia, JB Lippincott, 1994:475–487.
20. Driecer R, Williams RD: Renal parenchymal neoplasms. In Tanagho EA, McAninch JW (eds): Smith's General Urology, 14th ed. Norwalk, CT, Appleton & Lange, 1995:375–391.
21. Leder RA, Walther PJ: Radiologic imaging of cinoma: Its role in diagnosis, staging and management. In Vogelzang NJ, Scardino PT, Shipley WA, et al (eds): Comprehensive Textbook of Genitourinary Oncology. Baltimore, Williams & Williams, 1996:187–206.
22. Quesada J, Swanson DA, Gutterman JU: Phase II study of interferon alpha in metastatic cinoma: A progress report. J Clin Oncol 1985;3:1986.
23. Catalona WJ: Urothelial tumors of the urinary tract. In Walsh PC, Retik AB, Stamey TA, et al (eds): Campbell's Urology, 6th ed, vol 2. Philadelphia, WB Saunders, 1992:1094–1158.
24. Pisters LL, Wajsman Z: Surgery for invasive bladder cancer. In McKenna RJ, Murphy GP: Cancer Surgery. Philadelphia, JB Lippincott, 1994:455–473.
25. Carroll PR: Urothelial carcinoma cancers of the bladder, ureter and renal pelvis. In Tanagho EA, McAninch JW: Smith's General Urology, 14th ed. Norwalk, CT, Appleton & Lange, 1995:353.

Chapter 11

Testicular Cancer

Elizabeth Hossan, MS, RN, C-FNP,
Lawrence Hutchinson, MSN, RN, GNP, and
Robert J. Amato, DO

INTRODUCTION

Testicular cancer is a rare tumor, accounting for only 1% of all cancers in men, but it is the cancer that occurs most frequently in young adult men.[1] Fortunately, prevention and early detection of testicular cancer can decrease its mortality and morbidity rates. An increase in cure rates can be accomplished through education and training in self-examination, early detection, and continued improvement in management with chemotherapy. Testicular cancer is a disease that serves as a model of a curable solid tumor when managed with the combination of surgery, radiotherapy, and chemotherapy.[1]

EPIDEMIOLOGY

Testicular cancer, the most common tumor diagnosed in men between the ages of 15 and 34 years, accounts for 400 deaths per year in the United States.[2] The American Cancer Society (ACS) estimated that, in 1997 alone in the United States, 7600 males were diagnosed with testicular cancer.[2]

An increased incidence of testicular germ cell tumors has also been found in brothers, identical twins, and close male relatives such as uncles and grandfathers of patients with testicular cancer.[3]

The incidence of testicular cancer is increasing in white men, but its occurrence is very rare in black Americans and Asians.[4] Although there has been much speculation, the cause of testicular cancer is unknown. Age, endocrine and genetic abnormalities, trauma, and socioeconomic and occupational factors have been evaluated, but no epidemiologic studies have proved what single factor or combination of factors leads to the development of testicular cancer.[4] Cryptorchidism is the best documented risk factor for the development of testicular cancer; approximately 8.5% of patients diagnosed with testicular cancer have a history of this condition.[4] The risk of testicular cancer in males with cryptorchidism can be reduced by surgical repair (orchiopexy) before the boy reaches puberty. Orchiopexy is commonly performed before the age of 5 or 6 years to improve prospects for fertility. Inguinal hernia, which frequently exists with a cryptorchid testis, is another risk factor.[3] Finally, and for unknown reasons, primary tumors are more likely to be found in the right rather than the left testicle, but patients with a diagnosis of primary testicular cancer are at higher risk of a second primary tumor in the contralateral testis.[3]

GENETICS

A number of highly regulated expressive genes are needed for the testes to develop. These genes include transcription factors such as steroid hormone receptors and growth factors.[5] New data about the genetic basis of human male germ cell tumors have enabled construction of new and testable hypotheses regarding the development and differentiation of these tumors that may lead to a better understanding of them. Some findings include a genetic association of testicular cancer with Klinefelter syndrome (47XXY), which is particularly involved with primary mediastinal germ cell tumors, and Down syndrome (trisomy 21), which has been associated with an increased risk of germ cell tumors.[6] Other patients thought to be at increased risk for testicular cancer include true hermaphrodites and individuals with testicular feminization, müllerian syndrome, or cutaneous ichthyosis.[6]

PRESENTING HISTORY AND PHYSICAL EXAMINATION

As with any illness, the workup of a patient with a testicular mass begins with a thorough medical history. The most common symptom at the time of diagnosis is a painless swelling or enlargement of the testis. The second most common symptom is an acute painful testis, which can occur suddenly. This acute pain could represent torsion of a hidden mass, bleeding, or infarction of the tumor within the testis. A feeling of heaviness in the scrotum or a dull aching sensation in the lower abdomen or scrotum are other possible complaints in the clinical setting.[7]

Physical examination of the testis begins with the normal contralateral gonad. Careful palpation using the thumb and first two fingers of the examining hand is used to provide baseline information on the size and consistency of the normal testis. If it is unclear whether there is a mass in the testis, any firm or fixed area within the tunica albuginea should be considered suspicious until proven otherwise. Patients with any hard or firm nodular area on the testis should be referred to a urologist.

The physical examination also should include abdominal palpation for bulky nodal disease and inspection and auscultation of the chest for gynecomastia.[7] Approximately 3% of patients complain of breast tenderness resulting from the hormonal influence of the tumor.[7] Palpation of the supraclavicular area may reveal adenopathy if the disease has become metastatic. Metastatic disease may manifest as a mass in the left supraclavicular area, cough, hemoptysis, shortness of breath, chest pain, abdominal pain (bulky intra-abdominal disease), lower back pain (retroperitoneal disease involving psoas muscles or nerve roots), bone pain (skeletal metastasis), or other manifestations that affect the central nervous system, indicating its involvement. Gastrointestinal symptoms or an abdominal mass usually reflect extensive retroperitoneal disease. Weight loss is not uncommon.

The impact of delay in diagnosis of testicular cancer is substantial; if the disease is not detected and treated early, it continues to progress to higher grade, less treatable tumor stages. Common initial diagnoses include trauma, benign tumor, hydrocele, and infection.[7]

To reduce diagnostic delays, public education programs are important. These programs must emphasize the existence of the disease and the need for patients to consult health care providers quickly if a mass is suspected.[8] Education about testicular cancer should start with the midteenage group. Midlevel practitioners need to be reminded that testicular masses are malignant until proven otherwise, and neither the presence nor the absence of pain should keep them from considering a diagnosis of testicular cancer in patients presenting with these symptoms.[7]

HISTOLOGY, PATHOLOGY, AND RADIOLOGY

Dixon and Moore[9] and Mostofi and Price[10] proposed the current model for the development of germ cell tumors. During embryonal development, totipotential germ cells can travel down normal pathways and become spermatocytes. Carcinoma occurs when the totipotential germ cells travel down abnormal developmental pathways and become germ cell carcinomas.[11]

Table 11-1. Serum Markers for Testicular Cancer

PATHOLOGIC SUBTYPE	β-SUBUNIT OF HUMAN CHORIONIC GONADOTROPIN	α-FETOPROTEIN
Seminoma	+	−
Embryonal	+	+
Choriocarcinoma	+	−
Yolk sac (endodermal sinus tumor)	−	+
Teratoma	−	−

The two types of testicular cancer are nonseminomatous and seminomatous germ cell tumors. Both have tumor markers. A nonseminomatous germ cell tumor is indicated by an increase in the serum level of α-fetoprotein (AFP). A seminomatous germ cell tumor is indicated by an increase in the serum level of the β-subunit of human chorionic gonadotropin (β-hCG)[11] (Table 11–1).

Seminoma is the most common histologic subtype of testicular cancer, ac-counting for 35% to 40% of germ cell tumors. Embryonal carcinoma and a mixture of other pathologic subtypes make up more than 60% of all testicular germ cell tumors. The other pathologic subtypes include yolk sac tumor (also called endodermal sinus tumor), choriocarcinoma, immature teratoma, and ma-ture teratoma.[10]

A sonogram of the scrotum is an excellent tool with which to distinguish normal from abnormal scrotal contents and should be considered an extension of the physical examination. Computed tomography is currently the imaging modality of choice for the retroperitoneum.[12] A chest radiograph is helpful if the patient complains of hemoptysis or shortness of breath (Fig. 11–1).

DIFFERENTIAL DIAGNOSIS

A hard or firm nodular area on the testis should be considered malignant unless proved otherwise.[13] Other causes of testicular masses are listed in Table 11–2.[14] Transillumination is a simple method to help differentiate a hydrocele

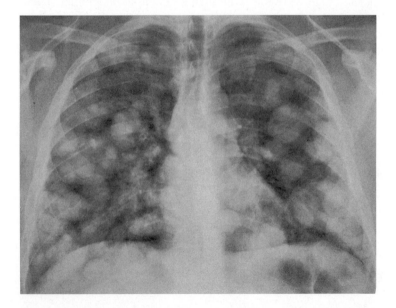

Figure 11-1. Chest radiograph of patient with choriocarcinoma meta-static to the lungs.

Table 11–2. Benign Causes of Testicular Symptoms

Orchitis	Infection or inflammation of the testes due to epididymitis/mumps
	Symptoms: pain and swelling of the testicle; fever; scrotum often reddened and edematous
Epididymitis	Infection
	Symptoms: pain in the groin and scrotum; edema, redness, tenderness of scrotum; chills, fever
Torsion of the appendix of the testes	Swelling of testes
	Symptoms: painful and enlarged testes usually seen in youths
Hydrocele	Abnormal accumulation of fluid in the scrotum and around the testicle
	Symptoms: none; swelling is usually painless
Varicocele	Engorgement of veins within the scrotum
	Symptoms: dragging sensation within the scrotum
Tuberculosis	Testicular involvement rarely seen until late stages of the disease
	Symptoms: none; usually a nontender mass involving the epididymis
Syphilitic orchitis (gumma)	Seen in tertiary stage of syphilis
	Symptoms: firm, hard testes, painless; serology positive for syphilis

From Hubbard SM, Jenkins J: An overview of current concepts in the management of patients with testicular tumors of germ cell origin: Part I. Pathophysiology, diagnosis, and staging. Cancer Nurs 1993;6:43.

from a solid lesion (Fig. 11–2). If doubt still exists, sonography of the testis helps to detect hydroceles, to differentiate a solid lesion from a cystic lesion, and to identify suspicious areas in the testicle.[15] Patients with testicular neoplasms may have pain from associated epididymitis or testicular torsion; hence, the presence of pain does not rule out malignancy.[13]

Young, active men are prime candidates for infection (epididymitis or orchitis) or trauma leading to torsion of the spermatic cord.[7] In acute epididymitis, it may or may not be possible to distinguish the enlarged, tender epididymis from the testis. In chronic epididymitis, the epididymis is enlarged and indurated. Acute orchitis is most often associated with mumps parotitis and causes the testis to become enlarged and painful. Torsion of the spermatic cord occurs most commonly in prepubescent boys and results in acute ischemia to the epididymis and testis. If acute pain has been present for several hours, scrotal exploration often is required for a definitive diagnosis.[15]

Transcrotal exploration or orchiectomy is contraindicated if a testicular neoplasm is suspected. The indicated method for obtaining a definitive diagnosis of testicular cancer is inguinal radical orchiectomy.[16] Because the lymphatic drainage of the testis is distinct from that of the scrotum, scrotal dissection in the presence of a testicular malignancy would place the patient at high risk for development of an inguinal metastasis or local recurrence[14] (Fig. 11–3).

If testicular neoplasm is the likely diagnosis, a blood specimen should be drawn before orchiectomy to determine baseline levels of tumor and nontumor markers in the serum.[13] As stated previously, AFP and β-hCG are proteins used as tumor markers for germ cell tumors. Isochromosome 12p is another tumor marker that is found in more than 80% of patients who have germ cell tumors.[6] This marker is not routinely used at the current time but may prove useful for identifying patients who have an unrecognized germ cell tumor.[6] The level of the enzyme lactate dehydrogenase, a nontumor marker, is used to indicate prognosis of germ cell tumors.[1, 6] Pretreatment values of AFP, β-hCG, and lactate dehydrogenase are increased in 70% to 80% of patients who have advanced disease.[17, 18] The half-lives of these three markers after orchiectomy are well documented, and all three have prognostic value in detecting the presence of metastatic disease and in assessing response to therapy.[19, 20]

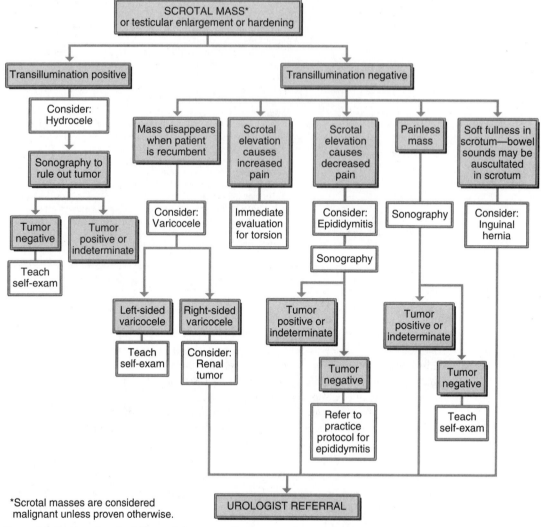

*Scrotal masses are considered
malignant unless proven otherwise.

Figure 11–2. Algorithm for differential diagnosis and treatment of a scrotal mass.

TREATMENT AND REFERRAL

A patient with a suspected testicular mass should be referred to a urologist for immediate confirmation and treatment to avoid additional morbidity. Once the existence of an intratesticular mass consistent with a testicular tumor has been established by physical examination, medical history, and scrotal sonography (if performed), radical inguinal orchiectomy should be arranged within 24 to 48 hours.[20] The focus of therapy is to limit morbidity by appropriate use of surveillance protocols and to minimize the amount and toxicity of therapy while maximizing cure rates.[12] Specific therapeutic options depend on the histologic diagnosis and stage of disease at presentation. Seminoma is radiosensitive and often is treated with modern megavolt radiotherapy to the primary areas of lymphatic drainage of the testis.[21]

Patients who have a stage I nonseminomatous germ cell tumor, which is a tumor confined to the testis, often undergo retroperitoneal lymph node dissection (retroperitoneal lymphadenectomy). The major disadvantage of this procedure is the induction of dry ejaculation caused by autonomic nerve dysfunction

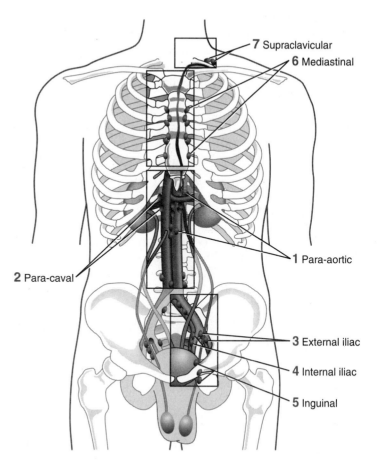

Figure 11–3. Lymphatic nodes draining the testes. Boxes indicate the radiation portals used in radiotherapy for testicular neoplasms. (From Hubbard SM, Jenkins J: An overview of current concepts in the management of patients with testicular tumors of germ cell origin. Part I: Pathophysiology, diagnosis, and staging. Cancer Nurs 1993;6:43.)

7 Supraclavicular
6 Mediastinal
1 Para-aortic
2 Para-caval
3 External iliac
4 Internal iliac
5 Inguinal

in the region of the aortic bifurcation.[22, 23] Surgeons experienced in more recently developed techniques of limited retroperitoneal lymph node dissection are sometimes able to preserve the patient's ability to ejaculate. However, any retroperitoneal lymph node dissection is a major surgical procedure and is necessary only if metastases are found or highly suspected. In a retrospective study done to encourage the use of nerve-sparing surgical techniques when possible, Donahue and Thornhill[24] found that up to two thirds of patients underwent retroperitoneal lymph node dissection unnecessarily because metastatic disease had not been identified.

Patients with stage II or III nonseminomatous testicular cancer are treated with combination chemotherapy, and, if indicated, surgical resection of residual disease. Advanced disease enters complete remission in approximately 85% of patients, and the relapse rate is low. Certain subsets of patients, such as those with extragonadal presentations (i.e., outside the testis) and those with high levels of biologic markers in the serum, have lower cure rates.[13]

POSTTREATMENT SURVEILLANCE

Current consensus is that the majority of patients with clinical stage I nonseminomatous germ cell tumors can be safely observed with a surveillance program.[25]

For patients who undergo radiotherapy for a stage I seminoma or chemotherapy for a metastatic seminoma or a nonseminomatous germ cell tumor and achieve complete remission of disease, the highest risk of recurrence is experienced in the first 2 years after the cessation of therapy. Compliance with the intensive follow-up required, particularly in patients in surveillance programs for low-stage disease, is often difficult in this young, mobile population.[14] Follow-up visits may be as frequent as monthly for men diagnosed with stage I nonseminomatous germ cell tumors who are in surveillance programs (Table 11–3).

Patients with testicular cancer who are in a surveillance program for stage I disease or have undergone retroperitoneal lymph node dissection for stage I nonseminomatous germ cell tumor, radiotherapy for stage I seminoma, or systemic chemotherapy for metastatic seminoma or nonseminomatous germ cell tumor should follow a regular schedule of clinical examination, computed tomography scanning, radiographs of the thorax, and serum marker analysis. Careful monitoring of the retroperitoneal area is particularly important if modern, less extensive procedures for retroperitoneal lymph node dissection are performed.[25]

Recurrent or progressive testicular cancer may spread by hematogenous dissemination to the lungs, liver, brain, gastrointestinal tract, or bone. Brain metastasis should be suspected in patients who have pulmonary disease and present with neurologic abnormalities.[14] Patients also should be screened for development of a second testicular tumor and taught testicular self-examination, because 2% to 5% of men with testicular cancer will have a tumor in the contralateral testis during their lifespan.[26, 27]

Table 11–3. Five-Year Posttreatment Surveillance Schedule

PATIENT STATUS	LABORATORY TESTS°	RADIOGRAPHY
Nonseminoma, stage I; after orchiectomy	AFP, hCG, LDH iso q 1 mo × 12 then q 3 mo × 4 then q 4 mo × 3 then q 6 mo × 4	CXR, CT abd/pelvis q 3 mo × 8 then q 4 mo × 3 then q 6 mo × 4 test US q year
Nonseminoma, stage I; after chemotherapy	Same as above; add CBC, diff, plt count, BUN/crt, liver function	Same as above
Nonseminoma, stage I; after retroperitoneal lymphadenectomy	AFP, hCG, LDH iso q 3 mo × 8 then q 4 mo × 3 then q 6 mo × 4	Same as above except CT abd/pelvis on alternate visits only
Nonseminoma, metastatic disease; after chemotherapy only	Same as above; add CBC, diff, plt count, BUN/crt, liver function	Same as stage I surveillance schedule
Nonseminoma: metastatic disease; after retroperitoneal lymphadenectomy	Same as above	Same as stage I surveillance schedule except CT abd/pelvis on alternate visits only
Seminoma, stage I; after radiation	AFP, hCG, LDH iso q 3 mo × 2 then q 6 mo × 2 then q yr × 3; CBC, diff, plt count first visit after radiation	CXR, CT abd/pelvis same as lab schedule; test US q year
Seminoma: metastatic disease; after chemotherapy	Same as nonseminoma metastatic disease after chemotherapy	Same as nonseminoma stage I surveillance

q, every; iso, isoenzymes; CXR, chest x-ray; abd, abdomen; US, ultrasound; diff, differential; plt, platelet; crt, creatinine; BUN, blood urea nitrogen.
°BUN and crt are drawn before CT abd/pelvis examination with contrast.

The most clinically significant chronic toxic effects after chemotherapy for testicular cancer are peripheral neurotoxicity, high-frequency hearing loss, a Raynaud-like phenomenon, and reduced spermatogenesis. Patients who survive testicular cancer also are at increased risk for the development of additional malignancies.[28]

SCREENING AND EARLY DETECTION

Morbidity and mortality rates from testicular cancer could be even further reduced by educating teenagers and young men about testicular self-examination.[4] The ACS reports that 90% of testicular cancers are discovered by the patient himself.[29] Testicular self-examination is a simple procedure that should be done after or during a shower or warm bath so that the scrotum is relaxed and the testes are easy to palpate. The individual should become familiar with the normal structures of the scrotum (testes, epididymides, and spermatic cord) so that changes can be detected.[30, 31] The ACS recommends that annual professional examination and monthly testicular self-examination be initiated during puberty. A thorough examination includes an estimation of the weight and equality of size of both testes. This is done by placing a testis in each hand and lifting and then gently pulling the testis anteriorly in the scrotal sac. Each testis and its anatomy, including epididymis and vas deferens, are palpated for any abnormality.

As discussed, differential diagnosis of scrotal masses can be difficult. The detection of any scrotal mass warrants prompt referral to a urologist.[32] Even a short delay may have a significant impact on the extent of disease if the patient is eventually diagnosed with testicular cancer. Patients who present with more advanced disease have a lower cure rate, require more therapy, and experience more side effects from treatment.

REFERENCES

1. Einhorn LH, Crawford DE, Shipley WU, et al: Testicular cancer. In DeVita VT, Helloman S, Rosenberg SA (eds): Cancer Principles & Practice of Oncology, 3rd ed. Philadelphia, JB Lippincott, 1989:1071–1093.
2. Landis SH, Murray T, Bolden S, Wingo PA: Cancer Statistics, 1998. CA Cancer J Clin 1998;48:6–29.
3. Frank IN, Graham SD, Nabors WL: Urologic and male genital cancers. In Halleb AI, Fink DJ, Murphy GP (eds): American Cancer Society Textbook of Clinical Oncology. Atlanta, American Cancer Society, 1991:283–286.
4. Oliver RTD: Epidemiology of testis cancer. In Vogelzang NV, Scardino PT, Shipley WU, et al (eds): Comprehensive Book of Genitourinary Oncology. Baltimore, Wilkins & Wilkins, 1996:923–932.
5. Lamb DT: Genes involved in testicular development and function. World J Urol 1995;13:227–284.
6. Loehrer PJ, Ahlering TE, Pollack A: Testicular cancer. In Pazdur R, Coia LR, Hoskins WJ, et al (eds): Cancer Management: A Multidisciplinary Approach. Medical, Surgical, and Radiation Oncology. Huntington, NY, PRR, 1996:401–416.
7. Kennedy BJ: Clinical signs and symptoms. In Vogelzang NV, Scardino PT, Shipley WU, et al (eds): Comprehensive Book of Genitourinary Oncology. Baltimore, Wilkins & Wilkins, 1996:921–923.
8. Wilson P: Testicular, prostate and penile cancers in primary care settings: The importance of early detection. Nurse Pract 1991;16:18–26.
9. Dixon FJ, Moore RA (eds): Atlas of Tumor Pathology. Washington, DC, Armed Forces Institute of Pathology, 1952:32.
10. Mostofi FK, Price ER Jr: Tumors of the male genital system. In Atlas of Tumor Pathology, 2nd series, fascicle 8. Washington, DC, Armed Forces Institute of Pathology, 1973.
11. Bower M, Rustin GJS: Serum tumor markers and their role in monitoring germ cell cancers of the

testis. In Vogelzang NV, Scardino PT, Shipley WU, et al (eds): Comprehensive Book of Genitourinary Oncology. Baltimore, Wilkins & Wilkins, 1996:968–981.

12. Watson DL, Kantoff PW, Richie JP: Staging and imaging of testis cancer. In Vogelzang NV, Scardino PT, Shipley WU, et al (eds): Comprehensive Book of Genitourinary Oncology. Baltimore, Wilkins & Wilkins, 1996:981–986.

13. Garnick MB: Testicular cancer. Semin Surg Oncol 1989;5:221–226.

14. Hubbard SM, Jenkins J: An overview of current concepts in the management of patients with testicular tumors of germ cell origin. Part II: Treatment strategies by histology and stage. Cancer Nurs 1983;6:125–139.

15. McGuire EJ: Male genitourinary system and hernia. In Judge RD, Zuidema GD, Fitzgerald FT (eds): Clinical Diagnosis: A Physiological Approach. Boston, Little, Brown, 1989:363–388.

16. Brock D, Fox S, Gosling G, et al: Testicular cancer. Semin Oncol Nurs 1993;9:224–236.

17. Bosl GJ, Geller NL, Cirrincione C, et al: Serum tumor markers in patients with metastatic germ cell tumors: A 10-year experience. Am J Med 1983;75:29–35.

18. Toner GC, Geller NL, Tan C, et al: Serum tumor marker half-life during chemotherapy allows early prediction of complete response and survival in nonseminomatous germ cell tumors. Cancer Res 1990;50:5904–5910.

19. Lange PH, Vogelzang NJ, Goldman A, et al: Marker half-life analysis as a prognostic tool in testicular cancer. J Urol 1982;128:708–711.

20. Moul JW, McLeod DG: Surgical management of testis cancer. In Vogelzang NV, Scardino PT, Shipley WU, et al (eds): Comprehensive Book of Genitourinary Oncology. Baltimore, Wilkins & Wilkins, 1996:902–1015.

21. Gregory C, Peckham MJ: Results of radiotherapy for stage II testicular seminoma. Radiother Oncol 1986;6:285–292.

22. Lang PH, Chang WY, Fraley EE: Fertility issues in the therapy of testicular tumors. Urol Clin North Am 1987;14:731–747.

23. Pizzocaro G: Management of stage I nonseminoma: Rationale for lymphadenectomy. In Horwich A (ed): Testicular Cancer: Investigation and Management. London, Chapman & Hall, 1991:167–173.

24. Donahue JP, Thornhill JA: Retroperitoneal lymphadenectomy in staging and treatment: The development of nerve-sparing techniques. In Horwich A (ed): Testicular Cancer: Investigation and Management. London, Chapman & Hall Medical, 1991:175–184.

25. Rorth M, Daugaard G: Observation and management for low stage seminoma and non-seminoma. In Vogelzang NV, Scardino PT, Shipley WU, et al (eds): Comprehensive Book of Genitourinary Oncology. Baltimore, Wilkins & Wilkins, 1996:1010–1021.

26. Osterlind A, Berthelsen JG, Abildgaad N, et al: Risk of bilateral testicular germ cell cancer in Denmark: 1960–1984. J Natl Cancer Inst 1991;83:1391–1395.

27. Bokemeyer C, Schmoll HJ, Schoffski P, et al: Bilateral testicular tumors: Prevalence and clinical implications. Eur J Cancer 1993;29a:874–876.

28. Aass N, Fossa SD, Raghavan D, Vogelzang NV: Late toxicity after chemotherapy of testis cancer. In Vogelzang NV, Scardino PT, Shipley WU, et al (eds): Comprehensive Book of Genitourinary Oncology. Baltimore, Wilkins & Wilkins, 1996:1090–1096.

29. Office of Cancer Communications: Testicular Cancer: Research Report, 1987. NIH Publication No. 87-654. Bethesda, MD, National Cancer Institute, 1987.

30. T.S.E. [Testicular Self Examination], American Cancer Society (pamphlet).

31. Murray BLS, Wilcox LV: Testicular self-examination. Am J Nurs 1978;78:2074–2075.

32. Haggery BJ: Prevention and differential of scrotal cancer. Nurse Pract 1983;8:45–52.

Chapter 12

Preinvasive Disease of the Female Genital Tract

Alma C. Sbach, MSN, RN, CS, FNP,
Gwendolyn Killiam Corrigan, MSN, RN, FNP,
and Michele Follen Mitchell, MD, MS

CERVICAL INTRAEPITHELIAL NEOPLASIA

Cervical intraepithelial neoplasia (CIN) is a preinvasive precursor to cervical cancer. Preinvasive cervical lesions exhibit a continuum of cellular alteration from the basement membrane to the surface of the cervix with no invasion of the basement membrane (Fig. 12–1).[1] The process begins as a generally well-differentiated neoplasm or mild dysplasia and ends as invasive carcinoma.[2]

Approximately 25% of preinvasive lesions of the cervix progress, although the rate of progression appears to differ with lesion severity.[3] For example, 14% of mild, moderate, and severe dysplasias progress to carcinoma in situ (CIS).[4] In turn, 36% of CIS lesions progress to invasive carcinoma.[4]

EPIDEMIOLOGY

The incidence of CIN (except for CIS) is unknown because cases are not reported. The estimated number of cases of CIS in the United States for 1995 was 65,000.[5] Nevertheless, CIN is far more common than cervical cancer, with estimates varying from 250,000 to more than 2 million cases per year,[6, 7] compared with an estimated 15,800 cases of cervical carcinoma in the United States for 1995.[5] Most cervical cancers diagnosed worldwide occur in developing countries where screening and treatment of preinvasive disease are uncommon.

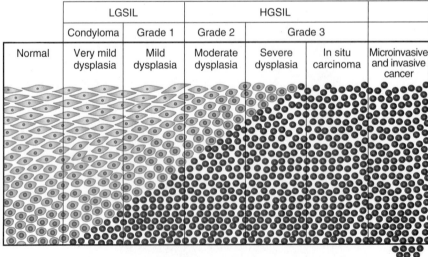

PRECURSORS TO INVASIVE CARCINOMA OF CERVIX
Cervical Intraepithelial Neoplasia

	LGSIL		HGSIL			
	Condyloma	Grade 1	Grade 2	Grade 3		
Normal	Very mild dysplasia	Mild dysplasia	Moderate dysplasia	Severe dysplasia	In situ carcinoma	Microinvasive and invasive cancer

Basement membrane

Figure 12–1. Schematic representation of cervical cancer precursors. Cervical intraepithelial neoplasia (CIN) grades 1, 2, and 3 correspond respectively to the traditional categories of very mild to mild dysplasia, moderate dysplasia, and severe dysplasia to carcinoma in situ. These categories are characterized by a progressive increase in the number of undifferentiated, malignant cells and a decrease in superficial cell differentiation paralleling the increasing severity of CIN. LGSIL, low-grade squamous intraepithelial lesion; HGSIL, high-grade squamous intraepithelial lesion. (Data from Ferenczy A: Cervical intraepithelial neoplasia. In Blaustein E (ed): Pathology of the Female Genital Tract, 2nd ed. New York, Springer-Verlag, 1982:158.)

In most developed countries, the incidence of cervical cancer has declined over the last 40 years owing to better screening and treatment of CIN or preinvasive disease and cervical cancers.

RISK FACTORS

The risk factors for preinvasive lesions of the cervix and for cervical cancer are similar (Table 12–1).[7] One common protective factor for both is the use of barrier methods of contraception, particularly the diaphragm.

Both CIN and cervical cancer have been linked to sexual factors. In many ways, CIN and cervical cancer behave like sexually transmitted diseases (STDs). Both CIN and cervical cancer have been linked consistently with human papillomavirus (HPV) infection. HPV appears as a strong risk factor across all types of epidemiologic studies. In the epidemiologic sense HPV is considered necessary but not sufficient for the development of cervical dysplasia.

CLASSIFICATION SYSTEMS

Screening and detection of CIN and of squamous intraepithelial lesions (SILs) of the cervix involve cervical cytology, or the Papanicolaou (Pap) smear. Several classification systems for Pap smears have been used. The Papanicolaou classifi-

Table 12–1. Risk Factors for Cervical Intraepithelial Neoplasia

	RISK FACTORS
CATEGORY	**MORE COMMON IN YOUNGER WOMEN OF REPRODUCTIVE AGE**
Sexual factors	Human papilloma virus (HPV) infection—more than 70 types
	HPV 16 is most common type worldwide and is high risk
	HPV 18, 45, and 56 are intermediate-risk types
	HPV 31, 33, 35, 51, 52, and 58 are intermediate-risk types
	HPV 6, 11, 42, 43, and 44 are low-risk types
	History of sexually transmitted diseases (STDs) other than HPV infection
	Male partners who have any of the following:
	History of STDs
	Multiple sex partners
	Previous partners with CIN or cervical cancer
	Intercourse with prostitutes
	Multiple (>1) sex partners
	Young age at first intercourse (<18 years of age)
Lifestyle factors	Cigarette smoking
Reproductive/contraceptive factors	High parity
	Long-term (5 yr) contraceptive use
Nutritional factors	Low vitamin A intake
	Low vitamin C intake
	Low folic acid intake
Socioeconomic or ethnic factors	Low socioeconomic status
	Membership in an ethnic minority population
Medical history	Immunosuppression

Data from Morris M, Tortolero-Luna G, Malpeca A, et al: Cervical intraepithelial neoplasia and cervical cancer. Obstet Gynecol Clin North Am 1996;23:347.

cation system was the first; it classified normal tissue through invasive cancer into five categories. The World Health Organization classified cervical cytology into different grades of dysplasia.[8] These categories do not, however, correlate with the current histopathologic classification systems, namely the Richart and Bethesda systems.[9-11] Richart's CIN system, introduced in the 1960s, is used for histologic diagnosis of preinvasive lesions. Most agencies now use the Bethesda System (TBS), introduced in 1988 and updated in 1991, for cytologic screening of Pap smears.[10, 11]

The TBS classification was developed by an expert panel convened by the National Cancer Institute (NCI) with the goal of standardizing Pap smear reports from cytology laboratories in the United States. Other goals were to define a uniform terminology, to outline criteria for Pap smear adequacy, and to develop a model that related Pap smear findings to the clinical management of the patient.[10] The panel determined that the Papanicolaou classification is not acceptable for use in Pap smear reports and that TBS should be used for cytopathology reports of the cervix and vagina.[10]

The categories used in TBS for squamous epithelial preinvasive lesions are *low-grade SIL* (HPV infection and CIN I) and *high-grade SIL* (CIN II, CIN III, and CIS).[10] In addition, a new category is called *atypical squamous cells of undetermined significance* (ASCUS). Today, many agencies use TBS for biopsy results also. For example, biopsy results may read "low-grade SIL, CIN I." Table 12-2 details the classification systems for CIN and gives general descriptions of the lesions identified.[12-14]

CLINICAL EVALUATION

PRESENTING HISTORY

Patients with CIN or SIL are asymptomatic. The condition is identified only after completion of a screening Pap smear.

MEDICAL HISTORY

Before the history is taken, all procedures should be explained, and the patient should give her informed consent. Any patient found to have an abnormal Pap smear should have a thorough medical history taken before the physical examination.

Important information to collect includes (1) past and present use of medications—especially contraceptives, hormone replacement therapy, vaginal preparations, antibiotics; (2) allergies to any drugs; (3) medical history—cancer, preinvasive or invasive cancer of the female genital tract, cardiovascular disease, hypertension, diabetes, asthma, and/or emphysema; (4) surgical history—cryosurgery, loop electrosurgery excision procedure (LEEP), laser surgery, conization, dilation and curettage, laparoscopy, and/or tubal ligation; (5) obstetric and gynecologic history—gravidity, parity, menstrual history, irregular vaginal bleeding, postmenopausal bleeding, Pap smear dates and results, vaginitis, pelvic inflammatory disease, and/or diethylstilbestrol exposure; (6) sexual history—date of first intercourse, number of partners for the patient and for her significant other, sexual orientation, and sexual activity or inactivity; (7) STDs—HPV infection, genital warts, gonorrhea, chlamydia, syphilis, human immunodeficiency virus (HIV) infection, *Trichomonas* infection, and/or herpes; (8) social history—past and present tobacco use, alcohol intake, and/or illegal drug use; (9) family history—cancer, heart disease, and/or diabetes; and (10) review of systems—abnormal vaginal discharge or bleeding, vaginal dryness, vulvar itching or lumps, and/or pelvic pain.

RISK FACTOR ANALYSIS

A risk factor analysis should be done as the medical history is taken to determine whether the patient is at low or high risk for CIN. Because screening interval, treatment plan, follow-up, and health education are all based on risk status, such analysis is important.

PHYSICAL EXAMINATION

A complete physical examination including a thorough pelvic examination should be done as follows. Inspect and palpate the external genital organs. Insert a vaginal speculum and repeat the Pap smear with a wooden spatula and cytobrush if the last Pap smear was obtained more than 6 weeks previously. (A current Pap smear is needed to correlate with the cervical biopsies, especially because the abnormality on the smear may have changed since the last smear.) The Pap smear should be done before any other cultures are taken. Never swab secretions from the cervix before obtaining the Pap smear unless they are copious. Exfoliated cells indicative of CIN or cancer may be removed.

Screen the patient for gonorrhea and chlamydia. Screening for the presence of HPV can be done after the other cultures have been taken (tests are available to detect HPV by type). Some experts advise its use for triage of patients with ASCUS or low-grade SIL Pap smears to determine the risk for development of CIN. Infection with a high-risk type of HPV indicates increased risk for invasive cervical cancer and an underlying lesion that is not benign but CIN. (NCI experts warn that, at present, HPV testing should be used only by health care providers who understand its limitations.[6])

Do a wet prep with potassium hydroxide and saline to check for vaginitis, if signs and symptoms warrant it. Before the colposcopic examination, remove the vaginal speculum and do a bimanual and rectovaginal examination to evaluate the internal organs and rectum for abnormalities (e.g., pregnancy, enlarged uterus, adnexal mass, pelvic inflammatory disease). Doing the bimanual and rectovaginal examination at this time, instead of after biopsies, is more comfortable for the patient and will not aggravate biopsy sites. Finally, reinsert the speculum to complete the colposcopic examination.

PAP SMEARS

The false-negative rate for Pap smears (i.e., when the smear is negative but the patient has disease) varies widely, from 10% to as high as 50%.[15] This rate is attributed to errors made in taking or preparing the slide (e.g., swabbing the

Table 12-2. Preinvasive Squamous Lesions of the Cervix

	NORMAL	ATYPIA (REACTIVE VS. DYSPLASTIC)	NONINVASIVE (PREMALIGNANT AND MALIGNANT) LESIONS			
Colposcopic photo						
Cytologic photo						
Histologic photo						

Histology	Well-oriented basal cell layer; full-thickness maturation; no nuclear atypia		Disorganized basal cell layer; cell maturation delayed to lower one-third thickness of squamous epithelium	Disorganized basal cell layer; cell maturation delayed to more than one-third, but less than two-thirds, the thickness of squamous epithelium	Disorganized basal cell layer; cell maturation delayed to more than two-thirds, but less than the full thickness of squamous epithelium	Full thickness squamous epithelium showing cellular atypia and no cell maturation
Cytology	Mature squamous cells		Nuclear enlargement; mild increase in nuclear-to-cytoplasmic ratio	Nuclear atypia; moderate increase in nuclear-to-cytoplasmic ratio	Nuclear atypia; marked increase in nuclear-to-cytoplasmic ratio	Nuclear atypia; alteration of nuclear-to-cytoplasmic ratio; syncytial grouping of cells
WHO terminology		Classification gave no terminology to use; individuals created various wordings, all meaning "atypia not classifiable"	Mild dysplasia	Moderate dysplasia	Severe dysplasia	CIS
Richart terminology, 1960s	Normal		CIN grade I	CIN grade II	CIN grade III	CIN grade III
The Bethesda System terminology, (NCI) 1988	Normal	ASCUS favor reactive process; ASCUS favor premalignant process (HPV or dysplasia)	LGSIL (includes CIN I and HPV)	HGSIL	HGSIL	HGSIL

Table courtesy of G. Staerkel, M.D., G. K. Corrigan, and N. Caraway, M.D., 1996.

Abbreviations: ASCUS, atypical squamous cells of undetermined significance; CIN, cervical intraepithelial neoplasia; LGSIL, low-grade squamous intraepithelial lesion; HGSIL, high-grade squamous intraepithelial lesion; HPV, human papilloma virus; CIS, carcinoma in situ.

*From Tedeschi C, Spitzer M: Home study course. The Colposcopist 1993;25(1):10.
†From Gunderson J, Noller LK: Home study course. The Colposcopist 1993;25(4):6.
‡From Spitzer M: Home study course. The Colposcopist 1995;27(1):6.

cervix before taking the Pap smear, not fixing the sample immediately), patient error (e.g., patient is menstruating or has douched, has used a vaginal preparation, or had sex within the previous 48 hours), and laboratory errors (e.g., misinterpretation). False-positive Pap smears (i.e., when the smear is positive but the patient does not have disease) may indicate atrophic changes, changes caused by radiation or chemotherapy, or infection in the cervix. The Pap smear should be done first with a spatula to sample the entire transformation zone, including the ectocervix, and then with a cytobrush to sample the endocervical canal (Table 12–3). Seven times more endocervical cells can be recovered with the use of the cytobrush.[16] An endocervical brush also can be used carefully during pregnancy, although this may cause minimal spotting.[16, 17]

Table 12–3. Performing the Pap Smear

Scheduling a patient	Advise patient to put nothing in the vagina for 48 hours before screening (i.e., no medications, spermicides, intercourse, douching).
	Do not schedule a Pap test during menses.
Patient education	Explain that the purpose of the Pap smear is screening and that it is not 100% accurate.
	Explain screening guidelines.
	Explain the procedure.
	Explain that the patient may have some spotting after the procedure.
	Explain importance of follow-up if there is an abnormal Pap smear.
Filling out the requisition	Review the questions on the requisition with the patient and complete the form.
	Explain that birth control pills, previous pelvic radiation, hormone replacement therapy, and pregnancy are all factors that may affect cells removed during the Pap smear.
	So that the pathologist may accurately assess the cells, provide date of patient's last menstrual cycle and accurate information.
Performing the pap smear	1. Have the Pap slide labeled correctly with patient name and number.
	2. Insert speculum to completely visualize cervix. Use no lubricant, since it will alter the Pap smear. Instead, use water, if necessary, to ease insertion.
	3. Do not swab discharge from the cervix unless there is a large amount.
	4. Take the spatula sample first, exerting firm but gentle pressure 360° twice, with spatula held in the free hand.
	5. Insert the cytobrush into the external cervical os so that all bristles are just inside the os. Turn the cytobrush only one-half turn. Rotating it more will usually cause bleeding. Adequate endocervical cell recovery occurs with this recommendation.
	6. Use a cotton swab moistened in saline (if the patient's vagina is dry) or the rounded end of the wooden spatula to collect a vaginal Pap smear.
	7. Quickly spread the sample taken with the spatula on the slide, taking care to spread collected material evenly from both sides of the spatula.
	8. Roll the cytobrush (or cotton swab for a vaginal smear) down the slide over the spatula sample.
	9. Spray or immerse sample in fixative immediately (95% alcohol can be used for bloody Pap smears).
	10. Allow slide to dry completely before transporting it to the laboratory or mailing.
	11. Take cultures for gonorrhea, chlamydia, or wet prep for vaginitis.
	12. Turn speculum to view vaginal tissue covered by speculum blades and then remove speculum.
	13. Perform bimanual and rectovaginal examination.

COLPOSCOPIC EXAMINATION

Colposcopy is a diagnostic technique used to evaluate the patient with an abnormal Pap smear. Specially trained physicians, nurse practitioners, nurse midwives, and physician assistants may perform colposcopy. A colposcope is used with binocular lenses that magnify the cervix 10 to 40 times. The purpose of the initial colposcopic examination is to rule out cancer; however, the final diagnosis rests on histology or biopsy of the cervix. (See colposcopic photos depicting CIN I, CIN II, and CIN III in Table 12–2.) It is helpful to give the patient ibuprofen (600 to 800 mg) 30 minutes before the procedure to help relieve pain related to cervical biopsies. Pancolposcopy is advised for the cervix, vagina, vulva, perineum, and perianal areas. Studies suggest that women with high-grade CIN/SIL of the cervix also are at risk for invasive carcinoma of the vagina, vulva, and anus, most likely because of contiguous spread of HPV.[18]

After the speculum is inserted, colposcopy of the cervix is done. Then, a solution of 3% to 6% acetic acid (vinegar) is applied, and colposcopy is repeated. Vinegar from the grocer's shelf (4% to 5% concentration) may be used. Caution should be used, however, because acetowhitening is not specific for HPV-related lesions or for vulvar intraepithelial neoplasia (VIN). Acetowhitened areas on the vulva may also indicate infection by *Candida* or herpes simplex, areas of coital trauma, or areas treated with caustic agents such as trichloroacetic acid or laser therapy.[19]

The procedure is as follows. Place 4×4-inch gauze sponges soaked with acetic acid on the vulvar and perianal skin. Tuck them around the speculum and leave them in place for 3 to 5 minutes. Evaluate the cervix first, then the vaginal fornices. Next inspect the vagina and turn the speculum so that the areas covered previously by the blades can be examined. Look for abnormalities such as acetowhitened epithelium and abnormal vascular patterns of punctation, mosaicism, or atypical vessels. Atypical vessels that look like spaghetti, hockey sticks, or corkscrews are the hallmarks of cancer. Standard protocol dictates that directed biopsies of the cervix and endocervical curettage be done on abnormal areas to assess the endocervical canal. An endocervical curettage is contraindicated, however, in the pregnant patient. Use benzocaine 20% spray or gel before taking biopsies of the cervix or vagina to control pain.

The colposcopist must also determine before biopsy whether the examination is satisfactory or unsatisfactory. If 360° of the squamocolumnar junction and the entire lesion can be seen, the colposcopy is deemed satisfactory. Different management regimens are used depending on whether the colposcopy is satisfactory or unsatisfactory. The entire medical history, physical examination, and colposcopic examination are then recorded on special forms and diagrams of the cervix, vulva, and vagina.

TREATMENT

After CIN has been diagnosed by cervical biopsy, management and treatment can begin (Table 12–4).[7, 20–23] Treatment should be individualized based on the patient's age, parity, previous treatment for CIN, desire for future fertility, current medical condition, and social condition; the location, severity, and extent of the cervical lesion; the results of Pap smears, cervical biopsies, and endocervical curettage; and the colposcopic impression. Patients with CIN I on cervical biopsy are often followed as most of these lesions will regress. Biopsy proven CIN II or III or CIS needs treatment. Triage protocols must be followed to

Text continued on page 198

Table 12–4. Treatment Methods for CIN of the Cervix*

TREATMENT	DEFINITION	HEALTH CARE PROVIDER	INDICATIONS	ADVANTAGES	DISADVANTAGES	RISKS	CURE RATE
Cryotherapy	Destruction of CIN by a cervical probe cooled with a refrigerant (e.g., nitrogen oxide): freeze (3 min), thaw (3 min), freeze (3 min)	Physician Midlevel provider°	All grades of CIN with adequate covering of lesion with the probe and good freeze May not be as effective for lesions extending into the endocervical canal more than 5–6 mm[23]	Office procedure Performed quickly Required skill level low Inexpensive Minimal pain Easy to teach and learn Used for many years[22]	No tissue specimen obtained SCJ recedes into the endocervical canal Slow to heal (3–4 wk) Heavy watery discharge for 2–3 wk Not suitable for large four-quadrant lesions or those extending into the vagina Not suitable for a cervix with irregular ectocervical contours[23]	Vasovagal response in some patients[23] Decreased amounts of cervical mucus in some patients[23] Cervical stenosis Infection Bleeding Recurrence of CIN	80%–90% in long-term follow-up[7]
Laser vaporization	Vaporization of CIN by directed beam of light from a carbon dioxide laser	Highly skilled physician required	CIN (usually high grade) VIN, VAIN, and PAIN	Office procedure Can be performed quickly Rapid healing (within 1 month) SCJ visible in most cases Less vaginal discharge than in cryotherapy Good for four-quadrant CIN with or without VAIN Not hampered by irregular contour of the cervix[22]	No tissue specimen obtained Difficult to teach and learn Required skill level high Equipment expensive Procedure expensive Provider needs high case load to maintain expertise Requires technical and safety training[22]	Bleeding Infection Cervical stenosis Cervical incompetence Recurrence of CIN	80%–90% in long-term follow-up[7]

Procedure	Description	Provider	Indications	Advantages		Complications	Success Rate
LEEP	Removal of CIN on the ectocervix only, with a wire loop (.8 mm standard depth) connected to electric current	Physician Midlevel provider proficient in colposcopy	CIN (usually high grade)	Can be done in office Tissue specimen obtained for pathologic confirmation Required skill level low Easy to teach and learn SCJ visible in most cases Rapid healing (within 1 mo) Can be used for large lesions on the cervix Minimal vaginal discharge[22]	Thermal artifact created on tissue specimen (artifact decreases as skill level increases[7])	Bleeding (incidence higher than in cryotherapy or laser vaporization) Infection Cervical stenosis Recurrence of CIN Cervical incompetence with repeat procedures	80%–95% in long-term follow-up studies[7]
LEEP cone	Removal of CIN on the ectocervix and removal of tissue from the endocervical canal (1.8–2.8 cm in depth) with wire loops connected to electric current	Physician Midlevel provider proficient in colposcopy	CIN See Table 12–5	Same as for LEEP	Same as for LEEP	Same as for LEEP	Varies depending on reason for therapy

Table continued on following page

Table 12-4. Treatment Methods for CIN of the Cervix* *Continued*

TREATMENT	DEFINITION	HEALTH CARE PROVIDER	INDICATIONS	ADVANTAGES	DISADVANTAGES	RISKS	CURE RATE
Laser cone	Removal of cervical tissue surrounding the endocervical canal using a beam of light from a carbon dioxide laser (1.8–2.8 cm in depth)	Highly skilled physician	CIN Treatment of choice if patient also has VAIN, VIN, or PAIN that requires treatment See Table 12–5	Tissue specimen obtained for pathologic confirmation Rapid healing (within 1 mo) SCJ visible in most cases Minimal vaginal discharge[22]	Thermal artifact created on tissue specimen, which makes it difficult for pathologist to read margins Although procedure can be done in an office, most are done in operating room under general anesthesia Difficult to teach and learn Required skill level higher than that for laser vaporization Requires good manual skills Provider needs high case load to maintain proficiency Requires technical and safety training	Bleeding Infection Cervical stenosis Cervical incompetence Recurrence of CIN	Varies depending on reason for therapy
Cold-knife cone (CKC)	A cone-shaped piece of tissue is removed from the cervix with a scalpel to evaluate the ectocervix and endocervical canal	Physician	See Table 12–5	Site of tissue removed can vary from patient to patient Specimen good for evaluating margins and making pathologic diagnosis	Expensive[22] High complication rates Requires good surgical skills Requires anesthesia Performed in operating room or outpatient surgery center[22]	Significant bleeding, immediate or delayed Cervical stenosis Cervical incompetence Infertility Infection Recurrence of CIN[7, 22]	Varies depending on reason for CKC

| Hysterectomy° | Removal of the uterus and, if indicated, the fallopian tubes and ovaries | Physician | Usually, other gynecologic conditions must exist (e.g., fibroids, prolapse, endometriosis, menorrhagia) CIN persists after ablative or excisional methods have failed Positive endocervical margins in a cone specimen Cervical stenosis and inability to adequately assess the endocervical canal post-treatment Significant cancer phobia[20] | Infection Bleeding Anesthetic complications Injury to the bowel, bladder, or ureter Thromboembolism Death[21] | Hysterectomy no guarantee that abnormal cells will not recur as VAIN |

°Not the primary method chosen for CIN.
Midlevel providers include nurse practitioners, nurse midwives, physician assistants, and clinical nurse specialists.
PAIN, perineal intraepithelial neoplasia.

Data from Lickrish GM: Cryotherapy for ectocervical neoplasia. In Wright VC, Lickrish GM, Shier EM (eds): Basic and Advanced Colposcopy; part II, 2nd ed. Houston, Biomedical Communications, 1995; Lickrish GM: Cryotherapy for cervical intraepithelial neoplasia. In Wright VC, Lickrish GM, Shier RM (eds): Basic and Advanced Colposcopy; part II, 2nd ed. Houston, Biomedical Communications, 1995; McDonald TW: Hysterectomy—indications, types, and alternatives. In Copeland LJ (ed): Textbook of Gynecology. Philadelphia, WB Saunders, 1993:779; Morris M, Tortolero-Luna G, Malpeca A, et al: Cervical intraepithelial neoplasia and cervical cancer. Obstet Gynecol Clin North Am 1996;23:347; and Wright TC, Richart RM, Ferenczy A: Electrosurgery for HPV-related Diseases of the Lower Genital Tract. New York, Arthur Vision, 1992.

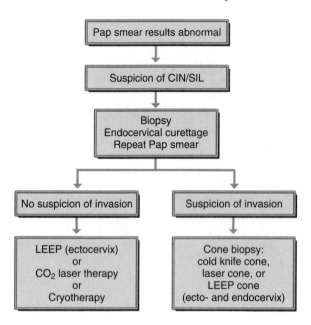

Figure 12–2. Treatment strategy for cervical intraepithelial neoplasia (CIN). SIL, squamous intraepithelial lesion; LEEP, loop electrosurgical excision procedure. (From Morris M, Tortolero-Luna G, Malpica A, et al: Cervical intraepithelial neoplasia and cervical cancer. Obstet Gynecol Clin North Am 1996;23:347–410).

reduce the chance of missing an invasive cancer. A management algorithm developed by Morris and colleagues[7] is described in Figure 12–2. Table 12–5 outlines criteria that must be fulfilled before lesions are treated with cryotherapy, laser therapy, or LEEP.[7, 23, 24] Table 12–6 gives the indications for a cervical conization.[7, 24] Not included here but under study are new treatments that use chemopreventive agents such as retinoids.[7]

MANAGEMENT OF ABNORMAL CYTOLOGY

REACTIVE OR REPARATIVE CHANGES

Cells showing reactive or reparative changes are not normal, but neither are they preinvasive. They may be seen in response to inflammation, cervical trauma, or pregnancy. No further workup is needed.

Table 12–5. Criteria for Cryosurgery, Laser Vaporization, and Loop Electrosurgical Excision Procedure of Cervical Intraepithelial Neoplasia

No evidence of invasive cancer on the Pap smear, colposcopy, or cervical biopsies
Satisfactory colposcopy (squamocolumnar junction seen 360° and entire lesion is seen)
Results of endocervical curettage normal
No discrepancy between Pap smear and biopsy; for example, Pap smear is HGSIL and cervical biopsy is LGSIL
Patient is compliant with follow-up
No evidence of adenocarcinoma in situ or adenocarcinoma
Patient not pregnant

Data from Cook E, Mitchell MF: Treatment of cervical intraepithelial neoplasia. Clinical Consultations in Obstetrics and Gynecology 1994;6(1):37; Lickrish GM: Cryotherapy for ectocervical neoplasia. In Wright VC, Lickrish GM, Shier EM (eds): Basic and Advanced Colposcopy, part II, 2nd ed. Houston, Biomedical Communications, 1995; and Morris M, Tortolero-Luna G, Malpeca A, et al: Cervical intraepithelial neoplasia and cervical cancer. Obstet Gynecol Clin North Am 1996;23:347.

Table 12–6. Indications for Cervical Cone Biopsy

Evidence of microinvasion, or invasion on Pap smear, cervical biopsy, or colposcopy.
Endocervical curettage positive for SIL/CIN.
Colposcopic examination unsatisfactory (squamocolumnar junction not seen 360° or entire lesion cannot be seen)
Patient is noncompliant
Discrepancy between Pap smear and biopsies
Adenocarcinoma in situ or adenocarcinoma of the cervix noted on cervical biopsies

Data from Cook E, Mitchell MF: Treatment of cervical intraepithelial neoplasia. Clinical Consultations in Obstetrics and Gynecology 1994;6:37; and Morris M, Tortolero-Luna G, Malpeca A, et al: Cervical intraepithelial neoplasia and cervical cancer. Obstet Gynecol Clin North Am 1996;23:347.

INFECTION

Vaginitis is common in many women. Pap smears in such cases may show (1) coccobacilli, indicating bacterial vaginosis; (2) *Candida albicans*; (3) *Trichomonas vaginalis*; (4) herpes simplex; (5) *Chlamydia trachomatis*; or (6) an obscuring inflammation. However, such findings do not necessarily signify infection.

To rule out infection, the following procedure is used. Correlate clinical signs and symptoms with the findings on the Pap smear, and, if indicated, have the patient return to the clinic for appropriate cultures and/or wet preps with potassium hydroxide and saline to reach a definitive diagnosis. Treat the patient with medication if needed, and have the patient return in 3 to 4 months for a follow-up Pap smear. Without a specific diagnosis, treatment with various antibiotic creams is not indicated.[6] If the Pap smear is normal, advise the patient to return for annual screening. If no infection is diagnosed by the tests described previously and if the repeat Pap smears continue to show signs of inflammation, refer the patient for colposcopy.[25] Underlying invasive cancer of the cervix with necrosis and inflammation can cause this type of smear.

SQUAMOUS CELL ABNORMALITIES

Low-Grade Squamous Intraepithelial Lesions

The inclusion of infection in the category of low-grade SIL and the overreading of low-grade SIL has led to a tremendous increase in the number of women with abnormal Pap smears. Treatment and follow-up of these patients is controversial, and management varies. The Interim Guidelines developed by the NCI specify two management options.[6] The first is to repeat Pap smears every 4 to 6 months for 2 years. The rationale behind this approach is that about 60% of cases diagnosed by cytology represent a process that will spontaneously revert to normal without therapy.[26] This is an appropriate option if the patient is not considered to be at high risk and will comply with follow-up. After three consecutive negative, satisfactory smears have been obtained during follow-up, the patient can return to annual screening. If any follow-up Pap smear is positive or abnormal, the patient should be referred for colposcopy, endocervical curettage, and directed biopsy. Patients must be carefully selected for this option and must be reliable. The second option is to refer the patient after one low-grade SIL-positive Pap smear for colposcopy and directed biopsy. The rationale for this decision rests on the high error rate of the Pap smear and the finding that about 15% of these lesions can progress to high-grade SIL.[26]

High-Grade Squamous Intraepithelial Lesions

The approach to a patient with high-grade SIL is straightforward. Such lesions are serious and require referral for colposcopy and directed biopsies. Though CIS often is thought to be an invasive disease because its name contains the word "carcinoma," it is in fact a preinvasive condition.

Atypical Squamous Cells of Undetermined Significance

ASCUS are cells that are more abnormal than cells seen in reactive or inflammatory lesions but they do not fulfill the criteria for low-grade SIL or high-grade SIL. In the TBS terminology, ASCUS must have abnormal nuclear characteristics without changes of koilocytotic stypic.[27] Such lesions must not correspond to the terms "atypia," "inflammatory atypia," or class II used in the now obsolete Papanicolaou classification.[28] Because there are no established cytologic criteria for the diagnosis of ASCUS, there has been a substantial increase in the number of Pap smears read as abnormal and labeled ASCUS.[28] ASCUS smears convey a 10% to 40% risk of underlying CIN, but most women with this cytology are normal.[28]

The clinical management of patients with ASCUS has been controversial; however, guidelines for clinicians have recently been published by the American Society of Colposcopy and Cervical Pathology (ASCCP) and the NCI.[6, 28] See Figures 12–3 and 12–4 for management algorithms, based on these guidelines, for patients with an abnormal Pap smear.[6, 28] The NCI is currently undertaking a multicenter, prospective clinical trial to evaluate different management strategies for ASCUS and low-grade SIL. The data gathered should help guide clinical management.

A diagnosis of ASCUS in a postmenopausal woman is different from that in a woman of reproductive age. In postmenopausal women, atrophic cells look like parabasal cells with a high nuclear-to-cytoplasmic ratio and may suggest SIL.[6] If the ASCUS smear is associated with severe inflammation, check for vaginitis and treat if indicated. In any woman considered to be at high risk for an STD, a screening culture for gonorrhea and chlamydia is recommended. Treat with vaginal estrogen cream before repeat cytology and colposcopy as long as no other signs and symptoms suggestive of cancer are present.[27] Make sure to assess the patient for contraindications for estrogen. The estrogen vaginal cream reverses the cell changes caused by atrophy.[27] Women taking oral estrogen replacement therapy may have vaginal atrophy and may benefit from topical therapy also. One recommended regimen is to put one-quarter to one-half applicator of estrogen vaginal cream in the vagina each night at bedtime for 2 weeks, followed by the same amount three times weekly for 2 to 3 months. If the repeat Pap smear remains abnormal after estrogen therapy, colposcopy should be considered.[6]

GLANDULAR CELL ABNORMALITIES

Endometrial Cells

The presence of endometrial cells or atypical endometrial cells on a Pap smear should alert the clinician to a possible problem. It is unclear what workup,

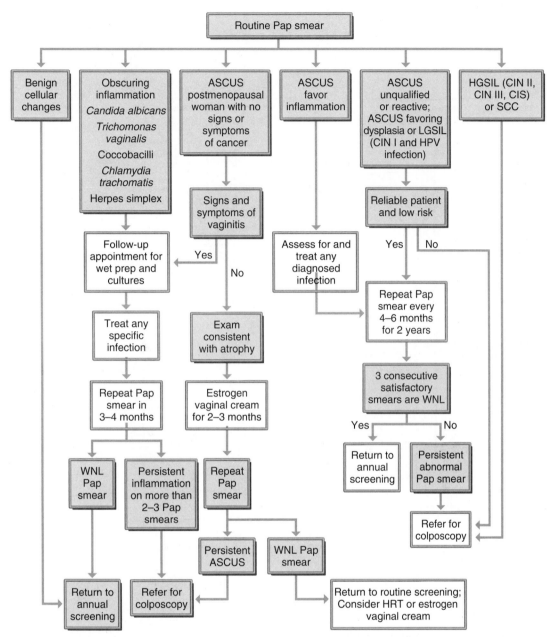

Figure 12–3. Management of squamous cell abnormalities on Pap smear. WNL, within normal limits; ASCUS, atypical squamous cells of undetermined significance; HRT, hormone replacement therapy; SIL, squamous intraepithelial lesion; LGSIL, low-grade squamous intraepithelial lesion; HGSIL, high-grade squamous intraepithelial lesion; HPV, human papilloma virus; SCC, squamous cell carcinoma; CIN, cervical intraepithelial neoplasia; CIS, carcinoma in situ. (Adapted from American Society for Colposcopy and Cervical Pathology Practice Committee: Management guidelines for follow-up of atypical squamous cells of undetermined significance (ASCUS). The Colposcopist 1996;27:1–15; and Kurman RJ, Henson DE, Herbst AL, et al: Interim guidelines for management of abnormal cervical cytology. JAMA 1994;271:1866–1869.)

if any, is needed. Burke and associates[29] recommend an endometrial biopsy and endocervical curettage when endometrial cells are seen in the Pap smear of a postmenopausal patient. The presence of endometrial cells or histiocytes is normal, however, if a Pap smear is taken on days 10 to 12 of the menstrual cycle.[30] These cells, called endometrial exodus cells, are necrotic cells sloughed from the menstrual endometrium. However, if such cells are seen on cytology

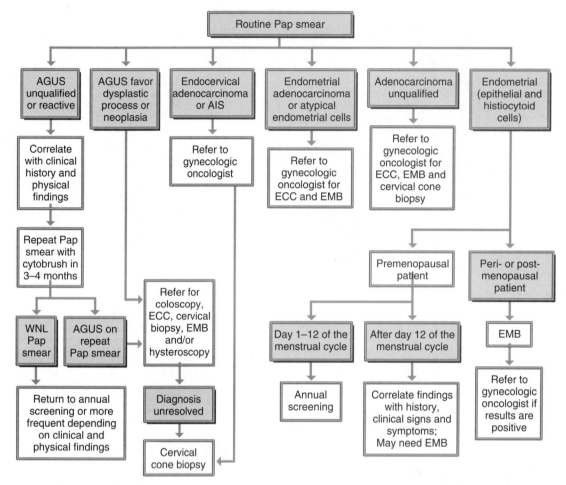

Figure 12–4. Management of glandular cell abnormalities on Pap smear. AGUS, Atypical glandular cells of undetermined significance; AIS, adenocarcinoma in situ; ECC, endocervical curettage; EMB, endometrial biopsy; other abbreviations as in Figure 12–3. (Adapted from American Society for Colposcopy and Cervical Pathology Practice Committee: Management guidelines for follow-up of atypical squamous cells of undetermined significance (ASCUS). The Colposcopist 1996;27:1–15; and Kurman RJ, Henson DE, Herbst AL, et al: Interim guidelines for management of abnormal cervical cytology. JAMA 1994;271:1866–1869.)

after days 10 to 12 of the menstrual cycle or on the Pap smear of a postmenopausal woman, further evaluation is warranted.[30] These cells may be indicative of endometrial polyps, endometrial hyperplasia, or adenocarcinoma.[31]

Atypical Glandular Cells of Undetermined Significance

Atypical glandular cells of undetermined significance (AGUS) may indicate a preinvasive or invasive condition in the endocervix, in the endometrium, or, rarely, in the fallopian tube or ovarian glandular tissue. Studies show that adenocarcinoma in situ and invasive adenocarcinoma of the cervix are being detected more frequently, especially in women younger than age 35.[6] AGUS identified on a Pap smear should be further qualified, if possible, as favoring a reactive, premalignant, or malignant condition.[6]

In primary care, a patient with an AGUS-positive Pap smear favoring a premalignant or malignant process should be referred to a trained colposcopist for a repeat smear, colposcopy, endocervical curettage (if not pregnant), cervical biopsies if a lesion is seen, endometrial biopsy, and possibly a hysteroscopy.[6] A persistent finding of AGUS that is not reconciled by these procedures usually requires a cone biopsy or dilatation and curettage of the uterus.[6] There is no consensus on when cytology reveals unqualified or reactive AGUS. One option is to repeat the Pap smear with a cytobrush in 2 to 3 months and, if AGUS persists, to refer the patient for colposcopy.[6]

FOLLOW-UP

One month after cryotherapy, laser therapy, LEEP, or cervical conization, the patient should return for a follow-up examination to check for healing of the cervix, to rule out cervical stenosis, and to check on the regularity of the menstrual cycle. Because 85% of CIN recurrences appear within 2 years of treatment, follow-up examinations are recommended every 4 to 6 months during this time.[24] To prevent errors in reading of the Pap smear, the first repeat Pap smear should not be done until 3 to 4 months after treatment because of reparative changes occurring in the cervix. A Pap smear and colposcopy are done at each visit, with repeat biopsy if indicated. If at the end of 2 years there has been no recurrence of the lesion, the patient can return to annual Pap smear screening. Because CIN or invasive disease of the vagina can occur in 1% to 3% of women treated by hysterectomy for high-grade CIN, all women treated in this fashion require lifetime follow-up with screening Pap smears.[20]

SCREENING AND EARLY DETECTION

The Pap smear is an excellent screening test. However, some populations are not being reached. Half of the women in this country who are diagnosed with cervical cancer have never had a Pap smear, and another 10% have not had one in the last 5 years, according to the National Institutes of Health (NIH) Consensus Development Conference on Cervical Cancer held in April 1996.[32] The NIH report also said that cervical cancer could be eradicated with universal screening programs but that for now it is a disease of the poor. Underscreened populations include the elderly, members of ethnic minority groups (especially Hispanics, African Americans, Native Americans, and American Eskimos), uninsured persons, and rural dwellers.[33] Mortality rates for blacks are twice those for whites. These populations can be reached by the development of culturally sensitive programs.

Early detection of CIN by the Pap smear and additional interventions such as colposcopy with directed biopsy and treatment can help prevent or delay progression to invasion. Cure rates of CIN reach 80% to 95% with one treatment and higher with a second treatment. On the other hand, treatment of cervical cancer is more costly, morbidity is high, and patients can eventually die of the cancer.

SCREENING GUIDELINES

A consensus recommendation has been adopted by the American Cancer Society, NCI, American College of Obstetricians and Gynecologists (ACOG),

American Medical Association, American Academy of Family Physicians, American Nurses Association, and American Medical Women's Association on advised intervals for Pap smear screening.[33] It is recommended that all women who are or have been sexually active, or who have reached the age of 18 years, should have an annual Pap smear. Pap smears may be performed less frequently at the discretion of the physician after three or more annual smears have been normal. However, the clinician should base the Pap test interval on the patient's risk factors for CIN and cervical cancer.[33] Guidelines based on risk factors have been published by ACOG.[34] ACOG suggests that when one or more of the following risk factors are present, more frequent smears should be done: (1) multiple sexual partners or a male partner who has had multiple partners; (2) initiation of intercourse at an early age; (3) a male sexual partner who has had other sexual partners with cervical cancer; (4) current or prior HPV infection; (5) current or prior herpes infection; (6) HIV positivity; (7) a history of other STDs; (8) immunosuppression; (9) tobacco and alcohol abuse; (10) a history of preinvasive or invasive cancer of the female genital tract; and (11) low socioeconomic status.

The consensus panel did not state at what age Pap smear screening should be discontinued. Recommendations vary by professional organization. Clinicians at the M.D. Anderson Cancer Center believe that screening with the Pap test should be continued for a lifetime. Women should continue having Pap smears even if they are no longer sexually active or have had a hysterectomy for a benign process. Having a Pap smear also allows the clinician to assess the patient for other disease processes such as cancers of the breast, lung, skin, colon, vagina, ovaries, uterus, and vulva; cardiovascular disease; and diabetes.

PREVENTION AND PATIENT COUNSELING

Table 12–7 outlines information to convey to patients for the prevention of CIN.

VULVAR INTRAEPITHELIAL NEOPLASIA

EPIDEMIOLOGY

Vulvar intraepithelial neoplasia (VIN) is not as common as CIN, though its incidence has risen from 1.2 to 2.1 cases per 100,000 women in the last 20

Table 12–7. Prevention and Patient Counseling for Cervical Intraepithelial Neoplasia/Squamous Intraepithelial Lesions

If appropriate, suggest that patient delay first sexual intercourse until age 20 years. Encourage monogamy.
Encourage use of barrier contraceptives to protect cervix (e.g., condoms, spermicides, female condom, or diaphragm).
Discourage smoking or, if patient smokes, encourage patient to stop.
Encourage regular Pap smears and pelvic examination beginning at age 18 years or after first sexual intercourse.
Inform patient of the risk factors for CIN/SIL.
Discuss the high-risk male who has had multiple partners or intercourse with prostitutes.
Encourage a healthy lifestyle of enough sleep, exercise, and nutritional food to keep the immune system functioning well.

Table 12–8. Risk Factors for Vulvar Intraepithelial Neoplasia

CATEGORY	RISK FACTOR
Sexual factors	Human papilloma virus infection
Reproductive and/or contraceptive factors	Oral contraceptive use
Lifestyle factors	Cigarette smoking
Medical history	History of or concurrent preinvasive or invasive disease of the cervix, vagina, or vulva
Socioeconomic/ethnic factors	Low educational level

Adapted from Edwards C, Tortolero-Luna G, Linares A: Vulvar intraepithelial neoplasia. Obstet Gynecol Clin North Am 1996;23:295.

years.[35] The increase has been largest in white women younger than 35 years of age.[35] Experts have theorized that the increase in VIN is probably linked to sexual factors such as HPV,[36] but there is no known cause.[37] There have been few studies on the natural history of VIN. However, in one study of 5 women who were observed for 2 to 8 years, all had disease that progressed to invasive carcinoma.[37] Table 12–8 describes risk factors for VIN.[38]

CLASSIFICATION SYSTEM

The CIN classification system has been adapted for preinvasive vulvar lesions, with cells characterized by "disordered maturation and nuclear abnormalities" classified as VIN.[39] Table 12–9 describes the VIN classification system.[40]

CLINICAL EVALUATION

PRESENTING HISTORY

Patients who are diagnosed with VIN may very well be asymptomatic. They also often complain of vulvar irritation and pruritus lasting for 6 months or longer. Vulvar lesions can be erythematous, ulcerative, or leukoplakic; they generally occur on the labia minora and are multifocal.[41] Preinvasive lesions are more likely to have one focus in older women. Pigmented lesions usually are

Table 12–9. Classification System for Vulvar Intraepithelial Neoplasia

CLASSIFICATION	DYSPLASIA	INVOLVEMENT
Preinvasive squamous lesions of the vulva		
VIN I	Mild	≤⅓ thickness
VIN II	Moderate	⅓ to ⅔ thickness
VIN III	Severe	>⅔ thickness
Carcinoma in situ		Full thickness involvement from the basement membrane to the surface of the squamous epithelium.

Adapted from Kaufman RH: Intraepithelial Neoplasia of the Vulva (Distinguished Professor Series). Gynecol Oncol 1995;56:8.

gray or brown with sharp borders.[38] See Figures 12–5 and 12–6 for examples of such lesions.

PHYSICAL EXAMINATION

As with CIN of the cervix, a complete medical history and physical examination should be done for the patient presenting with a vulvar lesion or vulvar itching. A comprehensive gynecologic examination also is necessary, including inspection of the vulva, a Pap smear, and bimanual and rectovaginal examination (as described previously). Inspection of the vulva is the most important technique for detecting abnormalities and should be done as follows. With the use of a good white light, start at one point and work through all the structures of the mons pubis, clitoral hood, clitoris, labia majora, labia minora, vestibule, introitus, perineum, and perianal and gluteal folds of the buttocks. Be sure to check hairy areas by separating pubic hairs to see the skin surface. Pay particular attention to areas where the patient has noted itching or irritation. Note any nevi or suspicious lesions.

COLPOSCOPIC EXAMINATION

If a suspicious lesion of the vulva is identified, colposcopy of the vulva, vagina, cervix, perineum, and perianal area is required, because intraepithelial disease

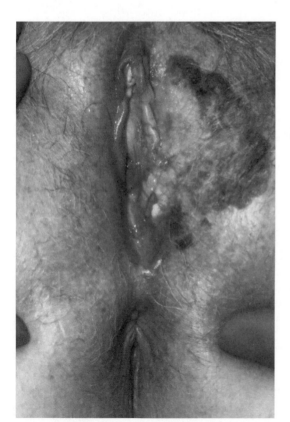

Figure 12–5. Carcinoma in situ in a 66-year-old woman. Irregular brown and black pigmentation, erythema, and acetowhite areas. (© The University of Texas M.D. Anderson Cancer Center.)

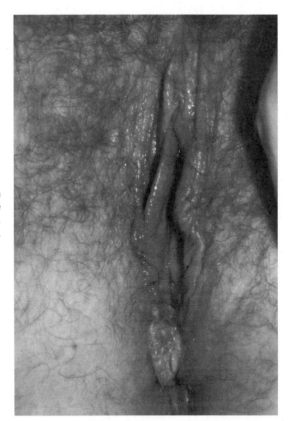

Figure 12–6. Carcinoma in situ in a 42-year-old woman: acetowhite thick area on posterior fourchette. (© The University of Texas M.D. Anderson Cancer Center.)

can be multicentric. Twenty-five percent to 50% of VIN lesions are associated with condyloma acuminatum, and 30% of patients with VIN have CIN of the cervix or vaginal intraepithelial neoplasia (VAIN).[42] Anoscopy may be done to rule out disease in the anal canal.[43]

In brief, colposcopy is done as follows: 4 × 4-inch gauze squares soaked in 3% to 6% acetic acid are placed on the vulva, perineum, and perianal areas for 3 to 5 minutes to outline and bring forth any subclinical lesions that are not grossly evident. Clinicians not trained in colposcopy may use a handheld lens (magnification, 200% to 300%) to assess lesions. During colposcopy, look for and assess hyperpigmented areas, abnormal-appearing nevi, acetowhitened epithelium, and any abnormal vascular patterns such as punctation, mosaicism, and atypical vessels. Because abnormal vascular patterns are not often seen on the vulva, a high-grade lesion is suspected when they are seen.

The most abnormal-appearing areas should be liberally biopsied to rule out invasive disease (see Table 12–10 for a recommended procedure).[44] Suspicious (white, red, or pigmented) lesions require biopsy.[40] When in doubt, biopsy. Condylomas should be biopsied before treatment if irregular pigmentation is present or if a lesion does not resolve with topical treatment, to rule out VIN or an invasive process. Patients with vulvar nevi that are asymmetric, have irregular borders, are more than one color, are larger than 6 mm, or are growing or changing in any way should be referred to a dermatologist for biopsy to rule out dysplastic changes or melanoma of the vulva. Document on the diagram of the vulva any lesions identified and where biopsies were taken. Once VIN is diagnosed by biopsy, the patient should be referred to a gynecologic oncologist or an obstetrician/gynecologist trained in colposcopy for treatment and follow-up.

Table 12–10. Procedure for Punch Biopsy of the Vulva

Patient preparation	Explain the procedure to the patient and answer any questions
	Ask about allergies to any medications or Betadine
	Have the patient sign the informed consent document
Indication	Suspicious lesion seen by gross inspection or colposcopy of the vulva
Supplies needed	Betadine solution swabs
	2×2-inch or 4×4-inch gauze squares
	Dental syringe holder (metal syringe holder)
	21-gauge needle
	Disposable cartridge of 2% lidocaine hydrochloride with epinephrine (1:50,000)
	Disposable Keye skin biopsy punch (3, 4, and 5 mm) (a Mini Townsend Tischler [cervical biopsy forceps] may be used for papular lesions)
	Small forceps and scissors
	Silver nitrate sticks or Monsel paste
	Specimen container with appropriate label
Technique	Clean the biopsy site with Betadine
	Dry the area with a gauze square if indicated
	Inject the 2% lidocaine hydrochloride with epinephrine, using the metal syringe holder
	Insert needle just below the epidermis and raise a wheal with the local anesthetic; use 1–2 mL of anesthetic since it will quickly dissipate because of the rich vascular and lymphatic supply to the vulva
	Local swelling caused by the anesthetic actually facilitates the biopsy
	Allow 60 seconds after the injection for anesthesia to take effect before performing biopsy
	Use disposable Keye punch (usually 3–4 mm) to biopsy a small circular plug of tissue
	Use only light pressure and a simple twisting motion
	Lay aside the instrument
	Lift the plug of tissue with a pickup forceps
	Cut the specimen at the base with scissors
	Place the plug in the specimen container with fixative
	Blot the biopsy site with a dry gauze sponge
	Stop bleeding by applying silver nitrate sticks or Monsel paste
Discharge instructions to patient	Advise patient to keep biopsy site clean and dry; no bandage is needed, and the patient can clean the area during the usual daily bath or shower
	Advise patient to check the wound daily; if it becomes red, swollen, or painful, call or return to the clinic
	Give patient written discharge instructions.
Documentation	Draw and label lesion on a vulvar diagram or on the progress note
	Describe the lesion, including size and color, on the progress note

Adapted from The University of Texas M.D. Anderson Cancer Center Colposcopy Clinic Protocol: Houston, © The University of Texas M.D. Anderson Cancer Center, 1994.

TREATMENT

Figure 12–7 illustrates a management pathway for VIN as described by Edwards and colleagues.[38] VIN I is histologically difficult to distinguish from HPV infection of the vulva.[19] If the patient with VIN I is reliable, she may be monitored carefully with Pap smears and colposcopic examinations of the vulva, cervix, and vagina every 6 months and rebiopsy if needed. VIN II, III, and CIS of the vulva should be treated.

New alternative therapies with chemopreventive agents such as retinyl acetate gel are under study. This type of agent has been used on other sites, including the cervix, to revert precancerous changes to normal.[45]

FOLLOW-UP

The schedule of follow-up appointments to check healing after surgery varies among health care providers. If possible, the patient should undergo a repeat

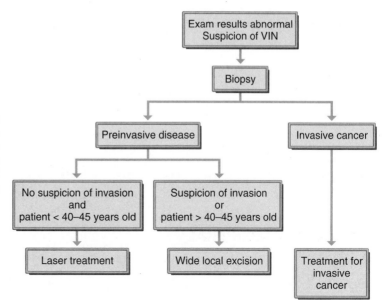

Figure 12–7. Treatment schema for vulvar intraepithelial neoplasia (VIN). (From Edwards C, Tortolero-Luna G, Linares A: Vulvar intraepithelial neoplasia. Obstet Gynecol Clin North Am 1996; 23:295–324.)

Pap smear and colposcopic examination of the vulva, vagina, and cervix every 6 months for 2 years. If examinations are negative after 2 years, annual screening may be resumed. However, because recurrence is common with VIN, patients require lifetime follow-up.

SCREENING AND EARLY DETECTION

All primary care practitioners are encouraged to thoroughly inspect the vulva and adjacent areas in all women when pelvic examinations are done. This is simply done, takes little time, and incurs no additional cost. Any suspicious areas should be biopsied. Because VIN and vulvar cancer are associated with significant morbidity, detecting lesions in their early stages is most important.

Table 12–11 outlines advice to give patients concerning early detection and patient counseling on VIN.[46]

Table 12–11. Prevention and Patient Counseling for Vulvar Intraepithelial Neoplasia

Discourage smoking or if the patient smokes encourage the patient to quit.
If appropriate suggest that patient delay first intercourse until age 20 years. Encourage monogamy.
Encourage use of barrier contraceptives to prevent sexually transmitted diseases (e.g., use condoms, diaphragms, or the female condom).
Stress the need for routine Pap smears and pelvic examinations.
Inform the patient of the risk factors for VIN.
Teach vulvar self-examination using inspection and palpation monthly.[46]
Teach signs and symptoms to look for (i.e., itching, irritation, burning, sore, lump, or new pigmentation).
Encourage seeing a health care provider early if signs and symptoms develop.
Teach good vulvar hygiene (i.e., wiping front to back, wearing cotton underwear, avoiding perfumes and deodorant products, no douching, avoiding tight clothing, using nonirritating soaps and washing powders to clean underclothes).

Adapted from Sandella J: Vulvar self exam (VSE). Oncology Nursing Forum 1987;14:71.

Table 12–12. Classification System for Vaginal Intraepithelial Neoplasia

CLASSIFICATION	DYSPLASIA	INVOLVEMENT
Preinvasive squamous lesions of the vagina		
VAIN I	Mild	≤⅓ thickness
VAIN II	Moderate	⅓ to ⅔ thickness
VAIN III	Severe	>⅔ thickness
Carcinoma in situ		Full-thickness involvement from the basement membrane to the surface of the squamous epithelium

Adapted from Wharton JT, Tortolero-Luna G, Linares A: Vaginal intraepithelial neoplasia and vaginal cancer. Obstet Gynecol Clin North Am 1996;23:325.

VAGINAL INTRAEPITHELIAL NEOPLASIA

EPIDEMIOLOGY

VAIN is uncommon both in the United States and worldwide. In the United States the incidence is estimated to be only about .2 to .3 cases per 100,000 women.[47] The cause of VAIN is unknown. Moreover, it is not possible to make generalizations on the natural history of VAIN because of the small number of cases and studies. However, in a study of 12 patients by Petrilli and coworkers,[48] disease was persistent in half of cases and repressed in the other half. Vaginal intraepithelial changes are graded by histology, using the VAIN classification system described in Table 12–12.[47] Risk factors for VAIN are listed in Table 12–13.[47]

CLINICAL EVALUATION

PRESENTING HISTORY

Patients with VAIN are almost always asymptomatic at presentation. Occasionally, postcoital bleeding and/or abnormal vaginal discharge may be noted.[47] VAIN is usually detected by an abnormal Pap smear. VAIN lesions are often multifocal erythematous or ulcerative lesions or leukoplakias that occur in the distal third of the vagina.[47] Patients with VAIN detected on a Pap smear should be referred

Table 12–13. Risk Factors for Vaginal Intraepithelial Neoplasia

CATEGORY	RISK FACTOR
Sexual factors	Human papillomavirus infection
Lifestyle factors	Cigarette smoking
Medical history	Hysterectomy at young age
	History of or concurrent preinvasive or invasive disease of the cervix, vagina, or vulva
	Previous abnormal Pap smear
Socioeconomic factors	Low educational level
	Low socioeconomic level

Adapted from Wharton JT, Tortolero-Luna G, Linares A: Vaginal intraepithelial neoplasia and vaginal cancer. Obstet Gynecol Clin North Am 1996;23:325.

to a gynecologic oncologist or obstetrician/gynecologist skilled in assessing and treating such patients to prevent unneeded surgery and loss of sexual function.

MEDICAL HISTORY AND PHYSICAL EXAMINATION

A complete medical history and physical examination are required when VAIN is found on a Pap smear. As with CIN and VIN, a thorough gynecologic examination should be done, including inspection of the vulva, vagina, and cervix; a Pap smear; a bimanual and rectovaginal examination; and palpation of the vagina. For details, refer to the clinical examinations described previously for CIN and VIN. A word of caution: most clinicians do not thoroughly *inspect* the vagina. (An example of a grossly visible vaginal lesion is shown in Fig. 12–8.)[49] Therefore, once the vaginal speculum is in place to take a Pap smear, look at the vaginal walls grossly under a good white light. The Pap smear should be taken from the cervix, if present, with a cytobrush and spatula. A vaginal smear should be done if the cervix has been surgically removed. Use a moistened cotton swab (if the vagina is dry) or the rounded end of the spatula to sample the cuff area and all four walls. Palpate the vaginal cuff along with the anterior, posterior, and lateral walls. Lesions not grossly visible may be identified as indurations or masses.

COLPOSCOPIC EXAMINATION

Colposcopy of the vulva, vagina, and cervix should be done when a patient presents with VAIN to rule out invasive cancer. First, colposcopically examine the cervix and then the vagina after liberal swabbing with 3% to 6% acetic acid. Vaginal lesions may appear as ulcerations or acetowhitened areas with or without vascular abnormalities such as punctation, mosaicism, and atypical vessels. Invasive cancer should be suspected when atypical vessels are seen. Because it is difficult to evaluate the vagina with its many folds, Lugol solution, which contains

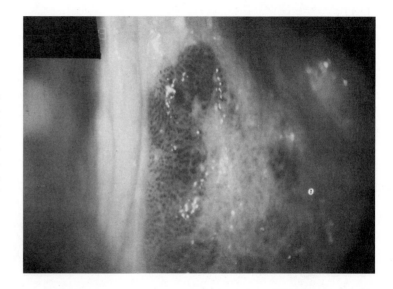

Figure 12–8. Anterior fornix of the vagina in a 38-year-old woman before the application of vinegar. A red, raised lesion is noted with punctation and atypical vessels. Superficial invasion was found on vaginal biopsy. (From Burke L, Abu-Jawdih GM: Home Study Course. The Colposcopist 1994;26:6–7.)

iodine, is often used to delineate lesions. Normal glycogenated tissue stains mahogany brown, whereas VAIN stains yellow. VAIN occurs most often on the anterior and posterior vaginal walls, which may be covered by the blades of the vaginal speculum; therefore, rotate the blades so as to visualize these areas after application of acetic acid and Lugol solution. Then, take colposcopically directed biopsies of the cervix and vagina. Because VAIN is often multifocal, take biopsies from several places to rule out invasion. As the speculum is removed, look at the vagina as it folds on itself. Finally, examine the vulva grossly and with the colposcope.

TREATMENT

Figure 12–9 provides a management algorithm for VAIN suggested by Wharton and associates.[47] VAIN I is often followed conservatively with estrogen vaginal cream if indicated. VAIN II and VAIN III require treatment.

FOLLOW-UP

Recurrences of VAIN are common. One recommendation for follow-up is to perform Pap smears and colposcopy every 4 to 6 months for 2 years, followed by annual screening if the results are normal. The patient should be counseled about the need for lifetime yearly Pap smears and pelvic examinations.

SCREENING AND EARLY DETECTION

VAIN is associated with high morbidity and alterations in sexual functioning. Early detection of VAIN with adequate treatment can help prevent cancer of

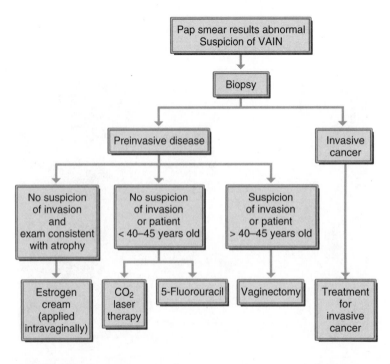

Figure 12–9. Treatment strategy for vaginal intraepithelial neoplasia (VAIN). (From Wharton JT, Torto-lero-Luna G, Linares A: Vaginal intraepithelial neoplasia and vaginal cancer. Obstet Gynecol Clin North Am 1996;23:325–345.)

Table 12–14. Prevention and Patient Counseling for Vaginal Intraepithelial Neoplasia

Discourage smoking; or if the patient smokes encourage patient to stop.
If appropriate, suggest that the patient delay first sexual intercourse until age 20. Encourage monogamy.
Encourage use of barrier contraceptives to protect the vagina and cervix (e.g., use condoms, diaphragms, the female condom, and spermicides).
Stress need for routine Pap smears and pelvic examinations beginning at age 18 years or after first sexual intercourse.
Inform patient of the risk factors for VAIN.
Teach signs and symptoms to look for (i.e., abnormal vaginal discharge, postcoital bleeding).
Encourage seeing health care provider early if signs and symptoms develop.

this site. Therefore, all primary care practitioners are encouraged to perform routine Pap smears and to inspect and palpate the vagina when pelvic examinations are done. Pap smear screening guidelines are given in the section on CIN.

See Table 12–14 for advice to give patients about prevention and care of VAIN.

REFERENCES

1. Ferenczy A: Cervical intraepithelial neoplasia. In Blaustein A (ed): Pathology of the Female Genital Tract, 2nd ed. New York, Springer-Verlag, 1982:158.
2. Ferenczy A, Wright TC: Anatomy and histology of the cervix. In Kurman RJ (ed): Blaustein's Pathology of the Female Genital Tract, 4th ed. New York, Springer-Verlag, 1994:185.
3. Rubin SC, Hoskin WJ: Cervical and preinvasive neoplasia. Philadelphia, Lippincott-Raven, 1996:10.
4. Mitchell MF, Hittelman WN, Hong WK, et al: The natural history of cervical intraepithelial neoplasia: Argument for intermediate end-point biomarkers. Cancer Epidemiol Biomarkers Prev 1994;3:619.
5. Wingo PA, Tong T, Bolden S, et al: Cancer Statistics 1995. CA Cancer J Clin 1995;45:12.
6. Kurman RJ, Henson DE, Herbst AL, et al: Interim guidelines for management of abnormal cervical cytology. JAMA 1994;271:1866–1860.
7. Morris M, Tortolero-Luna G, Malpica A, et al: Cervical intraepithelial neoplasia and cervical cancer. Obstet Gynecol Clin North Am 1996;23:347–410.
8. U.S. Department of Health and Human Services: Improving the Quality of Clinician Pap Smear Technique and Management, Client Pap Smear Education, and the Evaluation of Pap Smear Laboratory Testing: A Resource Guide for Title X Family Planning Projects. Washington, DC, U.S. Department of Health and Human Services, 1989.
9. Richart RM: Natural history of cervical intraepithelial neoplasia. Clin Obstet Gynecol 1968;10:748.
10. National Cancer Institute Workshop: The 1988 Bethesda System for reporting cervical/vaginal cytologic diagnoses. JAMA 1989;262:931.
11. National Cancer Institute Workshop: The Bethesda System for reporting cervical/vaginal cytologic diagnoses: Report of the 1991 Bethesda Workshop. JAMA 1992;267:1892.
12. Tedeschi C, Spitzer M: Home Study Course. The Colposcopist 1993;25:10–13.
13. Gunderson J, Noller LK: Home Study Course. The Colposcopist 1993;25:6–9.
14. Spitzer M: Home Study Course. The Colposcopist 1995;27:6–8.
15. Koss L: Cervical Pap smear. Cancer Supplement 1992;1:1406–1412.
16. American College of Obstetricians and Gynecologists. Cervical Cytology: Evaluation and Management of Abnormalities. Technical Bulletin No. 183. Washington, DC, American College of Obstetricians and Gynecologists, 1993.
17. Orr JW, Barrett JM, Orr PF, et al: The efficacy and safety of the cytobrush during pregnancy. Gynecol Oncol 1992;144:260–262.
18. Crum CP, Newkerk GR: Abnormal Pap smears, cancer risk, and HPV. Patient Care 15 June 1995:35–71.
19. Campion MJ, Ferris DG, diPaola FM, et al: Colposcopy of the vulva. In Modern Colposcopy: A Practical Approach. Augusta, GA, Educational Systems, 1991.
20. Lickrish GM: Hysterectomy for cervical intraepithelial neoplasia. In Wright VC, Lickrish GM, Shier RM (eds): Basic and Advanced Colposcopy, part II, 2nd ed. Houston, Biomedical Communications, 1995.
21. McDonald TW: Hysterectomy: Indications, types, and alternatives. In Copeland LJ (ed): Textbook of Gynecology. Philadelphia, WB Saunders, 1993:779–801.

22. Wright TC, Richart RM, Ferenczy A: Electrosurgery for HPV-related Diseases of the Lower Genital Tract. New York, Arthur Vision, 1992.
23. Lickrish GM: Cryotherapy for ectocervical neoplasia. In Wright VC, Lickrish GM, Shier EM (eds): Basic and Advanced Colposcopy, part II, 2nd ed. Houston, Biomedical Communications, 1995.
24. Cook E, Mitchell MF: Treatment of cervical intraepithelial neoplasia. Clinical Consultations in Obstetrics and Gynecology 1994;6:37–43.
25. Anderson M, Jordan J, Morse A, et al: Etiology and natural history of cervical carcinoma. In Integrated Colposcopy. St. Louis, CV Mosby, 1991:48.
26. Nasiell K, Roger V, Nasiell M: Behavior of mild cervical dysplasia during long term follow-up. Obstet Gynecol 1986;67:665–669.
27. Tortolero-Luna G, Linares A, Mitchell MF: Epidemiology of cervical intraepithelial neoplasia. Clinical Consultations in Obstetrics and Gynecology 1994;6:2–10.
28. American Society for Colposcopy and Cervical Pathology Practice Committee: Management guidelines for follow-up of atypical squamous cells of undetermined significance (ASCUS). The Colposcopist 1996;27:1–15.
29. Burke TW, Tortolero-Luna G, Malpica A, et al: Endometrial hyperplasia and endometrial cancer. Obstet Gynecol Clin North Am 1996;23:411–456.
30. Blaustein RL: Cytology of the female genital tract. In Blaustein A (ed): Pathology of the Female Genital Tract, 2nd ed. New York, Springer-Verlag, 1982:838–867.
31. Cherkis RC, Patten SF, Andrews TJ, et al: Significance of normal endometrial cells detected by cervical cytology. Obstet Gynecol 1988;71:242–244.
32. National Institutes of Health Consensus Development Conference Statement: Cervical Cancer. April 1–3, 1996. Bethesda, MD, National Institutes of Health, 1996.
33. Woolf SH: Screening for cervical cancer. In Guide to Clinical Preventive Services' Report of the U.S. Preventive Services Task Force, 2nd ed. Baltimore, Williams & Wilkins, 1996.
34. American College of Obstetricians and Gynecologists: Recommendations on Frequency of Pap Test Screening. ACOG Committee Opinion Number 152. Washington, DC, ACOG, March 1995.
35. Sturgeon SR, Brinton LA, Devesa SS, et al: In situ and invasive vulvar cancer incidence trends (1973–1987). Am J Obstet Gynecol 1992;166:1482.
36. Mack TM, Cosen W, Quinn MA: Epidemiology of cancers of the endometrium, ovary, vulva, and vagina. In Coppleson M (ed): Gynecologic Oncology: Fundamental Principles of Clinical Practices. New York, Churchill-Livingstone, 1992:44.
37. Jones RJ, McLean MR: Carcinoma in situ of the vulva: A review of 31 treated and five untreated cases. Obstet Gynecol 1986;68:499.
38. Edwards C, Tortolero-Luna G, Linares A: Vulvar intraepithelial neoplasia. Obstet Gynecol Clin North Am 1996;23:295–324.
39. Scully RE, Boniglio TA, Kurman RT, et al: Vulvar epithelial tumors and related lesions. In Histological Typing of Female Genital Tract Tumors, 2nd ed. Berlin, Springer-Verlag, 1994:64.
40. Kaufman RH: Intraepithelial neoplasia of the vulva. Distinguished Professor Series. Gynecol Oncol 1995;56:8–12.
41. Rhodes-Morris HE: Treatment of vulvar intraepithelial neoplasia and vaginal intraepithelial neoplasia. Clinical Consultations in Obstetrics and Gynecology 1994;6:44–53.
42. Burke L, Antonioli DA, Ducatman BS: Colposcopy Text and Atlas. Norwalk, Appleton & Lange, 1991.
43. Wright VC: Colposcopy of intraepithelial neoplasia of the vulva and adjacent sites: Differentiation from other lesions. In Wright VC, Lickrish GM, Shier RM (eds): Basic and Advanced Colposcopy, part I, 2nd ed. Houston, Biomedical Communications, 1995.
44. The University of Texas M.D. Anderson Cancer Center Colposcopy Clinic Protocol: Houston, The University of Texas M.D. Anderson Cancer Center, 1994.
45. Meyskens FL, Surwit E, Moon TE, et al: Enhancement of regression of cervical intraepithelial neoplasia II (moderate dysplasia) with topically applied all-trans-retinoic acid: A randomized trial. J Natl Cancer Institute 1994;86:539–543.
46. Sandella J: Vulvar self exam (VSE). Oncology Nursing Forum 1987;14:71–73.
47. Wharton JT, Tortolero-Luna G, Linares A: Vaginal intraepithelial neoplasia and vaginal cancer. Obstet Gynecol Clin North Am 1996;23:325–345.
48. Petrilli ES, Townsend DE, Morrow CP, et al: Vaginal intraepithelial neoplasia: Biologic aspects and treatment with topical 5-fluorouracil and the carbon dioxide laser. Am J Obstet Gynecol 1980;138:312.
49. Burke L, Abu-Jawdih GM: Home Study Course. The Colposcopist 1994;26:6–7.

Chapter 13

Invasive Gynecologic Cancers

Yvette DeJesus, MSN, RN, and Thomas Burke, MD

Overall, gynecologic cancers account for 13% of all cancers occurring in women and approximately 10% of all cancer deaths.[1] In 1997 an estimated 81,800 women were diagnosed with a gynecologic malignancy and approximately 26,500 women lost their lives as a result.[2] The probability for a woman to develop a cancer by the age of 39 years is approximately 2%, with an increase in probability as age increases. There is a 9% probability by the age of 59 years, a 23% probability by age 79, and a 39% probability by the end of life.[3] The current life expectancy for women extends 30 to 40 years after the onset of menopause, increasing the potential risk of developing a cancer.[4]

Invasive carcinomas of the genital tract typically penetrate the cellular basement membrane and possess the potential to metastasize to adjacent structures and throughout the body.[1] Carcinoma of the vulva accounts for a small percentage (3% to 5%) of all female genital tract cancers; vaginal carcinoma is likewise uncommon.[1] Cancer arising from the cervix is the second most common cancer among women worldwide, after breast cancer.[5] Endometrial (uterine) cancer is the eighth most common malignancy in women worldwide.[6] Despite the fact that ovarian cancer accounts for only 4% of cancers in women, it is the leading cause of death among women with gynecologic malignancies in the United States.[7]

This chapter covers carcinomas of the vulva, vagina, cervix, uterus, and ovary. To assist the health care provider in providing appropriate care and referring patients in a timely manner, the discussion of each disease site includes information on epidemiology, etiology, risk factors, pathology, symptoms, diagnosis, staging, prognosis, treatment, surveillance, prevention, and early detection through screening. A clear appreciation of these basic concepts is essential. Sound clinical judgment must be correlated with these concepts to provide quality patient care outcomes.

CARCINOMA OF THE VULVA

About 3% to 5% of all cancers of the female genital tract are carcinomas of the vulva, and squamous cell cancer accounts for 90% of vulvar cancers.[1] Cancer arising from the vulva is a rare tumor with an annual age-adjusted incidence of 1.6 cases per 100,000 women in the United States, accounting for only 1% of all malignancies in women.[8] This type of cancer tends to grow slowly; it spreads by direct extension and by lymphatic drainage through the inguinal, femoral, and pelvic lymph nodes.[1] Hematogenous spread is rare for vulvar carcinoma. Vulvar carcinoma is highly curable when it is diagnosed at an early stage, with survival depending primarily on the pathologic status of the inguinal nodes.[9] The treatment usually is surgical, although alternative methods that reduce disfigurement while improving survival are now being reported.[1]

EPIDEMIOLOGY

Vulvar cancer tends to occur in women of middle age and older. The median age for patients with vulvar carcinoma in situ is 44 years; for those with microinvasive carcinoma, it is 58 years; and for those with frank invasive carcinoma, it is 61 years. Most women with invasive carcinoma of the vulva are in their 60s and 70s, although the disease occasionally occurs in women younger than 40 years of age.[1] An increased incidence of this disease does not appear to be associated with any particular ethnic group. However, it has been reported that women of lower socioeconomic status have a vulvar cancer incidence three times that of women in the highest socioeconomic group.[1]

No etiologic agent has been identified; however, there is evidence associating an increased risk of vulvar cancer with particular factors. These include a history of certain sexually transmitted diseases, including condyloma acuminata; an increasing number of sexual partners; a weakened immune system; and a history of smoking.[10] Human papillomavirus (HPV) infection is present in 22% to 78% of women diagnosed with vulvar carcinoma; however, no specific cause-and-effect relation has been conclusively demonstrated.[11] There may be two types of vulvar carcinoma: an HPV-associated type in younger women and a non-HPV-associated type in the elderly.[11] Various medical conditions associated with this cancer include obesity, hypertension and diabetes mellitus, early age at menopause, nulliparity, and the presence of a second primary tumor (usually a preinvasive or invasive cervical carcinoma).[12] Some reports have suggested that leukoplakia and lichen sclerosis are precursors of vulvar carcinoma.[13]

NATURAL HISTORY AND PATTERN OF SPREAD

The slow growth pattern of vulvar carcinoma may indicate a preinvasive or invasive phase of disease. Growth occurs more slowly in tumors of the vulva than in those of the vagina or cervix. Although most cervical lesions are associated with an intraepithelial lesion, this is found in only one third of vulvar carcinomas.[14] The majority of vulvar cancers are unilateral, well-circumscribed lesions; are not associated with HPV; and arise in elderly women.[15] The stage of disease at the time of diagnosis is usually early, with the lesion measuring 2 cm or smaller and with a low incidence (approximately 10%) of lymph node metastasis.[14] The pattern of spread is influenced by the grade (degree of differentiation) and cell type of the carcinoma. Lesions that are well differentiated (grade 1) tend to spread along the surface with minimal invasion, whereas poorly differentiated (grade 3) lesions have a higher incidence of deep invasion and metastasis to the lymph nodes.[15]

PATHOLOGY

Approximately 90% of cases of vulvar carcinoma are of the invasive squamous cell type.[12] Grossly, these lesions are endophytic and ulcerated in one third of patients and exophytic in the rest.[1] Melanoma accounts for 2% to 9% of vulvar carcinomas, with depth of invasion directly related to the incidence of nodal metastasis and to survival.[1] Bartholin gland carcinomas are of different histologic types depending on their area of origin. If the lesion arises from the transitional epithelium of the duct, it is papillary; if from the orifice of the duct, squamous; and if from the gland itself, adenocarcinoma.[1]

CLINICAL PRESENTATION, DIAGNOSIS, STAGING, AND PROGNOSIS

Up to 20% of patients are asymptomatic, with the lesion detected during routine pelvic examination.[1] Women with vulvar carcinoma tend to delay seeking medical treatment because of embarrassment due to the intimate area of the body involved.[15] Consequently, a woman may have symptoms for 2 to 16 months before she is examined. Pruritus is the most common presenting complaint of patients found to have vulvar carcinoma.[15] It has been observed in about 70% of such patients and may be caused either by the carcinoma itself or by associated intraepithelial changes or benign conditions such as dystrophy.[13] The vulva comprises the mons pubis, labia majora, labia minora, prepuce, vestibule, clitoris, and perineum. Physical assessment of the vulva should focus on the labia majora, labia minora, clitoris, and Bartholin glands. Good visualization of these areas and the perineum is of utmost importance. The most common site of primary vulvar lesions is the labia, followed by the clitoris. Labia majora lesions are three times more common than are those of labia minora.[15] Delays in diagnosis of up to 12 months are common. The cause of the delay has been explained as twofold: the patient's refusal to seek medical attention and the health care provider's failure to examine the patient who has a complaint or to biopsy an obvious lesion.[15] When performing a biopsy of an obvious lesion, a wedge of the lesion along with surrounding normal tissue should be obtained. This allows for evaluation of the depth of invasion. A detailed description of the physical assessment of the vulva is presented in Chapter 12.

The most efficient way to diagnose vulvar cancer is to maintain a high index of suspicion and to biopsy questionable areas early.[1] Characteristics that merit further evaluation are lesions that are raised and appear fleshy, ulcerated, leukoplakic, or warty. Warty carcinoma has increased in incidence and now accounts for about 20% of vulvar carcinoma cases.[1] Definitive diagnosis of vulvar carcinoma is made by excisional biopsy.[13] Further diagnostic evaluation may include colposcopy, proctoscopy, cystoscopy, chest radiography, computed tomography (CT), and a biochemical profile if clinically indicated.[1] The system used to stage all gynecologic cancers was approved by the International Federation of Gynecology and Obstetrics (FIGO) in 1989. Staging incorporates the clinical findings from the initial assessment with the pathologic findings from the surgical procedure. Each stage of vulvar carcinoma is illustrated in Figure 13–1. Clinical lymph node assessment may be inaccurate, because microscopically positive nodes may go undetected; therefore, clinical and surgical staging results are compared for accuracy.[12] With timely and appropriate management of invasive vulvar carcinoma, the prognosis is good. In operable cases, the 5-year survival rate is approximately 70%. The survival rate correlates directly with the stage of disease at diagnosis.[12] Women with negative inguinal lymph nodes at diagnosis have a 5-year survival rate of about 90%; for those with positive nodes, the rate is 50%.[12] The next most important prognostic factor is the number of positive lymph nodes. A single microscopically positive node confers a relatively good prognosis regardless of the stage of disease, whereas the presence of three or more positive nodes is associated with a poor prognosis.[12] Patients with positive pelvic nodes have a 5-year survival rate of 15%.[12]

TREATMENT

In the past, the best treatment for invasive carcinoma of the vulva was considered to be radical surgery; responses to radiation therapy and chemother-

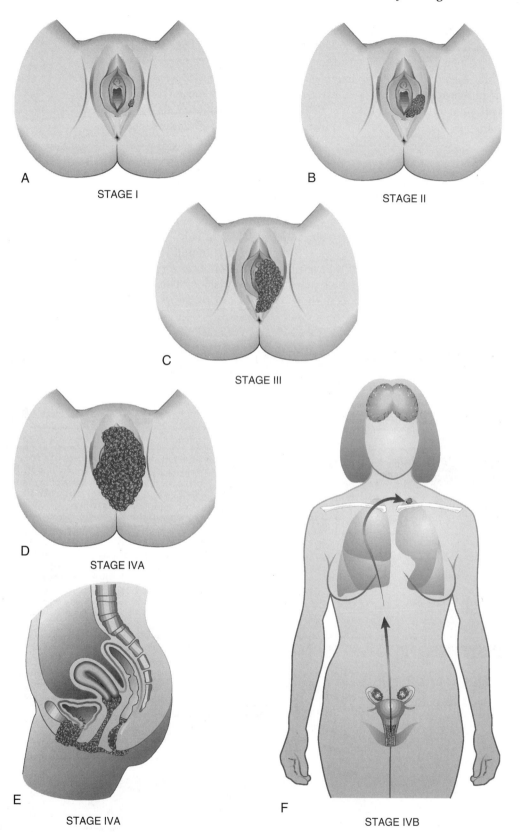

STAGE I

STAGE II

STAGE III

STAGE IVA

STAGE IVA

STAGE IVB

Figure 13–1. Carcinoma of the vulva by stage. (From Edwards CL, Tortolero-Luna G, Linares A, et al: Vulvar intraepithelial neoplasia and vulvar cancer. Obstet Gynecol Clin North Am 23:312, 313, 1996.)

apy were limited.[1] The current treatment approach is more conservative, with new focus on decreasing short-term and long-term morbidity. Treatment depends on the location and stage of the disease.[1] Figure 13–2 lists the treatments of choice for each stage of vulvar cancer along with recommended surveillance. An expanded role for radiation therapy is being explored. Its use in the treatment of small primary vulvar cancers is debatable, but radiation with or without chemotherapy may prove useful for advanced, inoperable vulvar carcinoma.[1]

CANCER PREVENTION AND EARLY DETECTION THROUGH SCREENING

Early detection and appropriate medical management of vulvar cancer are of paramount importance. These can be accomplished by programs that educate women about self-examination of the vulva and the importance of regular pelvic examinations to identify suspicious lesions at an early stage. The health care provider can provide important educational information to the patient (Table

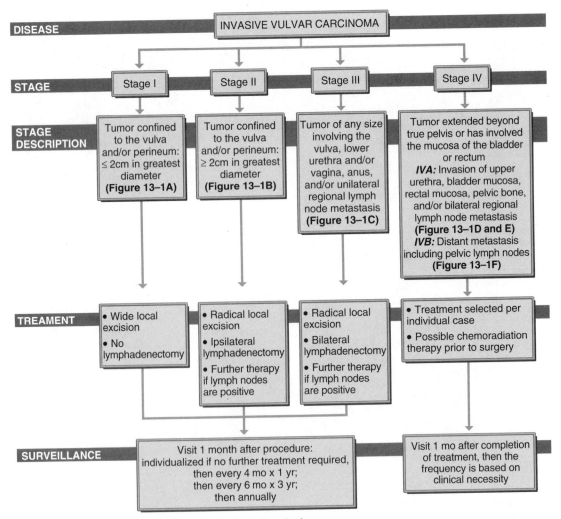

Figure 13–2. Treatment and surveillance of carcinoma of the vulva by stage.

Table 13–1. Vulvar Cancer Prevention and Detection: Advice to Health Care Providers

Background
  Associated with age, obesity, other anogenital cancers, HPV, other sexually transmitted
    diseases, and smoking
  Most common presenting symptom is vulvar pruritus
  Lesions may be hyperpigmented (usually brown or gray with sharply demarcated borders)
    or erythematous or ulcerated
Prevention education and early detection
  Teach vulvar self-examination
  Encourage smoking cessation
  Encourage prevention of sexually transmitted diseases
  Closely monitor high-risk women
  Perform complete vulvar inspection and biopsy early in treatment of persistent vulvar
    inflammation or pruritus
  Biopsy persistent vulvar condyloma if local therapy has failed
  No routine screening recommended except careful inspection of vulva in all patients
    when Pap smear is performed
  For equivocal lesions, apply acetic acid for approximately 5 min to reveal acetowhite
    epithelium to biopsy
  No proven chemoprevention agents

HPV, human papillomavirus; Pap, Papanicolaou.
From Edwards CL, Tortolero-Luna G, Linares A, et al: Vulvar intraepithelial neoplasia and vulvar cancer. Obstet Gynecol Clin North Am 23:320, 1996.

13–1). He or she can teach vulvar self-examinations, encourage smoking cessation, encourage prevention of sexually transmitted diseases, and encourage close monitoring of high-risk patients (age older than 70 years; history of smoking; history of cervical, vaginal, or perianal cancer or sexually transmitted disease).[14] The provider also can reinforce knowledge of the most common symptoms: persistent vulvar itching and irritation, vulvar lump (some patients), vaginal bleeding, and pain or discharge.[14] Providing this type of information allows the patient to participate in prevention and early detection behaviors that promote an early diagnosis[14] (Table 13–2).

CARCINOMA OF THE VAGINA

Carcinoma of the vagina is a primary malignancy that arises in the vagina but does not involve the cervix or vulva. Cancers that originate in the vagina are rare

Table 13–2. Vulvar Cancer Prevention and Detection: Advice to Patients

Major risk factors
  Known risk factors: age (>70 yr); smoking; history of cervical, vaginal, or perianal cancer,
    HPV, or sexually transmitted diseases
  Suspected risk factors: diet, infrequent pelvic examinations, infrequent Papanicolaou
    smears
Most common symptoms
  Persistent vulvar itching and irritation; vulvar lump (in some patients); vaginal bleeding,
    pain, or discharge
Prevention education and early detection
  Perform monthly vulvar self-examination (using hand mirror and flashlight)
  Report promptly changes in pigment or any round, red, or raised bumps
  Seek expert help for any persistent itching or irritation
  Stop smoking
  Avoid constricting undergarments and perfumes and dyes in the vulvar region
  Use barrier contraception (condoms or diaphragm) to prevent sexually transmitted
    diseases

HPV, human papillomavirus.
From Edwards CL, Tortolero-Luna G, Linares A, et al: Vulvar intraepithelial neoplasia and vulvar cancer. Obstet Gynecol Clin North Am 23:320, 1996.

and constitute only 1% to 2% of female genital malignancies.[1] Primary vaginal carcinomas usually are squamous cell cancers.[1] Vaginal carcinomas appear to follow the same biologic pattern as cervical carcinomas, but overall cure rates for the former are much lower and treatment-associated morbidity remains high.[12] Although vaginal carcinomas have the potential to be discovered at an early stage, during routine Papanicolaou (Pap) smears and pelvic examinations, most women present with disease that has already spread beyond the vagina.[12]

EPIDEMIOLOGY

The median age of patients with invasive vaginal cancer is the mid-70s. Over the last 20 years the incidence of vaginal carcinoma in the United States has been .42 per 100,000 women and has remained stable.[16] Vaginal cancer often is associated with other malignancies of the genital tract.[17] Associated risk factors for vaginal carcinoma (either in situ or invasive) are low family income, low educational level, a history of abnormal Pap smears, vaginal discharge or irritation, genital warts, early hysterectomy, and smoking.[19] Women who have had malignancies of the cervix or vulva have an increased risk of developing abnormalities of the vagina. About 30% of women with primary vaginal carcinoma have a history of invasive or in situ cervical cancer treated at least 5 years earlier; this is known as the "field effect" and recognizes the entire genital tract to be at risk.[18] Although carcinoma in situ of the vagina can occur up to 17 years after carcinoma in situ of the cervix, one third of cases are diagnosed within 2 years.

HPV also has been associated with vaginal carcinoma and has been proposed as an etiologic factor for cancer in the entire female genital tract; however, many women with HPV never develop malignancies.[11] Prior radiation therapy given for other gynecologic malignancies may also be a predisposing factor for primary vaginal carcinoma.[1] Clear cell adenocarcinoma of the vagina has been associated with exposure to diethylstilbestrol (DES) in utero. [17] DES appears to cross the placental barrier and to affect the müllerian ducts, leading to abnormalities of the upper vagina and cervix. The actual risk that a DES-exposed woman will develop clear cell adenocarcinoma is .14 to 1.4 per 1000 women through 24 years of age.[1]

NATURAL HISTORY AND PATTERN OF SPREAD

Vaginal carcinomas spread to adjacent structures by direct extension or from the lymphatics due to the absence of anatomical barriers. Tumors that involve the cervix or vulva are considered to be primary at those sites because they are more common than vaginal carcinoma.[17] Vaginal tumors that spread laterally may involve the parametrial, paracolpal, and pararectal tissues, with extension to the pelvic side walls.[19] Most vaginal carcinomas arise from the posterior wall of the upper third of the vagina. Approximately 52% of vaginal cancers are found in the upper third of the vagina, and 58% are found on the posterior wall.[19]

PATHOLOGY

Squamous cell carcinoma is the most common type of vaginal cancer, accounting for 75% to 85% of all cases.[19] These may appear grossly as endophytic and ulcerated tumors or as exophytic tumors protruding into the vaginal canal.[17] Microscopically, most are keratinizing epidermoid carcinomas with pleomorphic squamous cells that display lack of organization and loss of cellular cohesion.[1] The lesions may show dysplasia, carcinoma in situ, or invasion. The second most common cell type is adenocarcinoma. The most common adenocarcinoma subtype is clear cell carcinoma, which has been associated with exposure to DES in utero.[1, 17, 19]

CLINICAL PRESENTATION, DIAGNOSIS, STAGING, AND PROGNOSIS

The most common presenting symptom of invasive vaginal carcinoma is abnormal, painless vaginal bleeding, which occurs in 50% to 75% of cases.[19] The bleeding is usually postmenopausal, because this is the age group most often affected by the disease, but it also may occur after coitus. Thirty percent of patients seek medical attention because of a vaginal discharge. Five percent to 10% of affected women are asymptomatic, and the carcinoma is detected on routine examination and Pap smear.[12] Another 5% present with pelvic pain due to advanced disease.[12] There may also be complaints of bladder discomfort and frequent urination, because the bladder neck is located near the vagina.[12] Symptoms involving the bladder or rectum usually indicate advanced disease. The average duration of symptoms before diagnosis is 7.4 months.[1]

The medical history should include information on particular risk factors such as DES exposure.[12] Clinical assessment of the vagina is accomplished by careful examination and palpation. The health care provider should focus on early identification of lesions and visualization of all vaginal quadrants.[12] Lesions that are small and occur in the lower two thirds of the vagina often are missed on examination because the speculum blades can obscure the lesions. The speculum should be rotated carefully so that all four vaginal quadrants can be visualized, especially in the fornices.[12] Examination usually includes an initial Pap smear and a pelvic and rectal examination with palpation of the vagina and colposcopy. Any raised, irregular areas in the vagina should be biopsied.[12] The lesions observed are usually exophytic, fungating, and polypoid. They may also be endophytic. Ulceration of the surface may occur in advanced disease.[17]

A definitive diagnosis usually is made by biopsy of a gross lesion.[12] Exfoliative cytology studies are useful to detect early squamous cell carcinomas but not clear cell adenocarcinomas, because the latter often grow in submucosal locations. Colposcopy can provide adequate information to evaluate abnormal areas in the vagina.[19] The staging workup for vaginal carcinoma is clinical and includes careful inspection of the vagina and cervix, biopsy, bimanual examination, chest radiograph, and biochemical profile. Further evaluation may include abdominal and pelvic CT scans with contrast, barium enema, cytoscopy, proctoscopy, and magnetic resonance imaging if clinically indicated.[12]

The four stages of vaginal carcinoma are illustrated in Figure 13–3. In terms of prognosis, the overall survival rate for patients with vaginal carcinoma has decreased compared with the rates for patients with vulvar and cervical carcinomas.[20] One of the most important predictors of survival is stage of disease.

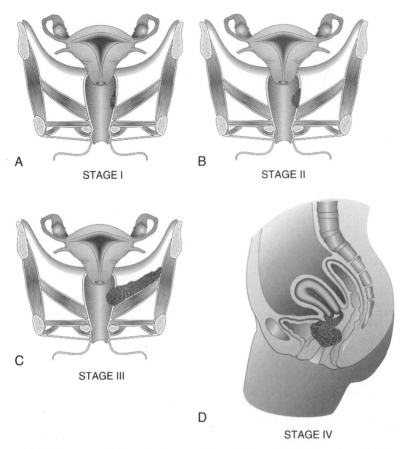

Figure 13–3. Carcinoma of the vagina by stage. (From Wharton JT, Tortolero-Luna G, Linares A, et al: Vaginal intraepithelial neoplasia and vaginal cancer. Obstet Gynecol Clin North Am 23:338, 339, 1996.)

Factors such as tumor size, cell type, patient age, or prior hysterectomy were shown not to influence survival rate.[20] The overall survival rate for patients with squamous cell carcinoma is about 45%: for stage I disease, 69%; stage II, 51%; stage III, 27%; and stage IV, 4.5%).[20]

TREATMENT

The primary treatment for vaginal carcinoma is radiation, with surgical resection used depending on the size and location of the lesion. Treatment choices should be individualized. Early-stage vaginal carcinoma can be treated with radical hysterectomy and upper vaginectomy; this option preserves sexual and ovarian function in young women.[17, 20] A more radical surgical approach is employed for more extensive disease. Radiation is the primary therapy used for advanced vaginal cancer, especially squamous cell carcinoma.[1] In these advanced cases, surgery is reserved for palliation of bleeding or management of vesicovaginal fistulas.[12] The specific treatments according to stage of disease are detailed in Figure 13–4.

AFTER-TREATMENT SURVEILLANCE

The after-treatment surveillance depends on the clinical necessity. Patients with early-stage lesions are monitored on a routine basis, such as every 3 months

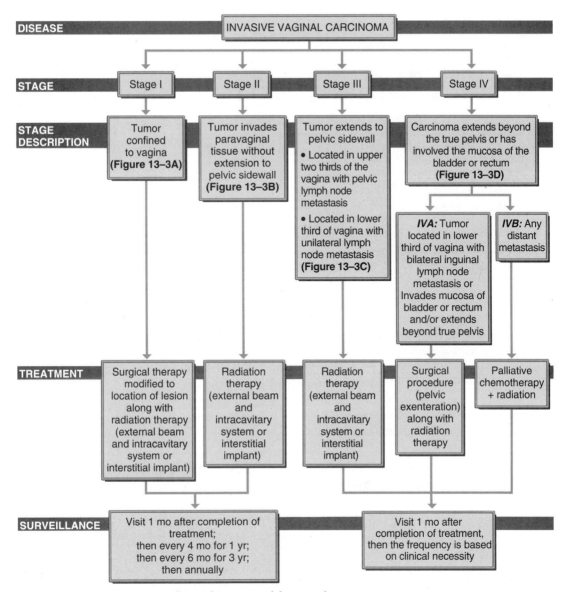

Figure 13–4. Treatment and surveillance of carcinoma of the vagina by stage.

for 2 years, then every 6 months for 3 years, and annually thereafter. The visit for patients with early lesions should consist of a complete physical assessment including pelvic examination and Pap smear. If further evaluation of a suspicious area is needed, a colposcopy should be performed.[19] Patients with advanced-stage lesions are monitored depending on the clinical necessity, for example, tumor-related complications (bleeding, fistula formulation, bowel obstruction) or pain management.[19]

CANCER PREVENTION AND EARLY DETECTION THROUGH SCREENING

In view of the fact that most women with vaginal carcinoma are asymptomatic until the disease is advanced, it is important for the primary care provider to

Table 13–3. Vaginal Cancer Prevention and Detection: Advice to Health Care Providers

Background
    Most cases of vaginal carcinoma are asymptomatic; there may be vaginal discharge or
        postcoital bleeding
    Tends to occur in patients who were previously treated with hysterectomy or radiation for
        cervical cancer
    Patients exposed to diethylstilbestrol are at increased risk
    Preinvasive lesions tend to be multifocal, invasive lesions unifocal
Prevention education and early detection
    Encourage regular Papanicolaou (Pap) smears
    Encourage smoking cessation
    Encourage prevention of sexually transmitted diseases
    In suspected cases, perform Pap smear and colposcopy (using acetic acid and Lugol
        staining as necessary) with full rotation of speculum
    No routine screening recommended except careful inspection of the vagina in all patients
        when Pap smear is performed
    No proven chemoprevention agents

From Wharton JT, Tortolero-Luna G, Linares A, et al: Vaginal intraepithelial neoplasia and vaginal cancer. Obstet Gynecol Clin North Am 23:343, 1996.

promote routine pelvic examinations and Pap smears. It is also essential to continue to provide cytologic screening to women who have had a hysterectomy, regardless of the indications.[17] Early detection can improve the patient's overall outcome in terms of diagnosis, treatment, and survival.[17] Involving patients in their own care, especially prevention and early detection, is essential. Information for the health care provider (Table 13–3) can be used as a quick point of reference for prevention and screening interventions. Information listed in Table 13–4 can be used for patient education efforts.

CARCINOMA OF THE CERVIX

Cervical carcinoma is the second most common malignancy among women worldwide.[5] In the United States, cervical cancer is the third most common malignancy of the genital tract and accounts for 12% of all cancers in women. Cervical carcinoma can be detected by an effective and inexpensive screening technique (Pap smear), leading to a favorable prognosis.[5] Since the 1950s, the incidence and mortality rates for this cancer have declined in most of the

Table 13–4. Vaginal Cancer Prevention and Detection: Advice to Patients

Major risk factors
    Known risk factors: age (>40 yr); history of invasive cervical carcinoma; previous
        exposure to diethylstilbestrol; hysterectomy for preinvasive disease; previous abnormal
        Pap smear
    Suspected risk factors: smoking; previous radiation therapy
Most common symptoms
    Usually no specific symptoms; occasionally there may vaginal bleeding or a foul discharge;
        pain
Prevention education and early detection
    Get routine Pap smears
    Stop smoking
    Use barrier contraception (condoms or diaphragms) to prevent sexually transmitted
        diseases
    Seek expert help for any abnormal vaginal bleeding or persistent vaginal odor or
        discharge

Pap, Papanicolaou.
From Wharton JT, Tortolero-Luna G, Linares A, et al: Vaginal intraepithelial neoplasia and vaginal cancer. Obstet Gynecol Clin North Am 23:343, 1996.

developing countries.[21] This decline has been attributed to screening with the Pap smear. Despite screening efforts, invasive cervical carcinoma remains a significant health care problem for women worldwide.[5]

EPIDEMIOLOGY

For 1997, it was estimated that 14,500 new cases and 4,800 deaths would occur from cervical cancer in the United States.[2] The mean age for women who develop cervical cancer is 52.2 years; there are two peak age groups, 35 to 39 years and 60 to 64 years.[22] The disease affects primarily women from the lower socioeconomic classes and women of Latin American culture,[23] perhaps because of lack of access to routine medical care in these populations.[5] Cervical cancer occurs infrequently among Jewish and European women. The low frequency in Jewish women has been attributed to the routine circumcision of Jewish men; however, a similar correlation has not been demonstrated in the partners of non-Jewish circumcised men.[23] Another consideration for the low incidence rate in Jewish women may be a genetic resistance to the development of cervical tumors.[23] The exact mechanism of cervical cancer development has not been demonstrated, but several risk factors confer a higher risk, including sexual activity at an early age, multiple sexual partners, partners who visit prostitutes, and a history of genital warts.[20, 23] Immunocompromised women also are at increased risk. Current data support the role of HPV infection as an important cofactor.[5] Other associated factors are cigarette smoking and decreased intake of vitamins A, C, and E, carotenoids, and folic acid.[5]

NATURAL HISTORY AND PATTERNS OF SPREAD

Squamous cell carcinoma usually arises from the squamocolumnar junction of the cervix and is preceded by cervical dysplasia and carcinoma in situ.[1] The time scale of this progression is debatable; reported intervals range from 1 to 20 years, although the 10-year interval is widely accepted.[1] When malignant epithelial cells break through the basement membrane to enter the stroma, invasive carcinoma occurs. With continued growth, the lesion becomes visible and progressively involves more cervical tissue with invasion of the lymphovascular spaces. Cervical cancer spreads by direct local extension into the paracervical tissue, the vagina, or the endometrium. When there is involvement of the lymphovascular spaces, the cancer is able to spread via the lymphatic channels as well as by hematogenous spread.[23]

Tumor dissemination usually follows an orderly pattern; however, on occasion a small cervical cancer may spread to lymph nodes, invade the bladder or rectum, or produce distant metastasis.[23] The most frequently seen metastatic sites of cervical cancer are the lungs, mediastinal and supraclavicular lymph nodes, bones, and liver.[23]

PATHOLOGY

The pathology of cervical carcinomas is divided into gross and microscopic characteristics. Neither in situ nor "occult" carcinoma of the cervix has gross abnormalities at presentation. Whereas visible lesions can be categorized as endophytic or exophytic, the microscopic characteristics deal with the morphologic changes and identify the cell type in which the carcinoma originated.[1] Most cervical carcinomas (90%) are squamous cell carcinomas.[1] Adenocarcinomas account for 10% to 15% of cervical carcinomas. There are other cell types, such as adenosquamous, clear cell, glassy cell, adenoid cystic, and mucoepidermoid carcinomas, but these are rarely seen.[24] Other rare primary cervical carcinomas include malignant melanoma and lymphoma, sarcomas, Hodgkin's disease, and verrucous carcinomas.[1]

CLINICAL PRESENTATION

The majority of women diagnosed with early-stage cervical cancer are asymptomatic; their disease is discovered on a routine Pap smear.[23] Symptoms of an early invasive cervical carcinoma can include vaginal discharge or vaginal bleeding, of which the most common type is postcoital spotting.[12] The classic symptom is intermenstrual bleeding in a premenopausal patient. Other commonly reported symptoms are heavy menstrual flow and metrorrhagia.[12] As the lesion increases in size, the vaginal discharge may become copious and serosanguinous and may have a foul odor.[1] Once a visible cervical lesion is noted, a biopsy is warranted to confirm the diagnosis, especially because Pap smear results in this setting may be negative for malignancy owing to the presence of inflammation and necrosis.[23]

A pelvic examination, a Pap smear, and a detailed medical and sexual history are needed to further evaluate a cervical lesion.[1] The pelvic examination is important to determine the size of the cervix and the lesion and whether disease is present in the vagina or parametrium. The cervix may appear bulky without any visible lesion. The normal cervix has a smooth, soft texture. Findings of a firm, fixed cervix on palpation could indicate invasive cervical carcinoma.[23] Any visible suspicious lesion warrants further evaluation. In addition to the pelvic and rectovaginal examination, a complete physical examination should be performed, with special attention to the lymph nodes.[23] Areas of primary concern are the supraclavicular, axillary, and inguinal regions, which are the most common sites of metastases.[23] Correlation of the medical history and physical findings is of utmost importance for obtaining an accurate diagnosis. A triad of clinical findings is almost always present with unresectable disease on the pelvic side wall; it consists of unilateral leg edema, sciatic pain, and ureteral obstruction.[12] The diagnosis of cervical cancer is suggested by an abnormal Pap smear or abnormal physical findings. The lesions may be exophytic, ulcerative, or plaque-like in appearance. Appropriate measurements of the lesion and whether the lesion extends to the pelvic side wall or invades the vagina are important to determine the clinical stage of disease at the time of presentation.[5]

Colposcopy is indicated for the patient with an abnormal Pap smear. Colposcopic findings indicative of invasive cervical carcinoma are a dense, acetowhite epithelium on the ectocervix and atypical blood vessel patterns including punctation and mosaicism. Biopsies should be obtained from the ectocervix and endocervix if the colposcopic findings suggest invasion. The clinical stage of the lesion at initial evaluation is the most important prognostic factor for invasive cervical carcinoma.[23] Each stage of disease is illustrated in Figure 13–5. Overall 5-year survival rates range from 95% to 100% for patients with stage IA cervical cancer, and 75% to 90% for those with stage IB, to 5% or less for those with stage IV disease.[12] The factors that affect prognosis in stage I (early invasive) disease are tumor size, histologic grade, percentage of cervical stromal invasion, and

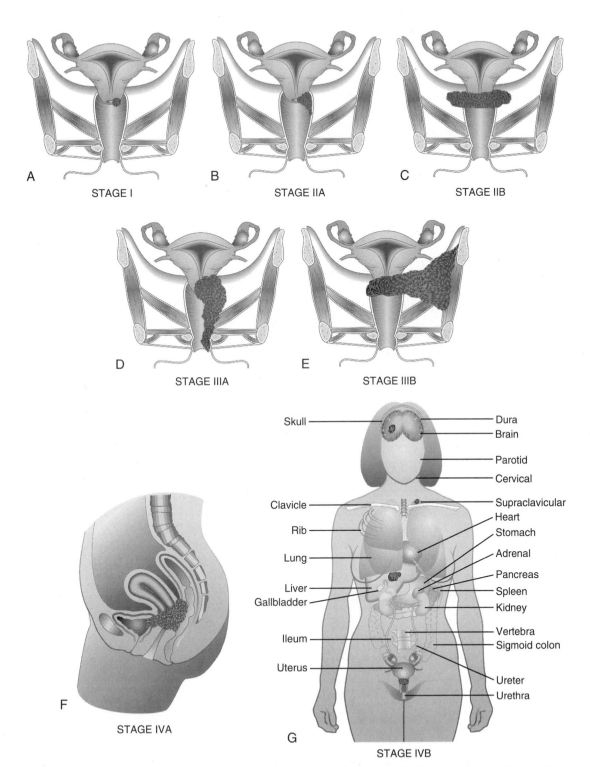

Figure 13–5. Carcinoma of the cervix by stage. (From Morris M, Tortolero-Luna G, Malpica A, et al: Cervical intraepithelial neoplasia and cervical cancer. Obstet Gynecol Clin North Am 23:382, 383, 1996.)

lymphovascular space involvement.[1] Lesions smaller than 2 cm in diameter that are superficially invasive, well differentiated, and without lymphovascular space involvement have a good prognosis.[1] For patients with stage I disease who have undergone a radical hysterectomy, additional poor prognostic factors include positive vaginal or parametrial margins and metastases to the pelvic lymph nodes.[12] For patients with stages II through IV disease, the main prognostic factors are size and histology of the primary tumor. Disease spread beyond the pelvis is associated with a significantly decreased overall survival rate.[1] The prognostic factors that yield the greatest information are tumor volume, endometrial tumor extension, and lymph node involvement.[1, 12] The prognosis may be affected if there is large tumor volume, extensive disease in the endometrium, or more than four positive lymph nodes.[1]

TREATMENT

As with other gynecologic malignancies, the appropriate treatment regimen for invasive cervical carcinoma is greatly affected by the stage of disease. Cell type is also a consideration.[14] Treatment may be individualized according to disease stage (Figure 13–6). Microinvasive cervical carcinoma may be treated by simple hysterectomy.[12] Certain treatment options, although associated with possible risks, can accommodate the patient's desire to maintain her fertility.[5, 12] In such cases, a simple cone biopsy (which involves removal of the cervical transformation zone) may be adequate treatment for patients who have superficial invasion of less than 3 mm, minimum lateral extension, no lymphovascular space involvement, and biopsy margins free of dysplasia and microinvasive carcinoma.[5] Follow-up for these patients should include a Pap smear every 3 months for 2 years, then twice a year. An abnormal smear is an indication for a repeat colposcopy.[5] Stage IB disease is treated by radical hysterectomy (removal of the uterus, cervix, and parametrial tissue) or radiation, depending on the patient's desire and tumor size. Once the cancer has spread beyond the cervix, external and intracavitary beam radiation therapy usually are combined. Stage II through IVA disease usually is managed by radiation therapy, except for a few stage IVA patients who can receive primary pelvic exenteration.[1] Stage IVB cervical carcinoma usually is treated by the combination of chemotherapy plus radiation therapy.[1] Chemotherapy traditionally has been used only palliatively for cervical cancer.[1, 5]

AFTER-TREATMENT SURVEILLANCE

Because tumor regression may continue for up to 3 months after completion of radiation therapy, response must be confirmed by monthly examinations during this period. Most recurrences appear within 2 years after treatment; patients should be evaluated every 6 months during this interval and less often thereafter.

Follow-up also should include a breast and vaginal and rectovaginal examination, an annual Pap smear and chest radiograph, and palpation of the supraclavicular and inguinal lymph nodes.[23] If not contraindicated, low-dose estrogen and a progestational agent should be used indefinitely.[23] Women who were diagnosed with an early-stage lesion should have a minimum of a Pap smear and endocervical curettage every 3 to 4 months for the first 2 years and thereafter every 6

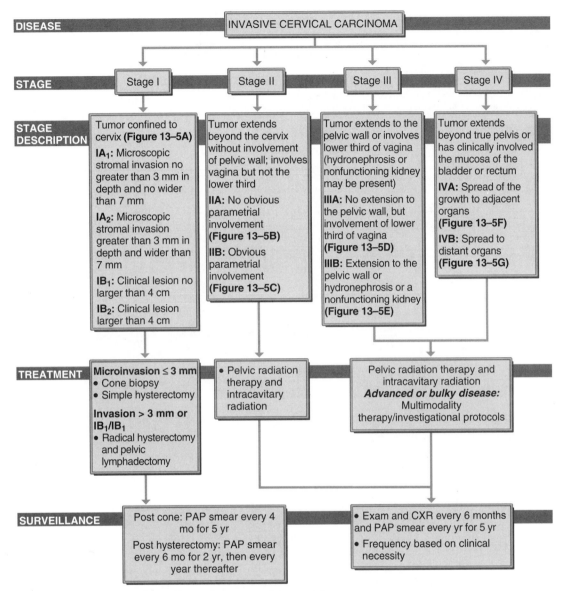

Figure 13–6. Treatment and surveillance of carcinoma of the cervix by stage.

months for another 3 years. If the treatment is for an invasive cervical cancer, the M.D. Anderson Cancer Center Guidelines for follow-up are:

First Year:
A physical examination including a pelvic examination every 3 months
A Pap smear once a year
A chest x-ray once a year

Second Year:
A physical examination including a pelvic examination every 4 months
A Pap smear once a year
A chest x-ray every 6 months

Third and Fourth Years:
A physical examination including a pelvic examination every 6 months
A Pap smear once a year
A chest x-ray every 6 months

Table 13–5. Cervical Cancer Prevention and Detection: Advice to Health Care Providers

Background
  Cervical cancer is on the rise
  Most patients are asymptomatic; patients may have postcoital bleeding, irregular menses, or abnormal discharge
  Risk factors include multiple sex partners, history of STD (especially HPV), smoking, early age at first intercourse, immunosuppression (including HIV)
Prevention and early detection
  Encourage routine Pap smears
  Encourage smoking cessation
  Encourage prevention of STD
  Monitor high-risk women closely
  Use colposcopy to evaluate patients with an abnormal Pap smear and biopsy gross cervical lesions

HPV, human papillomavirus; HIV, human immunodeficiency virus; Pap, Papanicolaou; STD, sexually transmitted diseases.
From Morris M, Tortolero-Luna G, Malpica A, et al: Cervical intraepithelial neoplasia and cervical cancer. Obstet Gynecol Clin North Am 23:399, 1996.

Fifth Year:
A physical examination including a pelvic examination every 6 months
A Pap smear once a year
A chest x-ray once a year

CANCER PREVENTION AND EARLY DETECTION THROUGH SCREENING

Cervical cytologic screening should be promoted. In every population studied, the use of the Pap smear has resulted in both a significant reduction in the incidence of invasive cervical carcinoma and a shift toward earlier-stage disease at diagnosis.[3] Increased screening and earlier detection have led to an increase in the number of new cases detected but also in decreased mortality.[15] Tables 13–5 and 13–6 have useful information for the health care provider and the patient, respectively, regarding prevention and early detection.

Table 13–6. Cervical Cancer Prevention and Detection: Advice to Patients

Major risk factors
  Known risk factors: higher risk for African-American and Hispanic women; low socioeconomic status; low age at first intercourse; multiple sex partners; history of HPV, suppressed immune system; previous abnormal Pap smear; exposure to DES
  Suspected risk factor: smoking
Most common symptoms
  Most patients are asymptomatic; may have abnormal vaginal bleeding, especially after intercourse; may have irregular menses (periods) or foul vaginal discharge
Prevention and early detection
  Get routine Pap smears
  Stop smoking
  Use barrier contraception (condoms or diaphragm) to prevent STD
  Seek expert help for any abnormal vaginal bleeding or discharge; be persistent

HPV, human papillomavirus; Pap, Papanicolaou; DES, diethylstilbestrol; STDs, sexually transmitted diseases.
From Morris M, Tortolero-Luna G, Malpica A, et al: Cervical intraepithelial neoplasia and cervical cancer. Obstet Gynecol Clin North Am 23:400, 1996.

CARCINOMA OF THE UTERUS

Carcinoma of the endometrium is the most common gynecologic malignancy in the United States; the American Cancer Society estimates that 34,900 cases occurred in 1997.[2] Endometrial carcinoma is the eighth most common cancer in women worldwide—after breast, cervix, colon and rectum, stomach, lung, ovary, and mouth and pharynx cancers—and the eighth leading cause of death from malignancy in women, with an estimated 6,000 deaths each year.[2] Factors affecting the incidence of endometrial carcinoma are the increase in the life expectancy of women, early diagnosis, and a decreased incidence of cervical cancer.[1] In approximately 75% of patients presenting with endometrial cancer, the disease is confined to the uterine corpus at the time of presentation. The uncorrected survival rate for these women is 75% or greater.[1] The treatment for this cancer has evolved over the years, from preoperative radiation therapy followed by a hysterectomy to, currently, hysterectomy and surgical staging followed by additional therapy depending on various risk factors.[1]

EPIDEMIOLOGY

Endometrial cancer is diagnosed primarily in postmenopausal women (mean age, 60 years), although 25% of cases occur in premenopausal patients, and 5% in patients younger than 40 years of age.[1, 25] The incidence of this disease tends to be higher in Western countries and very low in Eastern countries; higher in urban than in rural residents; and, in the United States, twice as high in white women compared with black women.[26] Because immigrant populations tend to assume the risk of native populations, environmental factors are considered to be important in the genesis of this disease.[26] Adenocarcinoma, the most prevalent histologic subtype, can arise from normal, atrophic, or hyperplastic endometrium.

Two mechanisms are thought to be active in the development of this disease. Some women have a history of exposure to unopposed estrogen, either endogenous or exogenous. In this setting, the tumors begin as endometrial hyperplasia and progress to carcinomas which are usually well differentiated and carry favorable prognosis.[26] In other women the carcinoma develops spontaneously; it does not appear to arise from atypical hyperplasia but rather from inert or atrophic endometrium. These tumors tend to have a more undifferentiated cell type and a poorer prognosis.[26] Endometrial cancer frequently occurs in women with a long-term history of unopposed estrogen exposure with the estrogen source occurring endogenously or by exogenous administration.[26] Most women who develop endometrial cancer are obese: in those who are 30 pounds overweight, the risk is increased threefold, and in those 50 or more pounds overweight, it is increased 10-fold.[26] A possible etiologic role for nutrition is indicated by the high rate of this disease in Western countries (where diets are high in animal fat) and the low rate in Eastern countries. Other known risk factors include nulliparity, diabetes mellitus (threefold higher risk), hypertension (1.5-fold higher risk), endometrial hyperplasia, and a family history of endometrial cancer. Use of the nonsteroidal antiestrogen tamoxifen, under study as preventive therapy for breast cancer, has been linked to a 6.4-fold increased risk of endometrial cancer, particularly if it is used for longer than 5 years.[22] The classic triad of risk factors for endometrial cancer consists of obesity, diabetes, and hypertension.[20, 22]

NATURAL HISTORY AND PATTERN OF SPREAD

Endometrial carcinoma may spread along the uterine cavity to the cervix, penetrate the uterine wall, or spread through the fallopian tubes. The cancer can spread locally to the broad ligament, ovary, vagina, or other pelvic organs. Malignant cells can spread through the lymphatics or, less commonly, through the bloodstream.[1] Depending on tumor histology, grade, and myometrial invasion, reported incidences of pelvic and para-aortic nodal metastases have ranged from 1% to 25%.[1] Extension or metastasis of endometrial cancer to the fallopian tubes or ovaries occurs in 5% to 10% of patients, to the cervix in 5% to 10%, and to the vagina in 7%.[1] Disease recurrence rates as high as 34% have been reported for patients with positive peritoneal cytology.[1]

PATHOLOGY

Carcinoma of the endometrium is easily diagnosed, although occasionally a well-differentiated carcinoma may be difficult to distinguish from advanced atypical hyperplasia. All carcinomas are classified according to the degree of architectural differentiation of the tumor. Endometrioid adenocarcinoma (Grade 1) is the most common form of endometrial cancer.[20] In these well-differentiated lesions, the cells are uniform and have a gland-like pattern.[1] The more uncommon cell types are clear cell carcinoma, secretory carcinoma, and squamous cell carcinoma. There are two varieties of papillary endometrial carcinoma: endometrioid papillary and serous papillary. Both have characteristics of a poorly differentiated carcinoma, with serous papillary carcinoma having the worse prognosis.[1]

CLINICAL PRESENTATION, DIAGNOSIS, STAGING, AND PROGNOSIS

In postmenopausal women, symptoms of early endometrial carcinoma are few.[26] About 90% of patients complain of abnormal vaginal discharge; 90% of these have abnormal bleeding, usually after menopause.[26] A small group of patients (usually thin, elderly, and estrogen deficient) have a purulent vaginal discharge without bleeding as a result of cervical stenosis; these patients also may develop hematometra.[12] Signs of more advanced disease include pelvic pressure and other signs of uterine enlargement or extrauterine tumor spread.[12, 26] Diagnosis of endometrial cancer is more difficult in the premenopausal patient. The health care provider should maintain a high index of suspicion when a woman in this group presents with prolonged, heavy menstrual periods or intermenstrual spotting.[12, 26] Abnormal vaginal bleeding or discharge can occur for many other reasons. The differential diagnosis of endometrial cancer should consider hormonal imbalance, exogenous estrogens, atrophic endometritis or vaginitis, endometrial or cervical polyps, endometrial hyperplasia, cervical cancer, trauma, and urethral carbuncle.[12] The patient with endometrial carcinoma usually is postmenopausal and obese, although about 35% are not obese and are without signs of hyperestrogenism.[22] There usually are no abnormal findings in early stages. If advanced disease is present, the abdominal examination may reveal ascites with palpable hepatic or omental nodules, which represent metastases.[12] The pelvic examination should focus on inspection and palpation of the vulva, vagina, and cervix to rule out metastases and exclude other causes of bleeding.[12] Usually, no significant uterine enlargement is present, but the uterus may be boggy in consistency.[12] A rectovaginal examination is important to determine clinical signs of advanced disease.[12]

All women whose medical history and physical findings are suspicious for endometrial cancer should undergo endocervical curettage and endometrial biopsy at the time of the office visit. Before the cervix is dilated, the endocervix should be curetted; then sounding of the uterus can be done, followed by dilation of the cervix and systematic curetting of the entire endometrial cavity. Sampling procedures such as endometrial biopsy or aspiration curettage plus endocervical sampling are diagnostically definitive if positive for cancer.[20] These techniques can avoid the use of general anesthesia. If the samplings do not yield sufficient diagnostic information, a formal dilation and curettage is warranted.[20] Patients diagnosed with endometrial carcinoma should have a thorough history, physical examination, and pelvic examination and a chest radiograph. Further evaluation with a CT scan, cystoscopy, and proctosigmoidoscopy may be performed if clinically indicated. Laboratory studies should include a complete blood count and biochemical profile including renal and liver function tests and possibly measurement of CA-125.[1]

The FIGO staging classification for corpus cancer was changed from a clinical to a surgical system in 1988.[1] Figure 13–7 illustrates the stages of carcinoma of the endometrium. Staging can be accomplished both clinically and surgically. Clinical staging is determined by the amount of tumor found after a simple diagnostic evaluation; patients considered medically inoperable are clinically staged.[1, 22] The surgical staging system requires evaluation of operative findings. Overall, the prognosis of endometrial adenocarcinoma is excellent if it is diagnosed early and treated with abdominal hysterectomy and bilateral salpingo-oophorectomy.[18] The most important prognostic factors are staging and tumor grade. Another prognostic factor is age at diagnosis; younger women who have less extensive, better-differentiated lesions have improved survival rates.[22] Other prognostic factors are histologic cell type, depth of myometrial invasion, occult extension to the cervix, and invasion of the vascular space. Extrauterine factors include adnexal metastases, intraperitoneal spread to other structures, positive peritoneal cytology, pelvic lymph node metastases, and aortic node involvement.[20, 22, 26] The 5-year survival rate for endometrial cancer stage I is 75.1%; stage II survival is 57.8%; stage III is 30%; and stage IV is 10.6%.[22]

TREATMENT

The therapeutic approach to endometrial cancer is determined by FIGO stage, histologic type and grade, depth of myometrial penetration, and the patient's medical condition.[1] Abdominal hysterectomy with bilateral salpingo-oophorectomy is the treatment of choice.[20] Radiation therapy has an adjuvant role in patients with high-risk, early-stage disease or advanced disease, and in patients with early disease who are medically unsuitable to undergo hysterectomy.[1] Figure 13–8 illustrates treatments and surveillance according to each stage of disease. Patients with stage I or II occult disease who are medically fit should undergo total abdominal hysterectomy and bilateral salpingo-oophorectomy. Adjuvant radiation can reduce the chance of pelvic recurrent disease.[7] There are several treatment regimens that can be selected if the patient's disease requires further treatment after surgery.

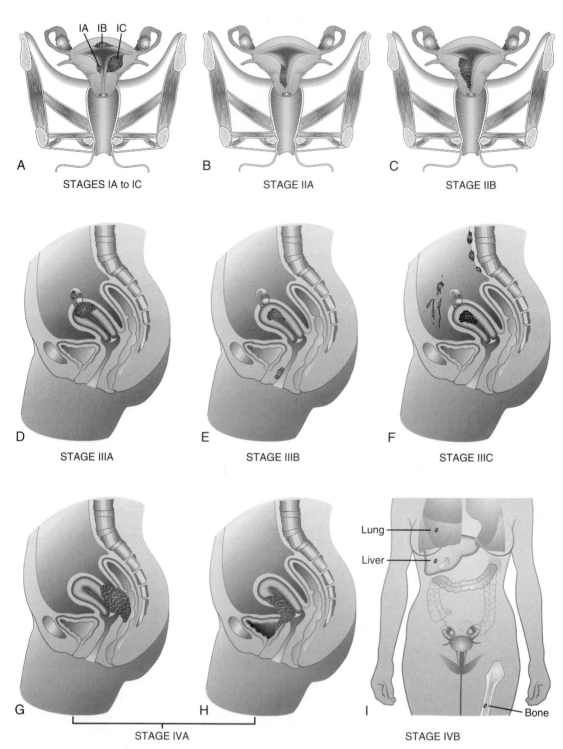

Figure 13–7. Carcinoma of the endometrium by stage. (From Burke TW, Tortolero-Luna G, Malpica A, et al: Endometrial hyperplasia and endometrial cancer. Obstet Gynecol Clin North Am 23:436, 437, 1996.)

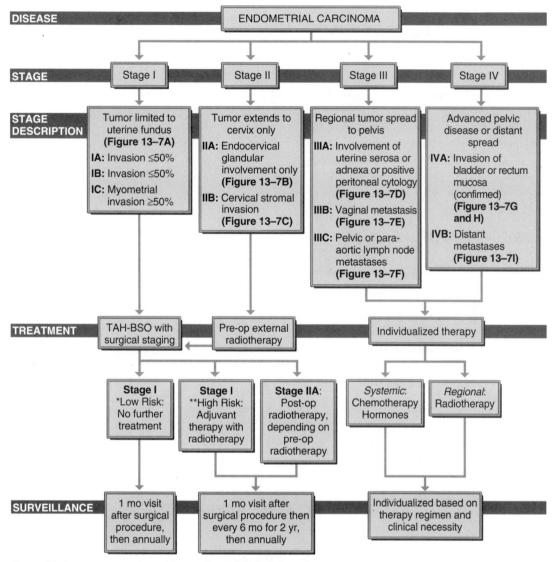

Figure 13–8. Treatment and surveillance of carcinoma of the endometrium by stage. Low-risk category includes stages IA, IB, and IC (grade 1) and stage IA (grade 2); high-risk category includes high grade and/or stage II, III, or IV. TAH-BSO, Total abdominal hysterectomy and bilateral salpingo-oophorectomy.

AFTER-TREATMENT SURVEILLANCE

After-treatment surveillance is dependent on whether further treatment is required. For patients in the low-risk category, a routine follow-up and examination 1 month after surgery, with subsequent annual well-woman examinations, is recommended.[20] High-risk patients require a follow-up examination 1 month after surgery, then a telephone follow-up call every 6 months for 2 years, as well as an annual well-woman examination.[20] If the patient's disease status requires adjuvant treatment such as chemotherapy or radiation, follow-up is individualized.[20]

CANCER PREVENTION AND EARLY DETECTION THROUGH SCREENING

Women with a history of endometrial cancer are at increased risk for developing a second malignancy, such as breast, ovarian, or colon cancer. These women should receive follow-up care that includes careful screening for new cancers and should continue to receive annual pelvic examinations and Pap smears. Screening for endometrial cancer has a role in asymptomatic patients who have no other indications for screening.[20, 26] Information for health care providers regarding prevention and detection of endometrial cancer is useful (Table 13–7). The patient should be kept informed of prevention and detection information (Table 13–8).

CARCINOMA OF THE OVARY

Epithelial ovarian cancer is responsible for more deaths among American women each year than all other gynecologic malignancies combined.[7, 24] The number of deaths from ovarian cancer continues to increase; however, therapeutic advances over the past few decades have begun to extrapolate into improved survival.[24] It is estimated that 75% or more of ovarian cancers are still diagnosed in advanced stages, which leads to a poor prognosis.[24] At comprehensive cancer centers throughout the country, the use of new drugs and innovative high-dose chemotherapy regimens with stem-cell support may make more favorable outcomes a reality.

EPIDEMIOLOGY

About one woman in 70 will develop ovarian cancer in her lifetime, and the disease accounts for about 1% of all deaths in women.[27] In the United States, approximately 26,800 new cases are diagnosed annually and about 14,200 ovarian

---

Table 13–7. Endometrial Cancer Prevention and Detection: Advice to Health Care Providers

Background
  Most common gynecologic malignancy
  Mortality rate is relatively low
  Most cases are confined to uterus at diagnosis (stage I)
  Oral contraceptives may decrease risk
Prevention education and early detection
  Patients receiving postmenopausal estrogen replacement with the uterus in situ should also receive progestational agent
  Continuous-dose estogen and progestin may be better tolerated than cyclical dosing
  No routine screening recommended
  Endometrial biopsy recommended for any postmenopausal woman with bleeding or premenopausal woman with heavy or irregular bleeding
  Endometrial biopsy recommended when endometrial cells seen in Pap smear for postmenopausal patient or when atypical glandular cells seen in Pap smear for premenopausal patient
  Endometrial evaluation, including biopsy, recommended for women still "menstruating" after age 50 years
  Periodic biopsy recommended for postmenopausal women taking estrogens

Pap, Papanicolaou.
From Burke TW, Tortolero-Luna G, Malpica A, et al: Endometrial hyperplasia and endometrial cancer. Obstet Gynecol Clin North Am 23:448, 1996.

Table 13-8. Endometrial Cancer Prevention and Detection: Advice to Patients

Major risk factors
    Known risk factors: age (>60 yr), obesity, exposure to unopposed estrogens (estrogens taken without taking a progestin hormone at the same time), diabetes, hypertension, menstrual irregularities, early age at menarche (first period) and at menopause, nulliparity (not having given birth), personal or family history of breast or colon cancer, use of drug tamoxifen
    Oral contraceptives (if they include progestin) may decrease risk
Most common symptom
    Bleeding after menopause or abnormal bleeding before menopause
Prevention education and early detection
    Maintain proper weight
    Seek expert help for any abnormal bleeding; be persistent

From Burke TW, Tortolero-Luna G, Malpica A, et al: Endometrial hyperplasia and endometrial cancer. Obstet Gynecol Clin North Am 23:449, 1996.

cancer deaths occur.[7, 24, 25] The disease occurs primarily in postmenopausal women, usually between 50 and 75 years of age. Ovarian cancer incidence increases with age and peaks at a rate of 54 per 100,000 persons in the 70- to 74-year-old age group.[7, 24] The median age at diagnosis is 63 years.[7] It appears that the incidence of this disease varies by race, although in many cases the effects of race are difficult to distinguish from the environmental effects of geography, culture, and socioeconomic status.[25] The U.S. age-adjusted rate of ovarian cancer among Caucasians is estimated at 14.2 per 100,000, significantly higher than the estimated rate of 9.3 per 100,000 among U.S. African Americans.[24, 25] The highest rates of ovarian cancer are found in industrialized countries and the lowest rates in underdeveloped nations. Japan, which has one of the world's lowest ovarian cancer rates, is a notable exception.[27] The estimated incidence of ovarian cancer in that country is 3.0 per 100,000.[25]

The cause of ovarian cancer remains unknown; however, a number of hormonal and reproductive, genetic, environmental, and dietary factors have been suggested to have a role.[7, 24, 25, 27] It appears that ovarian and breast cancers share some etiologic factors. Women with breast cancer have twice the risk of ovarian cancer, and those with ovarian cancer have a threefold to fourfold increased incidence of subsequent breast cancer.[27] Some clear associations have been noted between certain hormonal and reproductive factors and the risk of ovarian cancer. A higher incidence of epithelial ovarian cancer has been associated with a lower mean number of pregnancies, nulliparity, decreased fertility, and delayed childbearing.[7, 24, 25, 27] No association has yet been established between postmenopausal hormone replacement therapy and ovarian cancer development; however, evidence suggests that treatment with ovulation-inducing drugs, particularly for prolonged periods, may confer an increased risk.[25] Oral contraceptives have been demonstrated to have a marked protective effect against ovarian cancer, with users having a risk about half that of nonusers. The routine use of oral contraceptives may prevent as many as 2,000 cases of ovarian cancer in the United States annually.[25] This protective effect seems to persist years after discontinuation of these contraceptives.[25] It has for some time been recognized that women with a family history of gynecologic cancer, particularly ovarian or endometrial, are at increased risk for ovarian cancer.[25] More recently, three distinct autosomal-dominant gene syndromes of hereditary cancer involving the ovaries have been defined: site-specific ovarian cancer, breast-ovarian cancer syndrome, and Lynch II syndrome (a combination of Lynch I hereditary colon cancer and endometrial, breast, and ovarian cancer clusters in first- and second-degree relatives).[27] True hereditary ovarian cancer accounts for only 5% to 10% of all ovarian cancer cases.[25]

Epidemiologic evidence strongly suggests a role for environmental factors in the origin of ovarian cancer, but the data are inconclusive. Exposure to talc used as a dusting powder or to asbestos has been linked with an increased risk in some studies. The association of ovarian cancer risk with exposure to ionizing radiation has not been conclusively demonstrated.[25] Likewise, no clear effect of viral agents on ovarian cancer risk has been shown.[25] Dietary factors associated with an increased risk of ovarian cancer include a high consumption of animal fat and a high dietary intake of lactose in women with transferase abnormalities.[25, 27] No definitive risk has been associated with use of coffee, tobacco, or alcohol.[25, 27]

NATURAL HISTORY AND PATTERNS OF SPREAD

Most ovarian malignancies (80% to 90%) are epithelial carcinomas; the remainder arise from germ or stromal cells.[27] The surface epithelium or serosa of the ovaries gives rise to epithelial tumors.

Dissemination of epithelial tumors usually occurs by surface shedding, lymphatic spread, or hematogenous metastasis.[7] Tumors frequently spread by continuity and intraperitoneal dissemination. In disease that is clinically confined to one ovary, spread to the opposite ovary occurs in 6% to 13% of patients, and transperitoneal tumor implantation and lymphatic spread to the uterus and fallopian tubes occurs in 5% of patients.[27] The uterus is involved in 25% of patients with more advanced disease.[27] Transperitoneal dissemination is the most common type of extraovarian spread. This involves the shedding of free tumor cells from gross or microscopic tumor outgrowths on the primary tumor surface.[27] Exfoliated clonogenic cells attach to the peritoneal surfaces, form micrometastases, and continue to exfoliate clonogenic cells, which exit the peritoneal cavity via the diaphragmatic lymphatic channels.[27] Clearance is more extensive on the right side, where there is a flow of peritoneal fluid along the abdominal gutters into the submesothelial lymphatic capillaries of the diaphragm. Tumor cell obstruction of these lymphatics allows implantation on the omentum or at other sites or may cause accumulation of carcinomatous ascites.[27] Autopsy studies of patients who die of ovarian carcinoma almost always show omental involvement.[27] The ovarian lymphatic system is an important pathway of spread of this cancer.[27]

The most common sites of spread in ovarian cancer are the omentum, peritoneum, bowel surfaces, and retroperitoneal lymph nodes. Other organs sometimes involved, in order of decreasing frequency, are the liver, lungs, pleura, kidneys, bone, adrenals, bladder, and spleen.[27]

PATHOLOGY/HISTOLOGY

The ovary can give rise to a variety of neoplasms, each having a distinct embryologic origin and a differing histologic appearance. Most ovarian malignancies are epithelial in origin, arising from cells on the surface of the ovary; the remainder arise from the ovarian stroma or the ovarian primordial germ cells.[25] The type of tumor cell has less prognostic significance than do stage, volume of disease, and histologic grade. Epithelial tumors may be benign, malignant (invasive), or of low malignant potential (borderline malignant). Five- and 10-year survival rates of 93% and 91%, respectively, have been reported for patients with borderline tumors, compared with 34% and 29%, respectively, for patients with invasive epithelial carcinomas. Adenocarcinomas are also classified by degree of histologic differentiation. Tumors having clearcut glandular features are grade 1, or well differentiated; tumors made up mainly of solid sheets of tumor are grade 3, or poorly differentiated; tumors showing both glandular and solid areas are grade 2. There appears to be a rough correlation between the tumor's histologic grade and its biologic aggressiveness.[25]

Germ cell tumors account for fewer than 5% of ovarian malignancies, but they are important because they have an unusual natural history, occur in young women, and require different treatment from common epithelial ovarian cancers. Dysgerminoma, endodermal sinus tumor, and embryonal carcinoma are the most frequently encountered germ cell tumors; the latter two are highly aggressive and metastasize hematogenously.[27]

CLINICAL PRESENTATION, DIAGNOSIS, STAGING, AND PROGNOSIS

In its early stages, ovarian cancer may be a totally insidious disease, without specific signs or symptoms. Vague symptoms such as dyspepsia, nausea, and lower abdominal discomfort are frequently ignored by both the patient and her doctor.[27] The cancer may grow to 10 to 12 cm before its size produces symptoms of rectal pressure and urinary frequency.[27] Early ovarian cancers may be detected as a pelvic mass during a routine pelvic examination. Large pelvic masses may produce bladder or rectal symptoms such as constipation, urinary frequency, and pelvic pressure.[24, 25] Patients may have abdominal bloating or swelling if ascites is present.[25] The ascites can be detected by physical examination or imaging studies. Weight gain is noted although food intake has declined; both effects are secondary to fluid retention and to significant ascites. On occasion, there may be respiratory distress from a large pleural effusion.[25]

The ovary is situated in a spacious pelvic cavity and is loosely suspended by the ovarian and infundibulopelvic ligaments. All women with pelvic or abdominal symptoms, particularly perimenopausal or postmenopausal women, should undergo a thorough physical and pelvic examination, including careful evaluation of the adnexal area.[27] At initial assessment, a pelvic or pelvic-abdominal mass can be palpated in the majority of women with ovarian cancer.[4, 27] The physical examination should focus on a survey of the lymph nodes, which are occasional sites of metastases.[7, 24] Several characteristics of the pelvic mass may assist the health care provider in assessing the situation. A benign ovarian mass tends to be cystic, smooth, unilateral, and mobile, whereas a malignant mass tends to be solid, nodular, and immobile, or fixed.[4, 7, 24] Determining whether ascites is present could also assist in making the appropriate working diagnosis of a malignant mass. If ascites is present without a mass, other malignancies (e.g., colon, pancreas, stomach, breast, or liver cancer) should be considered.[4, 7, 24] If the abdominal examination reveals tumor nodules in the area of the umbilicus or midabdomen, it could represent metastasis to the omentum.[7, 24] The initial evaluation of a patient with suspected ovarian cancer should consist of CA-125 blood test, chest radiograph, and ultrasound. CT scan of abdomen and pelvis and a barium enema should be performed if clinically indicated.[7, 25, 27] Referral to a gynecologic oncology specialist for an extensive evaluation is of utmost importance for a definitive diagnosis and treatment plan.

The diagnosis usually is made by histopathologic study after exploratory laparotomy.[27] An adnexal mass in a premenarchal girl or in a postmenopausal woman usually warrants exploratory laparotomy, because functional ovarian cysts in these age groups should not occur and a mass may indicate malignancy. A palpable ovary in a postmenopausal woman may signal ovarian enlargement (especially greater than 4 to 6 cm), which should be checked by ultrasound.[27] During a woman's reproductive years, ovarian enlargement is usually benign. These patients can be monitored with a repeat pelvic examination and pelvic or vaginal probe, transvaginal ultrasound, and color-flow Doppler studies at 4- to 6-week intervals. Ultrasound can be used to assess intrapelvic disease.[27] As yet, tumor markers have not proved useful for detection of early ovarian tumors, although they have shown some value, particularly for detection of postoperative residual

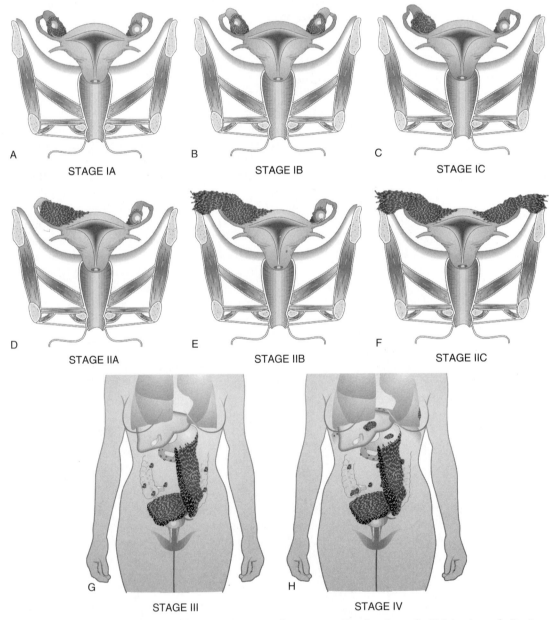

Figure 13–9. Carcinoma of the ovary by stage. (From Gershenson DM, Tortolero-Luna G, Malpica A, et al: Ovarian intraepithelial neoplasia and ovarian cancer. Obstet Gynecol Clin North Am 23:504, 505, 1996.)

Table 13–9. Ovarian Cancer Prevention and Detection: Advice to Health Care Providers

Background
   High mortality rate is due to difficulty of detecting in early stages; tends to be asymptomatic in early stages or to have nonspecific symptoms (vague abdominal discomfort, nausea, or gas)
   Risk factors include low parity; little oral contraceptive use; infertility; and most significantly, a strong family history of ovarian or related cancers
   Symptoms in early stages of diseases are nonspecific, such as abdominal discomfort, bloating, nausea, gas; in later stages, there may be abdominal swelling and pain
Prevention education and early detection
   No routine screening recommended
   In symptomatic women, perform rectovaginal pelvic examination to rule out ovarian mass
   Teach breast self-examination
   Closely monitor high-risk women, i.e., women with known or suspected family history of ovarian cancer; recommend use of oral hormone contraception when pregnancies not undertaken; evaluate early any pelvic symptoms; perform periodic mammography, breast examination, and fecal occult blood tests; refer patient to specialty center if screening tests become available
   Prophylactic oophorectomy after childbearing may be suggested for women at particularly high risk

From Gershenson DM, Tortolero-Luna G, Malpica A, et al: Ovarian intraepithelial neoplasia and ovarian cancer. Obstet Gynecol Clin North Am 23:529, 1996.

or recurrent disease. Carcinoembryonic antigen is elevated in more than half of patients with stage III epithelial ovarian cancer.[27] CA-125 is not useful as an ovarian cancer screening tool, because only about 50% of patients with clinically detectable ovarian cancer have increased levels of CA-125. However, CA-125 elevation may precede the appearance of ovarian cancer or its recurrence in patients receiving follow-up after primary therapy.[27] Other conditions associated with increased levels of CA-125 include liver disease and early pregnancy.[7, 24]

The FIGO staging system for ovarian cancer is illustrated in Figure 13–9. This system is based on the results of a properly performed exploratory laparotomy, which is of key importance in view of the problems with inadequate surgical staging.[25] The surgical staging of ovarian cancer is based on an understanding of the patterns of disease spread; staging must be thorough and systematic. Several factors affect the prognosis in ovarian cancer. Possibly the most important factor is disease stage; when properly determined, this factor has strong prognostic significance. The distribution of ovarian cancer cases by disease stage is 26% for stage I, 15% for stage II, 42% for stage III, and 17% for stage IV disease.[25] In general, the lower the volume of disease present at diagnosis, the more favorable the prognosis.[7, 24] The amount of residual tumor after the initial surgery is also of great importance in patients with advanced disease. Although the 5-year survival rate for patients with stage III disease and minimal or no residual tumor is 30% to 50%, stage III disease patients with a residual bulky tumor may have a 5-year survival rate of only 10%.[25] The histologic grade of the tumor has been found to have prognostic significance in early and advanced disease, but histologic cell type is of less significance.[25] Work is continuing to identify molecular markers that are prognostic for ovarian cancer. *ERBB2, p53, ras,* and other genes and oncogenes have been examined, but results have been variable.[25] Another factor demonstrated to have prognostic significance is the age of the patient. Considering all disease stages, the overall 5-year survival rate for women younger than 50 years old with ovarian cancer is 40%, compared with 15% for older women. However, a confounding variable affecting this difference may be that younger women have a higher incidence of low-grade tumors, which are

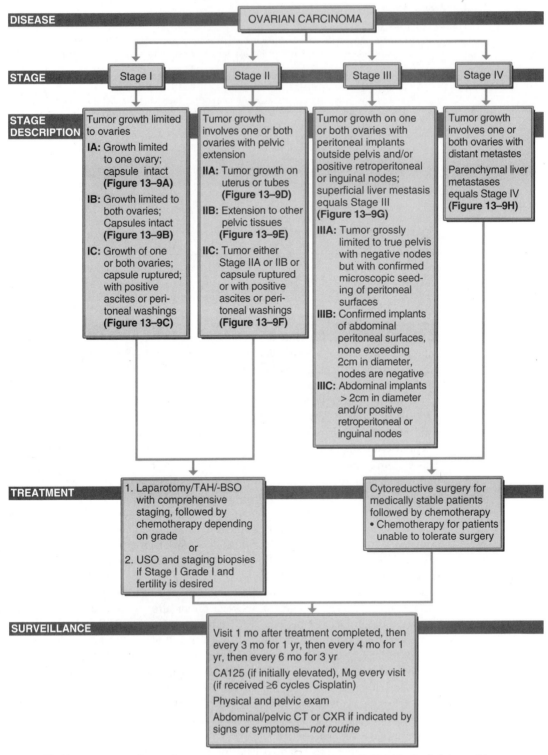

Figure 13–10. Treatment and surveillance of carcinoma of the ovary by stage. TAH-BSO, Total abdominal hysterectomy and bilateral salpingo-oophorectomy; BSO, bilateral salpingo-oophorectomy.

more amenable to treatment. A pretreatment Karnofsky performance status score of less than 70 is another finding associated with a shorter survival time.[7, 24]

TREATMENT

Surgery plays a pivotal role in the treatment of ovarian cancer and, when incorporated into a multidisciplinary regimen, affords the best chance of a favorable prognosis. Because ovarian cancer often involves dissemination of tumor throughout the abdominal cavity, surgery alone usually is not curative, and additional treatment is required.[25] Each stage of disease is treated by a different regimen. Figure 13–10 presents treatment plans according to the stage of disease. Postoperative chemotherapy is standard for all patients with advanced disease and for many with early-stage disease. Adjuvant chemotherapy, particularly with platinum- and paclitaxel-based regimens, can significantly prolong survival.[7, 25] Radiation therapy has a long history of use in ovarian carcinoma; nevertheless, data from comparative studies with chemotherapy are insufficient, and radiation therapy's current role—whether as upfront, combined modality, salvage, or palliative therapy—is unclear.[25]

AFTER-TREATMENT SURVEILLANCE

The surveillance plan must be individualized based on the stage of disease. For women with early-stage disease, routine examinations should be done every 3 months for 1 year, then every 4 months for 1 year, and then every 6 months for 1 year. After adjuvant treatment, an individualized approach must be considered pending clinical necessity.

CANCER PREVENTION AND EARLY DETECTION THROUGH SCREENING

No effective strategy exists for screening of the general population for ovarian cancer.[7] Helpful information on prevention and detection of ovarian cancer is available for both the health care provider (Table 13–9) and the patient (Table 13–10). Routine screening is not recommended, because the high rate of false-

---

Table 13–10. Ovarian Cancer Prevention and Detection: Advice to Patients

Major risk factors
    Known risk factors: Age (>60 yr); nulliparity or low parity (few or no live births);
       personal history of endometrial or breast cancer; family history of ovarian cancer
    Suspected risk factors: infertility
Most common symptoms
    Symptoms in early stages of disease are nonspecific, such as abdominal discomfort,
       bloating, nausea, gas
    In later stages, there may be abdominal swelling and pain
Prevention education and early detection
    Seek expert help for any persistent unexplained pelvic pain; be persistent
    If in high-risk group, get periodic gynecologic examinations and perform monthly breast
       self-examination
    Keep weight in healthy range to facilitate examination

From Gershenson DM, Tortolero-Luna G, Malpica A, et al: Ovarian intraepithelial neoplasia and ovarian cancer. Obstet Gynecol Clin North Am 23:530, 1996.

positive results leads to unnecessary invasive procedures.[25] A well-woman examination should be recommended as the annual follow-up procedure.

REFERENCES

1. Hoskins JW, Perez A, Young RC: Gynecologic tumors. In DeVita VT Jr, Hellman S, Rosenberg SA (eds): Cancer: Principles and Practice of Oncology, 4th ed. Philadelphia, JB Lippincott, 1993:1152–1225.
2. American Cancer Society. Cancer statistics. Cancer 1997;47:1.
3. Wingo PA, Tong T, Bolden S: Cancer statistics, 1995. CA Cancer J Clin 1995;45:8.
4. Ravnikar VA: Preface. Primary care of the mature woman. Obstet Gynecol Clin North Am 1994;21:9.
5. Morris, M, Tortolero-Luna G, Malpica A, et al: Cervical intraepithelial neoplasia and cervical cancer. Obstet Gynecol Clin North Am 1996;23:2.
6. Parkin DM, Pisani P, Ferlay J: Estimates of the worldwide incidence of eighteen major cancers in 1985. Int J Cancer 1993;54:594.
7. Gershenson DM, Tortolero-Luna G, Malpica A, et al: Ovarian intraepithelial neoplasia and ovarian cancer. Obstet Gynecol Clin North Am 1996;23:2.
8. Ansink AC, Heintz AP: Epidemiology and etiology of squamous cell carcinoma of the vulva. Eur J Obstet Gynaecol Reprod Biol 1993;48:111.
9. Homesley HD, Bundy BN, Sedlis A, et al: Assessment of current International Federation of Gynecology and Obstetrics staging of vulvar carcinoma relative to prognostic factors for survival. Am J Obstet Gynecol 1991;164:997–1004.
10. Gazaway PM, Huggins GR: Early detection of gynecological malignancy. In Barker LR, Burton JR, Zieve PD (eds): Principles of Ambulatory Medicine. Baltimore, Williams & Wilkins, 1995:1394.
11. Mitchell MF, Prasad CJ, Sila E, et al: Second genital primary squamous neoplasms in vulvarcarcinoma: Viral and histopathologic correlates. Obstet Gynecol 1993;81:13.
12. Berek JS, Hacker NF: Practical Gynecologic Oncology, rev. ed. Baltimore, Williams & Wilkins, 1989.
13. Gordan AN: Vulvar neoplasms. In Copeland LJ (ed): Textbook of Gynecology. Philadelphia, WB Saunders, 1993:1096–1116.
14. Edwards CL, Tortolero-Luna G, Linares A, et al: Vulvar intraepithelial neoplasia and vulvar cancer. Obstet Gynecol Clin North Am 1996;23:(2).
15. Walczak JR, Lkemm PR: Gynecologic cancers. In Groenwald SL, Hansen Frogge M, Goodman M, Henke-Yarbro C (eds): Cancer Nursing Principles and Practice. Boston, Jones and Bartlett, 1993:1065.
16. Henson D, Tarone R: An epidemiologic study of cancer of the cervix, vagina, and vulva based on the Third National Cancer Survey in the United States. Am J Obstet Gynecol 1977;129:525.
17. Wharton JT, Tortolero-Luna G, Linares A, et al: Vaginal intraepithelial neoplasia and vaginal cancer. Obstet Gynecol Clin North Am 1996;23:(2).
18. Burke T, Morris M: Cervical cancer. In Copeland LJ (ed): Textbook of Gynecology. Philadelphia, WB Saunders, 1993:989–1013.
19. Perez CA, Gershell DJ, McGuire WP, Morris M: Vagina. In WJ Hoskins, CA Perez, RC Young (eds): Principles and Practice of Gynecologic Oncology. Philadelphia, JB Lippincott, 1997:753–784.
20. Burke TW, Tortolero-Luna G, Malpica A, et al: Endometrial hyperplasia and endometrial cancer. Obstet Gynecol Clin North Am 1996;23:(2).
21. Coleman MP, Esteve J, Damiecki P, et al: Trends in cancer incidence and mortality. IARC Sci Publ 1993;121:1.
22. Barakat RR, Park RC, Grigsby PW, Muss HD, Norris HJ: Corpus epithelial tumors. In WJ Hoskins, CA Perez, RC Young (eds): Principles and Practice of Gynecologic Oncology. Philadelphia, JB Lippincott, 1997:859–896.
23. Stehman FB, Perez CA, Kurman RJ, Thigpen JT: Uterine cervix. In WJ Hoskins, CA Perez, RC Young (eds): Principles and Practice of Gynecologic Oncology. Philadelphia, JB Lippincott, 1997:785–858.
24. Ozols RF, Rubin SC, Thomas G, Robboy S: Epithelial ovarian cancer. In WJ Hoskins, CA Perez, RC Young (eds): Principles and Practice of Gynecologic Oncology. Philadelphia, JB Lippincott, 1997:919–986.
25. Rubin SC, Fennelly D, Randall ME: Ovarian cancer. In Pazdur R, Coia LR, Hoskins WJ, Wagman LD (eds): Cancer Management: A Multidisciplinary Approach. Huntington, NY, PRR, 1996:185–204.
26. Barakat RR, Greven K, Muss HB: Endometrial cancer. In Pazdur R, Coia LR, Hoskins WJ, Wagman LD (eds): Cancer Management: A Multidisciplinary Approach. Huntington, NY, PRR, 1996:168–184.
27. Young RC, Perez CA, Hoskins WJ: Cancer of the ovary. In DeVita VT Jr, Hellman S, Rosenberg SA (eds): Cancer: Principles and Practice of Oncology, 4th ed. Philadelphia, JB Lippincott, 1993:1226–1264.

Chapter 14

Bone Tumors

Laura A. Murphy-Fertak, BS, PA-C, and
Alan W. Yasko, MD

Primary bone tumors are rare. Because of their rarity, few clinicians consider them in the differential diagnosis of musculoskeletal complaints. These tumors are best managed with a multidisciplinary team of experts from the fields of orthopedic surgical oncology, pediatric and adult medical oncology, pathology, radiology, physical medicine, and nursing. Current treatment approaches have evolved over the past several decades with the emergence of effective chemotherapy regimens for malignant tumors, advances in diagnostic imaging technology, and improvements in reconstructive techniques. Recent advances in the treatment of these tumors and continued encouraging results reflect the success of the team approach for optimization of patient outcome.

The following is an overview of common benign and malignant bone tumors, their clinical and radiographic presentation and treatment.

EVALUATION, DIAGNOSIS, AND STAGING

Bone tumors are an extremely heterogeneous group of neoplasms (Table 14–1). The diagnosis of bone tumors is based on clinical, radiographic, and histologic evaluation. The patient history and physical examination are critical for assembling a differential diagnosis for patients who present with musculoskeletal complaints. Most patients seek medical attention because of pain. The character of the pain varies depending on the pathologic process, the site and extent of involvement, and the presence of impending or established pathologic fracture. Pain is usually localized, dull and continuous, deep-seated, present at rest and at night, and is usually exacerbated by motion or weight bearing of the affected limb. Commonly, recent trauma prompts medical attention, at which time the underlying neoplasm is detected. Localized soft tissue swelling, when present, is usually associated with tenderness and a palpable firm, deep, fixed mass. Perilesional inflammation induced by the tumor may result in soft tissue edema, synovitis, and joint effusion that may compromise the range of motion of the affected extremity.

The initial evaluation of any presenting musculoskeletal complaint should

Table 14-1. Common Bone Tumors

TUMOR	BENIGN	MALIGNANT
Bone	Osteoid osteoma Osteoblastoma	Osteosarcoma
Cartilage	Osteochondroma Enchondroma Chondroblastoma	Chondrosarcoma
Fibrous	Nonossifying fibroma Fibrous dysplasia	Malignant fibrous histiocytoma
Miscellaneous	Giant cell tumor Hemangioma Langerhans cell histiocytosis (eosinophilic granuloma) Unicameral bone cyst Aneurysmal bone cyst	Ewing's sarcoma Chordoma Adamantinoma Lymphoma Multiple myeloma
Imitators of bone tumors	Osteomyelitis Paget's disease of bone Stress fracture Brown tumor Bone infarct	

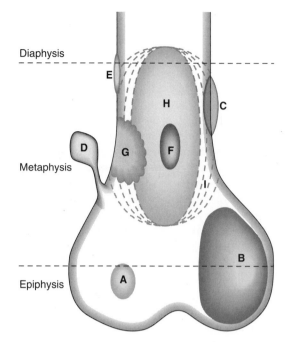

Figure 14–1. Benign bone tumors. *A,* chondroblastoma; *B,* giant cell tumor; *C,* aneurysmal bone cyst; *D,* osteochondroma; *E,* osteoid osteoma; *F,* enchondroma; *G,* nonossifying fibroma; *H,* fibrous dysplasia; *I,* unicameral bone cyst.

include conventional radiographs. Biplanar radiographs reveal the anatomic location of the abnormality within the affected bone and its relation to adjacent bone, the joint and soft tissue structures, the pattern of bone destruction (Figs. 14–1 and 14–2), the characteristics of a periosteal reaction, matrix production

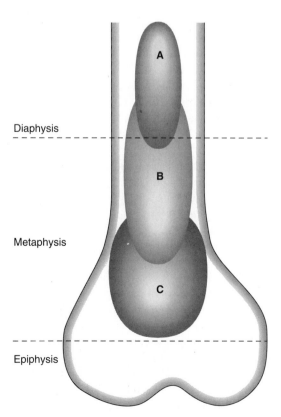

Figure 14–2. Malignant tumors. *A,* Ewing's sarcoma; *B,* chondrosarcoma; *C,* osteosarcoma. Metastatic bone disease may occur at any location.

within the lesion, and the presence of a soft tissue mass. Commonly the diagnosis of a primary neoplasm can be made presumptively on the basis of this clinical and radiographic evaluation; however, other studies are usually indicated to define more clearly the local and systemic extent of disease. These staging studies usually include computed tomography (CT) and magnetic resonance imaging (MRI) of the affected bone, a technetium 99m bone scan, and a chest radiograph and CT scan of the chest (for patients with malignant neoplasms).

The CT scan provides valuable information regarding the response of the bone to the tumor and provides excellent detail of tumor-induced changes in the cortical and cancellous bone and extent of mineralization within the lesion and surrounding soft tissues. MRI complements the CT scan by demonstrating the relational anatomy between normal and diseased tissues. The extent of bone marrow and soft tissue involvement are optimally visualized by this technique. The relation of the tumor to adjacent neural, vascular, and joint structures are best delineated by MRI. Cross-sectional images afforded by CT and MRI are critical to delineate the local extent of the disease for tumors arising in the spine and pelvis.

Technetium 99m bone scans are performed primarily to screen the skeleton for other osseous sites of involvement and early detection of skeletal metastases for malignant lesions. A radiographic skeletal survey is more appropriate than a bone scan to screen the skeleton for certain diseases, such as hereditary multiple exostosis and Langerhans cell histiocytosis (LCH). Chest radiographs are necessary to complete the staging evaluation for all bone sarcomas and certain benign tumors to detect pulmonary metastases. A CT is performed on all patients with high-grade bone sarcomas.

Peripheral blood studies have limited value in the evaluation of patients with primary bone neoplasms. Commonly, alkaline phosphatase and lactate dehydrogenase are elevated in osteosarcoma and Ewing's sarcoma, respectively. A sedimentation rate and leukocyte count may be helpful in patients for whom osteomyelitis is in the differential diagnosis.

The biopsy is a critical step in the diagnosis of primary bone neoplasms. Essential for a successful biopsy is a working knowledge of bone neoplasms and their treatment. The biopsy may be performed as a surgical (open) or percutaneous (closed) procedure. Currently, most tumors are biopsied by a surgical procedure. The biopsy must be placed appropriately and performed properly to optimize the yield of diagnostic tissue and not compromise the definitive surgical procedure for malignant tumors. Longitudinal skin incisions, limited tissue flaps, meticulous hemostasis, and avoidance of the joint and the plane of adjacent neurovascular structures are recommended. Biopsy-related problems occur more frequently when the biopsy is performed at the referring institution than when it is performed at the center where the definitive surgical resection is to be performed.[1]

Experience with percutaneous biopsy at large referral centers has resulted in a growing application of fine-needle aspiration and cutting core biopsy for the diagnosis of bone lesions. This minimally invasive procedure has been shown to be a safe, highly accurate, and economic diagnostic method when performed by experts in percutaneous musculoskeletal biopsy techniques. The accuracy of percutaneous biopsy has reached 90% in some centers[2] but remains highly variable overall, reflecting the level of clinical experience and cytopathologic expertise available to diagnose these rare neoplasms. The tissue specimen may be processed for standard histologic and cytologic preparations, immunohistochemical studies, electron microscopy, flow cytometry, and molecular studies as indicated. The histopathologic diagnosis should always be interpreted in the context of the clinical presentation and radiographic features of the primary lesion.

Bone tumors are staged by the system of the Musculoskeletal Tumor Society (Table 14–2).[3] For malignant tumors, the stage is determined by tumor grade (I, low-grade; II, high-grade), tumor extent (A, intraosseous involvement only; B, extraosseous extension), and presence of distant metastases (III). Patients with localized tumor may have stage IA, IB, IIA, or IIB disease. The presence of metastasis, regardless of the extent of the local disease, represents stage III disease. For benign tumors, the stage of the lesion is determined by its level of activity as defined by its radiographic characteristics: latent (stage 1), active (stage 2), and aggressive (stage 3).

The management approach to bone tumors depends largely on the diagnosis. Most high-grade malignant primary bone tumors require a multimodality treatment strategy which includes chemotherapy, surgery, and, occasionally, radiotherapy. Benign tumors usually are treated by surgery alone. The primary objective in the treatment of metastatic lesions to bone and multiple myeloma is palliation.

BENIGN BONE TUMORS

Benign tumors may arise from any cellular constituent in bone, including osteogenic, chondrogenic, histiocytic, and fibrohistiocytic elements. The treatment recommendations for benign bone tumors reflect the diverse biology of these tumors, from behavior characterized by relative quiescence to destructive aggressiveness. Treatment must be individualized for each patient based on the patient's age, the site and extent of involvement, and the proximity to growth plates and joint structures. In general the objectives of treatment of benign bone neoplasms are (1) local tumor control; (2) preservation of bone stock, growth plates, and adjacent joint; and (3) maintenance of normal extremity function. Intralesional excision by curettage is satisfactory to provide local tumor control in almost all patients. Reconstruction alternatives of the resultant osseous defect include autogenous bone graft, allograft preparations, bone cement (polymethylmethacrylate), and, more recently, bone graft substitutes.

The surgical staging system adopted by the Musculoskeletal Tumor Society defines three stages for benign bone tumors. Stage 1 benign tumors are latent lesions that demonstrate limited local growth and have no metastatic potential. They commonly are asymptomatic and often are discovered incidentally. These lesions may be observed or treated by intralesional excision with curettage. Stage 2 benign tumors are active lesions. They usually cause symptoms that prompt medical evaluation. The treatment usually is intralesional excision by curettage.

Table 14–2. Surgical Staging of Bone Sarcomas

STAGE	HISTOLOGIC GRADE	TUMOR EXTENT
IA	Low grade	Tumor is contained within bone
IB	Low grade	Tumor extends into soft tissues
IIA	High grade	Tumor is contained within bone
IIB	High grade	Tumor extends into soft tissues
III	Any grade	Metastatic disease is present

Data from Enneking WF, Spanier SS, Goodman MA: A system for the surgical staging of musculoskeletal sarcoma. Clin Orthop 1980;153:106–120.

These lesions may recur locally. Stage 3 benign tumors are aggressive lesions that often destroy the adjacent osseous tissue and extend into the surrounding soft tissues. Distant metastases can develop in rare instances. The most reliable means of achieving local control is by en bloc excision. This usually necessitates sacrifice of adjacent normal bone stock or resection of an adjacent joint, or both. To obviate such disability, curettage and an effective adjuvant therapy may be used, recognizing that the potential for recurrence is increased over that which would be obtained by an en bloc excision.

OSTEOCHONDROMA

Osteochondromas are the most common primary benign lesions of bone.[4] Osteochondromas are not neoplastic but rather represent an aberrancy of growth cartilage which results in a protruding bony mass. At presentation, most osteochondromas appear as a solitary mass; a peak incidence is observed in skeletally immature patients during the second decade. Males are more commonly affected than females. Osteochondromas arise in the region of growth plates in the long bones, pelvis, and spine. The most common sites include the distal femur, proximal humerus, proximal tibia, and proximal femur. They usually are asymptomatic unless there is associated nerve compression, mechanical irritation of overlying soft tissues, or bursa formation. Plain films show a bony excrescence arising near the end of a long bone in the metaphysis near the growth plate that projects away from the joint (Fig. 14–3). A CT scan is helpful to confirm bony continuity of the medullary canal of the bone with the osteochondroma. Osteochondromas may be pedunculated (narrow, stalked) or sessile (flat, broad). Osteochondromas exhibit growth in concordance with the skeletal growth pattern of the patient. They cease to grow when the patient reaches skeletal maturity. Growth of an osteochondroma after maturity may indicate malignant transformation of the cartilage component to a chondrosarcoma (<1% of cases).[4] Chondrosarcomatous transformation usually occurs in the third or fourth decade and is observed most commonly in osteochondromas of the pelvis.

Most extremity osteochondromas are treated by observation only. Surgery is

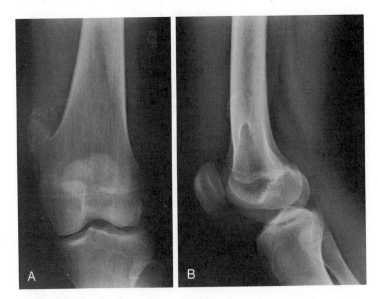

Figure 14–3. Osteochondroma. Anteroposterior (*A*) and lateral (*B*) radiographs of an osteochondroma involving the distal femur. The osteochondroma projects away from the joint. The intramedullary canal of the distal femur is in continuity with that of the osteochondroma (© The University of Texas M. D. Anderson Cancer Center.)

recommended if an osteochondroma is symptomatic, if it involves the bones of the pelvis, or if the clinician suspects chondrosarcomatous transformation. Patients can present with multiple osteochondromas (multiple hereditary exostosis). This is an autosomal dominant condition with a prevalence of at least 1 in 50,000. The risk of chondrosarcomatous transformation in these patients is approximately 1%.

OSTEOID OSTEOMA

Osteoid osteomas are bone-forming lesions that account for approximately 13% of benign bone tumors.[4] Osteoid osteomas most commonly occur in patients between the ages of 10 and 15 years; approximately 90% are found in patients younger than 30 years of age. The male-to-female ratio is 2:1. Any bone may be involved, but more than 50% of these tumors occur in the femur or tibia. Local pain, characteristically occurring at night and associated with swelling and tenderness, is a common presenting symptom. Frequently the pain is relieved with salicylates. Plain radiographs typically show a central, well-demarcated, oval or round, lucent nidus (<1 cm) surrounded by a variable amount of dense, sclerotic, reactive bone (Fig. 14–4). A CT scan may delineate the nidus better than plain films. Treatment includes surgical excision of the nidus. Recurrence is rare unless the nidus is incompletely excised.[5] Nonsurgical treatment with long-standing oral nonsteroidal anti-inflammatory agents has been reported as an alternative to surgical excision, but years may be required for successful treatment. [6]

OSTEOBLASTOMA

Osteoblastomas, although histologically similar to osteoid osteomas, are much less common. They account for approximately 3% of benign bone tumors.[4] The age and sex distributions are similar to those of osteoid osteoma. Osteoblastomas have a predilection for the axial skeleton (posterior elements of the spine) and the long bones. Typically, patients present with insidious, dull pain that is less severe than that observed with osteoid osteomas. Symptomatic relief with salicylates is inconsistent. Plain radiographs usually reveal a radiolucent, eccentric, well circumscribed, expansile lesion (>2 cm). Osteoblastomas have less reactive bone formation than do osteoid osteomas. A CT scan delineates the lesion more precisely. The treatment is surgical excision by curettage with or without autologous bone grafting. The recurrence rate is 5% to 10%.[5]

GIANT CELL TUMOR

Giant cell tumors (GCTs) account for approximately 20% of benign bone tumors.[4] GCTs occur most frequently in the third decade and have a 3:2 predominance in females. The distal femur and proximal tibia are the sites of approximately 50% of GCTs, followed by the distal radius and proximal humerus. Signs and symptoms include pain, localized soft tissue swelling, and occasionally a joint effusion. Plain radiographs usually demonstrate an eccentric, lytic lesion

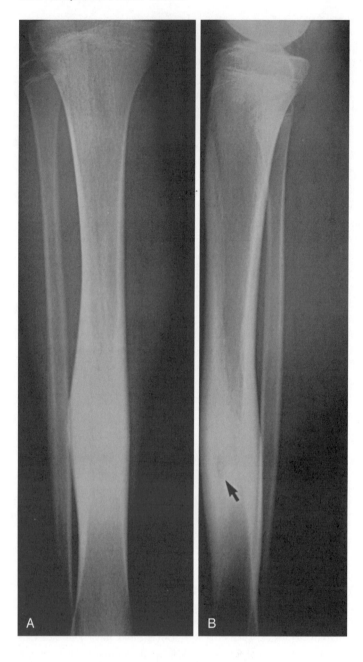

Figure 14–4. Osteoid osteoma. Antero-posterior *(A)* and lateral *(B)* radiograph of the tibia and fibula. Arrow on the lateral view marks the lytic nidus within the shaft of the tibia. Note the cortical reaction resulting in marked new bone formation about the osteoid osteoma nidus. (© The University of Texas M. D. Anderson Cancer Center.)

in the metaphyseal-epiphyseal region which extends to the subchondral bone underlying the articular cartilage of the adjacent joint (Fig. 14–5). There may be cortical expansion, thinning, and soft tissue extension. Treatment usually consists of surgical excision by curettage; the resultant cavitary defect is reconstructed with bone cement. Because these tumors exhibit locally aggressive behavior characterized by a high local recurrence rate, physical or chemical adjuvant therapies have been used to improve local tumor control. If extensive bone destruction has occurred, resection of the involved bone and adjacent joint may be necessary; the bond defect and joint are reconstructed with a segmental prosthesis, osteoarticular allograft, or segmental allograft for joint fusion (arthrodesis). For unresectable lesions, (e.g., patients with extensive sacral tumors), transcatheter arterial embolization or radiotherapy may be used.

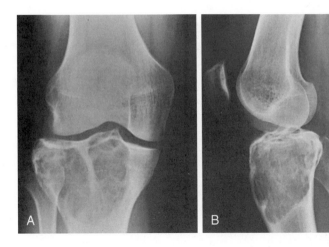

Figure 14–5. Giant cell tumor. Anteroposterior *(A)* and lateral *(B)* radiographs of the proximal tibia. The large, lytic lesion involves the metaphysis and epiphysis and extends to subchondral bone. Although the cortex is expanded and thinned, there is no evidence of cortical disruption or soft-tissue mass. (© The University of Texas M. D. Anderson Cancer Center.)

The aggressive behavior of these tumors can result in a high local recurrence rate. The overwhelming majority recur during the first 2 years after treatment. Recurrence may develop either in bone or in the surrounding soft tissues. Pulmonary metastases occur in approximately 3% of patients.

ENCHONDROMA

Enchondromas account for approximately 13% of benign bone tumors.[4] Enchondromas are usually detected in patients between the ages of 30 and 50 years; there is no gender predominance. Enchondromas are the most common benign bone tumors of the hand, and patients with a lesion in this site often present with a pathologic fracture. The distal femur and humerus are other common sites. Enchondromas usually are centrally located within the medullary canal in the metaphysis or diaphysis of long bones. The lesion is geographic (easily definable on plain films) and commonly has a calcified matrix. The adjacent cortex may be expanded, thinned, or scalloped, reflecting biologic activity (Fig. 14–6). Usually enchondromas are discovered incidentally during the evaluation of an unrelated problem. Localized pain, when present, is usually dull and aching. Diagnostic imaging studies include plain films and CT scan of the affected bone. Patients with asymptomatic lesions should be observed in annual follow-up with plain radiographs. For symptomatic lesions, curettage and cementation or bone grafting is recommended. Recurrence is unusual unless the lesion has not been completely excised. The differential diagnosis includes low-grade chondrosarcoma, which may be difficult to assess until the total specimen is analyzed. Ollier's disease is a nonhereditary condition characterized by multiple enchondromas, usually with unilateral or single-extremity skeletal involvement. Maffucci's syndrome is a nonhereditary, congenital disorder of enchondromatosis and hemangiomas.

CHONDROBLASTOMA

Chondroblastomas comprise approximately 5% of all benign bone tumors.[4] The great majority of patients are between the ages of 5 and 25 years at

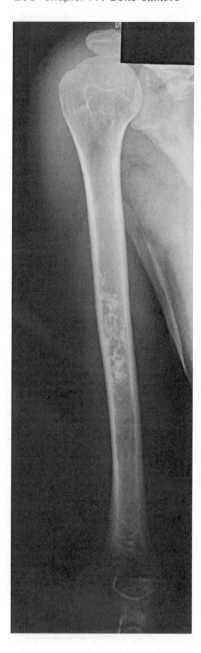

Figure 14–6. Enchondroma. Anteroposterior radiograph of the humerus. The lesion was an incidental finding. Note the central location of the calcified cartilage in the diaphysis. There is no evidence of bone destruction, suggestive of an inactive lesion. (© The University of Texas M. D. Anderson Cancer Center.)

diagnosis, with a peak in the second decade. Males are affected more commonly than females, in a ratio of approximately 2:1. The distal femur, proximal tibia, and proximal humerus are commonly involved. Chondroblastomas arise in the epiphyses of the long bones. Signs and symptoms include localized pain, soft tissue swelling, and effusion in the adjacent joint with associated decreased range of motion. The lesion may be present for months before diagnosis. Diagnostic studies include plain films and a CT scan. Radiographically, chondroblastomas are lytic lesions with a characteristic calcified matrix (Fig. 14–7). The recommended treatment consists of curettage and bone grafting. The recurrence rate is approximately 10% after appropriate treatment.[7]

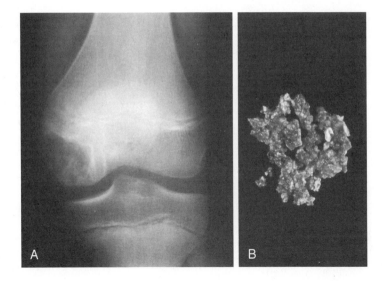

Figure 14–7. Chondroblastoma. *A*, Anteroposterior radiograph of a skeletally immature distal femur. There is a sharply demarcated, lytic lesion involving the epiphysis. *B*, The gross pathologic specimen. (© The University of Texas M. D. Anderson Cancer Center.)

NONOSSIFYING FIBROMA

Nonossifying fibromas account for approximately 5% of benign bone tumors.[4] Nonossifying fibromas are part of a spectrum of benign fibrous lesions, which range from small fibrous cortical defects to benign fibrous histiocytomas. They occur predominantly in the second decade of life, with a male predominance. The long bones of the lower extremity are most commonly affected, including the distal femur, distal tibia, and proximal tibia. Plain films demonstrate the well-defined, eccentric, lytic lesion arising in the metaphysis, characterized by a lobular pattern of bone destruction with a sclerotic, reactive border. The cortex usually is expanded and thinned (Fig. 14–8). Most patients have no symptoms unless a fracture develops. Observation is the preferred treatment, because most

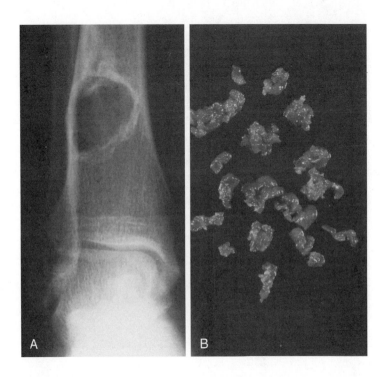

Figure 14–8. Nonossifying fibroma. *A*, Anteroposterior radiograph of lytic lesion in the metaphysis of the distal tibia. The lesion is well-marginated and eccentric within the bone. Often these lesions have a "soap-bubble" appearance. *B*, the gross pathologic specimen. (© The University of Texas M. D. Anderson Cancer Center.)

nonossifying fibromas heal spontaneously with skeletal maturity. Healing may be stimulated by a pathologic fracture. If the lesion is symptomatic or a pathologic fracture develops, curettage and bone grafting may be the appropriate intervention.

UNICAMERAL BONE CYST

Unicameral or simple bone cysts are benign, nonneoplastic, fluid-filled lesions that develop primarily in children. The mean age at presentation is 10 years, and 80% to 90% of these lesions occur before age 20. Males predominate over females in a ratio of 2:1 to 3:1. The great majority of cysts develop in the proximal humerus and proximal femur. Patients usually are asymptomatic unless a fracture develops. Plain films characteristically show a central, lytic lesion involving the metaphysis. Intralesional septations (partitioned segments) may be evident on radiographs. The cortex usually is thinned and symmetrically expanded. The lesion may have the "fallen fragment" sign, which is a fragment of cortical bone in the dependent portion of the lesion that has broken off. Serous or serosanguineous fluid seen on aspiration is diagnostic (Fig. 14–9). Unicameral bone cysts rarely heal spontaneously. Most are treated by percutaneous aspiration of the cystic fluid and intralesional injection of corticosteroids under fluoroscopic guidance after healing of any pathologic fracture. Persistence of the lesion after treatment is common, and multiple injections may be required to achieve healing. Rarely, curettage and bone grafting are required for the recalcitrant cyst.[8]

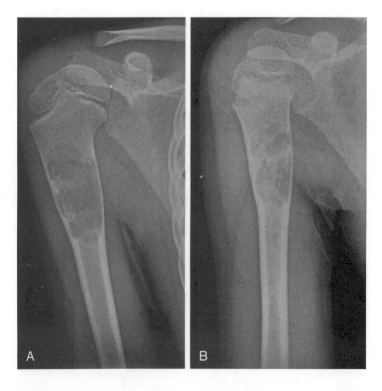

A   B

Figure 14–9. Unicameral bone cyst. Anteroposterior (A) and lateral (B) radiographs of the proximal humerus. The fluid-filled cyst is lytic and is located in the metaphysis. Septations (divided segments) are apparent. A pathologic fracture usually prompts medical attention and detection of the cyst. (© The University of Texas M. D. Anderson Cancer Center.)

ANEURYSMAL BONE CYST

Aneurysmal bone cysts are hemorrhagic cystic lesions that can develop de novo as primary lesions of bone or arise secondarily in association with another benign lesion such as osteoblastoma, chondroblastoma, GCT, or fibrous dysplasia. Eighty percent are detected before the age of 20 years, and they occur equally in males and females. Seventy percent to 80% of aneurysmal bone cysts occur in the distal femur, proximal tibia, and posterior elements of the spine. Localized pain and swelling are the common symptoms. Plain radiographs characteristically demonstrate a metaphyseal, lytic, eccentric, and well-marginated lesion. Cortical expansion and thinning (ballooning) are common (Fig. 14–10). Current treatment includes curettage and bone grafting. The 20% recurrence rate after appropriate treatment mandates that close surveillance be maintained.[9, 10]

LOCALIZED LANGERHANS CELL HISTIOCYTOSIS

Localized LCH, also called eosinophilic granuloma, is a rare, benign condition of bone of unknown cause which is characterized by a clonal proliferation of Langerhans-type histiocytes. Patients usually present during the first decade of life, with a 2:1 male predominance. Common sites of involvement include the skull, ribs, scapulae, vertebrae, pelvis, and long bones. Vertebral involvement may result in a compression fracture (vertebra plana). LCH may affect one or more bones; the ratio of single (monostotic) to multiple (polyostotic) bone involvement is 2:1. Patients usually present with local pain and swelling of several months' duration. A limp may be associated with a lesion affecting a bone in the lower extremity. The radiographic presentation may be variable, but the films usually show a lytic, well-defined lesion involving the medullary region with or without a soft tissue mass. LCH has been reported to occasionally resolve spontaneously, although without treatment it may progress and place the

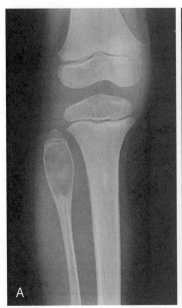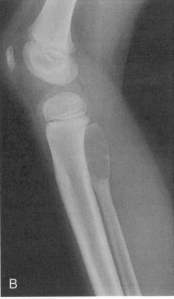

Figure 14–10. Aneurysmal bone cyst. Anteroposterior *(A)* and lateral *(B)* radiographs of the proximal fibula in a skeletally immature patient. The lesion is metaphyseal and gives the appearance of a blowout lesion caused by cortical thinning and expansion. (© The University of Texas M. D. Anderson Cancer Center.)

affected bone at risk for fracture. Treatment for painful lesions is variable and may include curettage with or without bone grafting, radiation therapy, or intralesional injection of corticosteroids.[11] The multifocal forms (Hand-Schüller-Christian disease and Letterer-Siwe disease), which may be associated with diabetes insipidus, hepatosplenomegaly, and adenopathy, carry a much worse prognosis. Treatment may include chemotherapy consisting of methotrexate, prednisone, and vinblastine.

FIBROUS DYSPLASIA

Fibrous dysplasia is a developmental anomaly characterized by defective enchondral bone maturation. It usually occurs in the skeletally immature patient and manifests in late childhood or adolescence with either a solitary, monostotic lesion or, less frequently, polyostotic lesions. Its incidence is the same in both genders. The proximal femur is the most common site in monostotic disease. Fibrous dysplasia is radiographically characterized by a well-defined, central or eccentric, lytic to opaque "ground-glass" lesion.[6] Cortical expansion and thinning may be present. Patients with polyostotic involvement may experience multiple small fractures of the femoral neck that result in a "shepherd's crook" deformity that may be associated with precocious puberty and skin lesions (Albright's syndrome). Most lesions are asymptomatic and require no intervention. For impending fractures, pathologic fractures, pain, or progressive deformity, curettage and allogeneic bone grafting with or without internal fixation may be necessary. Repeated surgical procedures may be needed if the disease progresses or the bone graft is resorbed.[12]

MALIGNANT TUMORS OF BONE

OSTEOSARCOMA

Osteosarcomas, the most common of the malignant primary tumors of bone, account for approximately 20% of all bone sarcomas.[4] The reported incidence is 2 to 3 cases per 1 million population per year. Osteosarcoma is a malignant spindle cell tumor that produces osteoid or bone. Approximately 95% of all osteosarcomas are primary tumors that develop de novo within a bone without evidence of a pre-existing lesion or prior treatment of the affected bone with radiation. It is more common in males and peaks during the second decade. The appearance of osteosarcoma is coincident with the period of rapid skeletal growth. Any bone and any site within a given bone can be affected. The metaphyseal region of the long bones is the primary site of occurrence (90%); the distal femur and proximal tibia account for 50% of the sites, followed by the proximal humerus, proximal femur, and pelvis.

Pain is an almost universal complaint. Local swelling and a soft tissue mass are common. Constitutional symptoms are rare. On physical examination, patients may also have tenderness to palpation or associated warmth, erythema, striae, or engorged veins in the region of the tumor. Laboratory assessment may indicate increased alkaline phosphatase and lactic dehydrogenase levels. Staging studies include plain films, MRI, and CT scan of the affected bone. The lung is the most common site of metastasis. A chest radiograph, chest CT, and bone scan are performed to screen for pulmonary and bone metastases. Plain radiographs characteristically reveal a bone-forming, nondiscrete lesion in the metaphysis of a long bone (Fig. 14–11). Cortical destruction usually is present, with an interrupted periosteal reaction and associated soft tissue mass. The MRI also delineates the extent of marrow involvement and the presence of skip metastasis (a separate site of tumor within the same bone). Ten percent to 20% of patients present with pulmonary metastases.[13]

There are many variants of osteosarcoma. The three histologic subtypes of conventional osteosarcoma are osteoblastic (most common), chondroblastic, and fibroblastic. Other variants include telangiectatic (lytic), well-differentiated intramedullary, and surface (periosteal, parosteal, dedifferentiated parosteal, and high-grade surface) osteosarcomas. Secondary osteosarcomas include radiation-induced osteosarcoma and Paget's sarcoma.

Low-grade variants (well-differentiated intramedullary and parosteal osteosarcoma) require only surgery for treatment. All high-grade variants of osteosarcoma are managed with chemotherapy and surgery. Chemotherapy regimens vary, but all consist of a combination of two or more of the known active agents against osteosarcoma, including doxorubicin, cisplatin, methotrexate, and ifosfamide. In

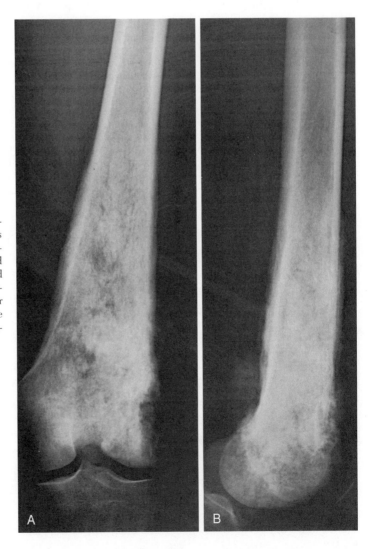

Figure 14–11. Osteosarcoma. Anteroposterior *(A)* and lateral *(B)* radiographs of the distal femur. This metaphyseal-epiphyseal lesion demonstrates a mixed pattern of bone destruction characterized by bone formation and lysis. An interrupted periosteal reaction and posterior soft-tissue mass are apparent. (© The University of Texas M. D. Anderson Cancer Center.)

general, three to four cycles of chemotherapy are administered preoperatively. Surgical excision is performed by either amputation or a limb-sparing surgical procedure. The method of reconstruction must be individualized and usually is accomplished with a prosthesis, allograft, or arthrodesis.[14] Local tumor control can be accomplished successfully in more than 90% of patients when oncologic surgical principles are followed appropriately.[15]

After surgery, an assessment of the tumor response (degree of tumor necrosis in response to preoperatively administered chemotherapy) is made on the resected specimen. The percentage of necrosis determines the postoperative chemotherapy regimen. The response of the tumor to chemotherapy is considered favorable if greater than 90% necrosis is observed and unfavorable if there is less than 90% necrosis. This histologically measured response to chemotherapy is the most powerful prognostic variable for patient survival. Limb-salvage procedures have not adversely impacted patient survival when performed appropriately.

Current 5-year survival rates for patients with localized disease have increased from historical levels (without chemotherapy) of 15% to 20% to 60% to 75% with chemotherapy.[16, 17] Patients with metastatic disease at presentation (10% to 20% of patients) have a poor prognosis, with a 5-year survival rate of 11%.[13] Approximately 30% to 40% of patients who subsequently develop pulmonary metastases can be salvaged with reinduction chemotherapy and surgery.

EWING'S SARCOMA

Ewing's sarcoma is the second most common primary malignant tumor of bone in children and the third most common overall. It accounts for approximately 6% of malignant bone tumors.[4] Ewing's sarcoma can occur at any age, but its peak incidence is in the second decade. Ewing's sarcoma occurs more commonly in males and is rarely diagnosed in American or African Blacks. Any bone can be involved, but the majority of tumors develop in the pelvis and lower extremity. The femur is the most common site of long bone involvement. Other common sites are the ribs and proximal humerus. Ewing's sarcoma can occur in the metaphysis of a long bone but most frequently involves the diaphysis.

The most common presenting symptom is pain. Localized soft tissue swelling is commonly associated with the pain. Occasionally constitutional symptoms, including fever, malaise, and weight loss, may be observed. In approximately 5% to 10% of patients, a pathologic fracture develops.[18]

Radiographically, Ewing's sarcomas usually exhibit a permeative pattern of bony destruction with poorly defined margins. Bone lysis, sclerosis, or a mixed pattern of bone destruction and sclerosis may be observed. The periosteal reactions associated with Ewing's sarcoma are variable, but the lamellated reaction, described as an "onion skin" appearance, is common (Fig. 14–12). A soft tissue mass is frequently present and usually large. The lung is the most common site of metastasis. The recommended staging studies include plain radiographs and MRI and CT scans for the local disease and a chest radiograph, CT scan of the chest, bone scan, and bone marrow aspiration and biopsy to detect the presence of distant disease.

Laboratory studies may demonstrate elevated alkaline phosphatase and lactic dehydrogenase values and an increased erythrocyte sedimentation rate. Anemia and leukocytosis also may be observed.

Chemotherapy is the mainstay of treatment for Ewing's sarcoma. The agents

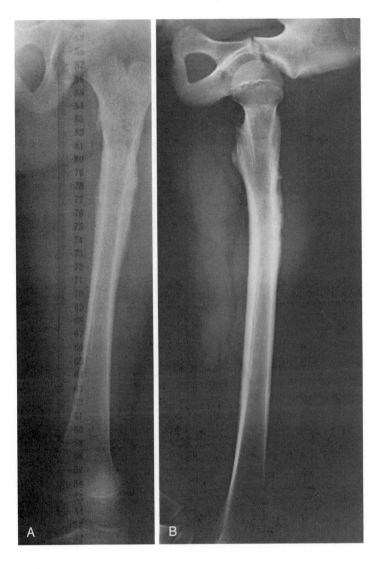

Figure 14–12. Ewing's sarcoma. Anteroposterior *(A)* and frog lateral *(B)* radiographs of the femur in a skeletally immature patient. The lesion involves the proximal diaphysis and metaphysis. Permeative bone destruction and interrupted periosteal reaction are characteristic of a malignant bone tumor. (© The University of Texas M. D. Anderson Cancer Center.)

include vincristine, actinomycin D, cyclophosphamide, doxorubicin, ifosfamide, and etoposide. Tumor necrosis greater than 90% is a favorable prognostic sign. The local treatment of Ewing's sarcoma usually includes surgery, radiotherapy, or both. The role of surgery has expanded, and surgery is currently recommended for all resectable lesions. Radiation therapy is recommended for patients with unresectable tumors or if the surgical margin of resection is unsatisfactory.[19] Five-year survival rates have been reported to be approximately 70% for patients with localized nonpelvic disease[20] and approximately 50% for patients with pelvis tumors.[21] Patients who have pulmonary metastases at presentation have a low survival rate.

CHONDROSARCOMA

Chondrosarcomas are the second most common primary malignant bone tumors, accounting for approximately 10% of all cases.[4] These tumors can arise de novo as primary neoplasms or occur secondarily in association with another benign process (e.g., osteochondroma, enchondroma). Primary chondrosarcomas occur in adults most commonly during the fifth and sixth decades, whereas secondary chondrosarcomas usually occur during the third decade, with both having a 2:1 predominance in men. Common sites of involvement include the pelvis, proximal femur, proximal humerus, distal femur, scapula, and ribs. Pain and swelling are the usual presenting complaints. Although the radiographic findings vary, a calcified matrix component is consistently noted within the tumor (Fig. 14–13). Bone lysis, cortical expansion and thickening with endosteal scalloping, and a soft tissue mass are characteristically associated with chondrosarcoma. Bone changes about the lesion can be delineated with a CT scan and the intramedullary and soft tissue involvement with an MRI scan.

Chondrosarcomas may be low-grade (lowest propensity to metastasize), intermediate-grade, high-grade, or dedifferentiated (highest propensity to metastasize). Chondrosarcomas are neither chemosensitive nor radiosensitive, making surgery the mainstay of treatment. Surgical procedures range from curettage and cementation for low-grade tumors to wide local excision for tumors of higher grade. Long-term survival is excellent among patients with low-grade chondrosarcomas but approaches zero for those with dedifferentiated chondrosarcomas.[22]

MALIGNANT SYSTEMIC TUMORS OF BONE

MULTIPLE MYELOMA

Multiple myeloma is a disseminated malignant proliferation of monoclonal plasma cells that represents the most common primary neoplasm of bone. It accounts for approximately 50% of all malignant bone tumors and approximately 1% of all cancer deaths.[23] The peak incidence of the disease is during the sixth and seventh decades of life. Males are more commonly affected than females.

The clinical features of multiple myeloma are variable. About 20% of patients

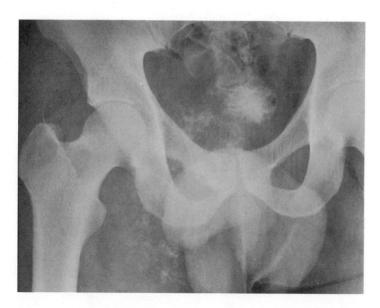

Figure 14–13. Chondrosarcoma. Anteroposterior radiograph of the pelvis showing a large calcified mass arising from the right superior pubic ramus with intrapelvic and extrapelvic soft-tissue extension. (© The University of Texas M. D. Anderson Cancer Center.)

are diagnosed incidentally during routine screening examinations on the basis of an elevated serum protein. The clinical signs supportive of the diagnosis include lytic bone lesions, anemia, hypercalcemia, renal insufficiency, and a history of recurrent infections. The diagnosis requires the presence of bone marrow plasmacytosis and a monoclonal protein in urine and/or serum.[24] Laboratory studies should include a complete blood count with differential, platelet count, serial chemistry panel, serum protein electrophoresis, 24-hour urine protein and electrophoresis, and quantitative immunoglobulins. Bone marrow aspiration and a skeletal radiographic survey complete the evaluation.

The most common presenting symptom of multiple myeloma is bone pain. Common sites of involvement are bones that contain hematopoietic marrow, including the vertebrae, ribs, pelvis, and skull. The classic radiographic description is a well-defined, lytic, "punched-out" lesion with little or no periosteal reaction. Diffuse vertebral osteopenia and compression fractures are commonly observed. Solitary plasmacytomas make up approximately 3% of plasma cell neoplasms.[24]

The treatment and prognosis depend on tumor burden at diagnosis. Systemic treatment with melphalan and prednisone is standard therapy for patients with low or intermediate risk. Multiagent chemotherapy with vincristine, doxorubicin, and dexamethasone is used for high-risk patients. Radiation therapy and/or surgery is used for localized disease (plasmacytoma) and for pain palliation in patients with disseminated disease. The surgical management includes stabilization of impending or established long bone or vertebral fractures. The 5-year survival rate is approximately 25%. Only about 5% to 10% of patients live longer than 10 years.[24]

METASTATIC BONE DISEASE

The skeleton is the third most common site of metastatic carcinoma, exceeded only by lung and liver. Metastatic bone disease can be a devastating consequence of advanced cancer that threatens the structural integrity of the skeletal system. Incapacitating bone pain may persist despite local and systemic therapies as a result of significant bone destruction, joint instability, mechanical insufficiency, and fracture. Primary tumors of the breast, prostate, lung, and kidney account for approximately 75% of all cases. Autopsy-based analyses of the distributions of bone metastases demonstrate that the most favored sites are the vertebrae, pelvis, femur, and bones of the upper extremity. Metastases distal to the elbow or knee are rare.

The evaluation of a patient with a known malignancy and bone pain begins with the physical examination and basic radiographic studies. For a newly discovered, undiagnosed bone lesion, the evaluation should include plain radiographs of the symptomatic site; chest radiographs; technetium bone scan; CT scans of the chest, abdomen, and pelvis; mammography (for women); digital rectal examination; urinalysis; a complete blood count, serum chemistries, and serum protein electrophoresis; and prostate-specific antigen determination (for men).

A painful bone lesion may be the first sign of a primary carcinoma, which should be suspected in any patient older than 40 years of age who presents with a bone lesion. Long bone or vertebral fractures with or without spinal cord compression also may be the first indication of advanced disease. Bone metastases may be lytic, blastic, or mixed. Lesions from the lung, kidney, or thyroid

(Fig. 14–14) are usually lytic. Blastic metastases are commonly associated with advanced carcinomas of the breast or prostate (Fig. 14–15). A biopsy is indicated if no primary tumor is detected or if the temporal relation between the bone lesion and a known primary carcinoma is not well established.

Contemporary management of patients with bone metastases requires a multi-disciplinary approach to optimize therapy options and coordinate their sequencing. Systemic therapy of the primary carcinoma is the mainstay of advanced disease management. Local irradiation is the most common therapy for a painful bone lesion. Surgical intervention can be an effective therapy to palliate pain, reduce patient anxiety, improve patient mobility and function, facilitate nursing care, preempt fracture, and control local tumor when nonsurgical therapies fail. Rarely, surgical resection is performed with curative intent (e.g., a solitary bone metastasis from renal cell carcinoma). There are no strict criteria for surgical treatment, and therapeutic decisions must be made on an individual basis. In general, surgery is recommended for patients with an established or impending pathologic fracture, spinal instability, or spinal cord compression.

IMITATORS OF BONE TUMORS

OSTEOMYELITIS

Inflammatory lesions may mimic neoplasia both clinically and radiographically. Patients with infection of bone (osteomyelitis) may have symptoms that are similar to those observed in patients with a bone tumor. Infection is much more common than neoplasia. Acute hematogenous osteomyelitis usually can be diagnosed presumptively on the basis of the patient's history and the radiographic

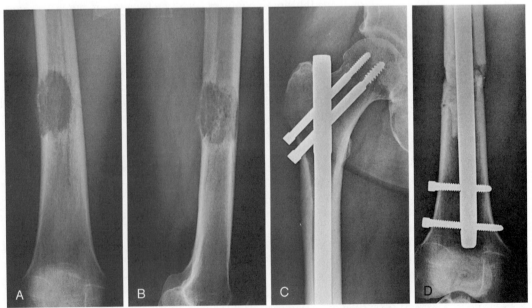

Figure 14–14. Metastatic renal cell carcinoma. Preoperative (*A* and *B*) and postoperative (*C* and *D*) radiographs of the femur reveal a lytic lesion with marked bone destruction placing the bone at risk for fracture. Treatment included curettage of the metastatic lesion and bone stabilization with an intramedullary rod and bone cement. (© The University of Texas M. D. Anderson Cancer Center.)

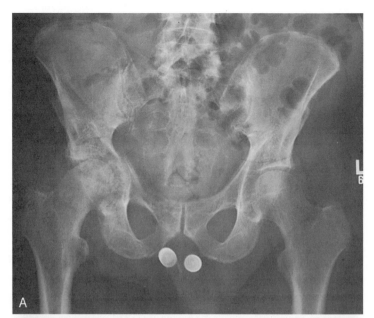
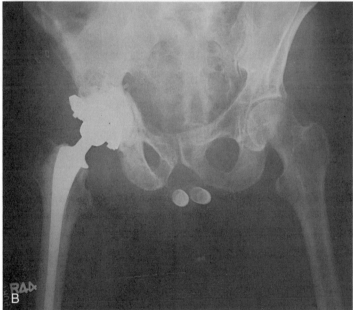

Figure 14–15. Metastatic prostate carcinoma. Anteroposterior preoperative *(A)* and postoperative *(B)* films of the pelvis in a patient with blastic metastases and pathologic fracture of the right acetabulum. A total hip arthroplasty with cement fixation was performed. (© The University of Texas M. D. Anderson Cancer Center.)

findings and confirmed by biopsy and culture. Usually patients present with localized pain, soft tissue swelling, and fever, and they often provide a history of recent febrile illness or frank infection. Blood studies reveal a leukocytosis and increased erythrocyte sedimentation rate. Patients with subacute or chronic osteomyelitis commonly present with a less specific history and nondiagnostic radiographic and laboratory findings.

Plain films commonly show a poorly marginated lesion that is associated with a permeative pattern of bone destruction and adjacent soft tissue swelling. Commonly a serpiginous, lucent track within the bone is observed radiographically. Usually there is periosteal reaction with new bone formation. Subacute and chronic osteomyelitis may appear radiographically to be less aggressive, with cortical thickening and sclerosis characteristic of a long-standing process. Dense fragments of bone (sequestra) may be seen within areas of bone destruction in these patients. Patients with a long-standing draining sinus can develop squamous cell carcinoma along the sinus track. Because the radiographic and clinical findings of osteomyelitis may overlap with those of a bone tumor, all biopsy material should be sent for microbiologic culture as well as pathology studies.

PAGET'S DISEASE

Paget's disease is a condition of unknown cause that affects primarily middle-aged and older persons, with a slight male predominance. It represents an uncoupling of normal bone resorption and formation and appears either as a monostotic process or in a polyostotic form. Common bony sites of involvement include the pelvis, femur, skull, tibia, and vertebrae. The most common symptom is bone pain. Fracture through pagetic bone occurs only occasionally but is a serious complication. The radiographic findings reflect the phase of involvement at the time of presentation. The initial or osteolytic phase is characterized by excessive localized bone resorption. A mixed lytic and blastic phase follows. The inactive or blastic phase represents the later stage of the condition. Radiographic findings include bone lysis and/or bony sclerosis, bone expansion, and thickened bony trabeculae and cortex. A technetium bone scan is performed to survey the skeleton to assess the extent of osseous involvement. Laboratory studies commonly reveal increased levels of alkaline phosphatase and 24-hour urine hydroxyproline (a marker for increased bone turnover). Treatment usually is directed at palliation of the associated pain. Commonly administered agents include bisphosphonates and calcitonin. Benign GCTs may arise within pagetic bone and usually demonstrate a remarkable sensitivity to systemic glucocorticoid treatment. Neoplastic degeneration of pagetic bone is rare, occurring in fewer than 1% of patients, and usually manifests clinically with increased pain and radiographically with cortical destruction and an associated soft tissue mass.

STRESS FRACTURES

Stress fractures, commonly observed in young patients, are associated with a history of repetitive trauma such as jogging or marching. Symptoms include local pain and swelling. Sites include the femur, tibia, and bones of the feet. Plain films may be unrevealing initially. The emergence of focal new bone formation; a smooth, uninterrupted periosteal reaction; and a transverse-oriented incomplete fracture line (or bony condensation) strongly support the diagnosis of a stress fracture. A technetium bone scan demonstrates increased activity focally. An MRI scan can provide supportive findings such as evidence of surrounding bone marrow and soft tissue edema and characteristically delineates the fracture line.

Treatment is directed at relieving the pain and protecting the bone until healing has occurred; this is done by immobilization of the bone, restriction of activity and weight bearing, and administration of analgesics. Serial plain films demonstrate healing coincident with resolution of pain. Internal stabilization may be required for patients whose fractures are refractory to nonsurgical treatment.

BROWN TUMOR

Overt skeletal manifestations of hyperparathyroidism occur infrequently but can appear as distinct intramedullary lytic lesions of bone designated as brown tumors. These lesions are focal areas of bone resorption that result from the diffuse demineralization of the skeleton caused by the disease. Brown tumors may be solitary or multifocal. Radiographically they may appear as lytic lesions, usually in association with indistinct margins and cortical expansion. The diagnosis is based on increased serum calcium, increased parathyroid hormone, and decreased serum phosphorus. Treatment is directed at the cause of the hyperparathyroidism, which in 80% of cases is a benign solitary adenoma. Protection of the bony lesion may be necessary to avoid fracture until healing has occurred.

BONE INFARCTS

Bone infarcts commonly are incidental findings. Patients at risk for development of infarcts include caisson workers, alcoholics, and patients with sickle cell anemia. Infarcts usually develop in the metaphyseal regions of the proximal tibia, distal femur, and ilium. Plain films show an area of lucency surrounded by a rim of calcification. A technetium bone scan may demonstrate increased uptake associated with the lesion. A CT scan may be helpful in distinguishing this condition from a cartilaginous neoplasm, which more commonly has a more uniformly distributed pattern of calcification. Usually no treatment is necessary. Rarely, a sarcoma arises in association with a bone infarct. Bone lysis and progressive pain are the hallmarks of malignant transformation.

CONCLUSION

Primary neoplasms of bone are rare. Their range of histologic characteristics is wide, as is their span of biologic behavior. Because of their rarity, evaluation and treatment of these tumors are optimally performed at a medical center staffed with a multidisciplinary team of experts in musculoskeletal oncology, including an orthopedic oncologist, bone pathologist, medical oncologist, and radiotherapist. The biopsy should be performed at the clinic or center where the patient is to be treated to avoid misdiagnoses and biopsy-related problems. Physician assistants and advanced practice nurses trained in oncology are an integral part of the multidisciplinary team.

REFERENCES

1. Mankin HJ, Mankin CJ, Simon MA: The hazards of biopsy, revisited. J Bone Joint Surg Am 1996;78:656.
2. Ayala AG, Ro JY, Fanning CV, et al: Core needle biopsy and fine-needle aspiration in the diagnosis of bone and soft-tissue lesions. Hematol Oncol Clin North Am 1995;9:633.
3. Enneking WF, Spanier SS, Goodman, MA: A system for the surgical staging of musculoskeletal sarcoma. Clin Orthop 1980;153:106.
4. Unni KK: Dahlin's Bone Tumors: General Aspects and Data on 11,087 cases, 5th ed. Philadelphia, Lippincott-Raven, 1996.
5. Frassica FJ, Waltrip RL, Sponseller PD, Ma LD, McCarthy EF Jr: Clinicopathologic features and

treatment of osteoid osteoma and osteoblastoma in children and adolescents. Orthop Clin North Am 1996;27:559–574.

6. Kneisl JS, Simon MA: Medical management compared with operative treatment for osteoid osteoma. J Bone Joint Surg Am 1992;74:179–185.

7. Springfield DS, Capanna R, Gherlinzoni F, et al: Chondroblastoma: A review of seventy cases. J Bone Joint Surg Am 1985;67:748–755.

8. Capanna R, Campanacci DA, Manfrini M: Unicameral and aneurysmal bone cysts. Orthop Clin North Am 1996;27:605–614.

9. Campanacci M, Capanna R, Picci P: Unicameral and aneurysmal bone cysts. Clin Orthop 1986;204:25–36.

10. Vergel De Dios AM, Bond JR, Shives TC, McLeod RA, Unni KK: Aneurysmal bone cyst: A clinicopathologic study of 238 cases. Cancer 1992;69:2921–2931.

11. Yasko AW, Fanning CV, Ayala AG, et al: Percutaneous techniques for the diagnosis and treatment of localized Langerhans-cell histiocytosis (eosinophilic granuloma of bone). J Bone Joint Surg 1998;80-A:219–228.

12. Stephenson RB, London MD, Hankin FM, et al: Fibrous dysplasia: An analysis of options for treatment. J Bone Joint Surg Am 1987;69:400–409.

13. Meyers PA, Heller G, Healey J, et al: Osteogenic sarcoma with clinically detectable metastasis at initial presentation. J Clin Oncol 1993;11:449–453.

14. Yasko AW, Johnson ME: Surgical management of primary bone sarcomas. Hematol Oncol Clin North Am 1995;9:719.

15. Simon MA, Aschliman MA, Thomas N, et al: Limb-salvage treatment versus amputation for osteosarcoma of the distal end of the femur. J Bone Joint Surg Am 1986;68:1331.

16. Hudson M, Jaffe MR, Jaffe N, et al: Pediatric osteosarcoma: Therapeutic strategies, results, and prognostic factors derived from a 10-year experience. J Clin Oncol 1990;8:1988–1997.

17. Meyers PA, Heller G, Healey J, et al: Chemotherapy for nonmetastatic osteogenic sarcoma: The Memorial Sloan-Kettering experience. J Clin Oncol 1992;10:5–15.

18. Vlasak R, Sim F: Ewing's sarcoma. Orthop Clin North Am 1996;27:591.

19. Wilkins R, Pritchard D, Burgert E, et al: Ewing's sarcoma of bone: Experience with 140 patients. Cancer 1986;58:2551.

20. Burgert EO Jr, Nesbit EM, Garnsey LA, et al: Multimodality therapy for the management of nonpelvic localized Ewing's sarcoma of bone: Intergroup study IESS-II. J Clin Oncol 1990;8:1517–1524.

21. Frassica FJ, Frassica DA, Pritchard DJ, et al: Ewing's sarcoma of the pelvis. J Bone Joint Surg Am 1993;75:1457–1465.

22. Healey JH, Lane JM: Chondrosarcoma. Clin Orthop 1986;204:119–129.

23. Alexanian R, Dimopoulos M: Management of multiple myeloma. Semin Hematol 1995;32:20.

24. Weber D: Multiple myeloma and other plasma-cell dyscrasias. In Pazdur R (ed): Medical Oncology: A Comprehensive Review, 2nd ed. New York, PRR, 1995:127.

Chapter 15

Soft Tissue Sarcoma

Paula Respondek, MS, PA-C, and
Peter W. T. Pisters, MD

INTRODUCTION

Soft tissue sarcomas are a group of rare malignant tumors that are anatomically and histologically diverse. Soft tissue sarcomas are most commonly found in the extremities, with the second most common site being the retroperitoneum. More than 30 different histologic subtypes of soft tissue sarcomas exist. They are classified according to their tissue of origin. Most arise from the mesoderm, except for malignant peripheral nerve sheath tumors, which arise from the ectoderm. Soft tissue sarcomas are classified separately from osteosarcomas and Ewing's sarcomas, which originate from bone, and from Kaposi's sarcoma, which arises from the dermis.

EPIDEMIOLOGY

Soft tissue sarcomas are rare tumors, accounting for approximately 1% of newly diagnosed cancers in the United States each year. Annually in the United States, approximately 7000 new cases are diagnosed and approximately 4300 patients die of this disease.[1] There is a slight male predominance, with a male-to-female ratio of 1.1:1.0. The race distribution is similar to that of the general population of the United States. In contrast to most other malignancies, which are more prevalent among elderly patients, soft tissue sarcoma occurs in patients of all ages.[2]

GENETICS

The cause of soft tissue sarcomas is unknown, but environmental factors, previous exposure to radiation, and chronic lymphedema have been associated with an increased risk of developing these tumors. Environmental factors that have been linked to sarcomas include occupational exposure to chemical products such as herbicides and asbestos.[3] Previous exposure to radiation is a predisposing factor that can lead to the development of soft tissue sarcomas up to 10 years later. For example, sarcoma may develop in the chest wall of a patient treated with irradiation for breast cancer years after the completion of radiotherapy.[4] Chronic lymphedema that develops after surgery or that is related to filiariasis has also been associated with the subsequent development of soft tissue sarcomas in the affected extremity. Affected patients can present with lymphangiosarcomas up to 10 years after the development of lymphedema.[5]

Several genetic syndromes are associated with soft tissue sarcomas. Gardner's syndrome, which is associated with familial polyposis, has also been associated with desmoid tumors.[6] Neurofibromatosis or von Recklinghausen's disease has been associated with malignant peripheral nerve sheath tumors such as neurofibrosarcomas.[7] The Li-Fraumeni syndrome, which has been described as a germline defect of the *p53* gene, has also been associated with an increased incidence of soft tissue sarcomas.[8]

A history of trauma to an affected area is frequently part of the medical history at presentation, but no specific relation has been documented between trauma to soft tissues and subsequent development of soft tissue neoplasms.

PATHOLOGY

The specific histopathologic diagnosis of an individual sarcoma is important because it influences the scope of the staging evaluation and the treatment plan. There are more than 30 different histologic subtypes of soft tissue sarcoma, and these tumors can be found anywhere in the body where soft tissues are located. The soft tissues where sarcomas may arise include adipose tissue, muscle tissue, connective tissue, nerve tissue, fibrous tissue, synovial tissue, and blood and lymph vessels. Sarcomas are named from the tissue from which they are thought to be derived. For example, liposarcoma, one of the most common histologic subtypes, is a tumor that is derived from adipose tissue. The histologic subtypes of soft tissue sarcomas differ by anatomic site, as outlined in Table 15–1.[9] A pathologist experienced in the diagnosis of malignant soft tissue tumors is required for an accurate diagnosis, because soft tissue sarcomas are quite rare and, even among expert pathologists, there is considerable discordance in the assignment of grade and histopathologic subtype.[10]

Although histologic subtype is important for classification of a particular soft tissue tumor, histologic grade is a better prognostic indicator of the aggressiveness of the sarcoma.[11] These tumors are commonly graded as low-, intermediate-, or high-grade based on light microscopic criteria.[12] Low-grade sarcomas rarely spread to distant sites, whereas high-grade sarcomas have an increased propensity to metastasize. The most common site for distant metastasis of soft tissue sarcomas is the lungs.

Low-, intermediate-, and high-grade sarcomas can recur locally after completion of treatment. For patients treated with an appropriate multimodality approach, the risk of local recurrence is relatively low (<15% for soft tissue sarcoma of an extremity).[13] Patients who have a history of locally recurrent sarcoma and those who have a positive microscopic surgical margin are at higher risk for local recurrence.[11]

Soft tissue sarcomas are most commonly staged with the system devised and modified by the American Joint Committee on Cancer (AJCC). The AJCC staging system for soft tissue sarcomas is outlined in Table 15–2. This staging system uses the tumor, node, metastasis (TNM) criteria and also includes histologic grade (G) as a staging criterion.[14] The histologic grade of the tumor is very important in stratifying patients for risk of distant recurrence and death. Tumors of 5 cm or less are classified as T1, and those larger than 5 cm are classified as T2. Sarcomas larger than 5 cm are associated with a higher risk of distant recurrence and a poorer prognosis for survival.[11] Lymph node involvement is

Table 15–1. Common Histologic Subtypes of Soft Tissue Sarcomas

	OCCURRENCE BY SITE (%)		
	EXTREMITY		
TYPE	LOWER	UPPER	*RETROPERITONEAL*
Liposarcoma	30	14	41
Malignant fibrous histiocytoma	22	26	5
Leiomyosarcoma	7	7	29
Fibrosarcoma	7	18	6
Other	20	13	15
Synovial sarcoma	14	11	—
Malignant peripheral nerve tumors	—	11	4

Data from Pisters PWT, Brennan MF: Sarcomas of soft tissue. In Abeloff M, Armitage J, Lichter A, et al (eds): Clinical Oncology. New York, Churchill Livingstone, 1995:1799–1803.

Table 15-2. AJCC Sarcoma Staging System

STAGE	DESCRIPTION			
G	Tumor grade			
	GX	Grade cannot be assessed		
	G1	Well differentiated		
	G2	Moderately differentiated		
	G3	Poorly differentiated		
	G4	Undifferentiated		
T	Primary tumor site			
	TX	Primary size cannot be assessed		
	T0	No evidence of tumor		
	T1	≤ 5 cm		
	T1a	Superficial to muscular fascia		
	T1b	Deep to muscular fascia		
	T2	> 5 cm		
	T2a	Superficial to muscular fascia		
	T2b	Deep to muscular fascia		
N	Regional lymph node status			
	NX	Regional nodes cannot be assessed		
	N0	No regional lymph node metastasis		
	N1	Regional lymph node metastasis		
M	Distant metastasis			
	MX	Presence of distant metastasis cannot be assessed		
	M0	No distant metastasis		
	M1	Distant metastasis		

STAGE	G	T	N	M
IA	G1,G2	T1a, T1b	N0	M0
IB	G1,G2	T2a	N0	M0
IIA	G1,G2	T2b	N0	M0
IIB	G3,G4	T1a,T1b	N0	M0
IIC	G3,G4	T2a	N0	M0
III	G3,G4	T2b	N0	M0
IV	Any G	Any T	N1	M0
IV	Any G	Any T	Any N	M1

Used with permission of the American Joint Committee on Cancer (AJCC), Chicago, Illinois. The original source for this material is the AJCC Manual for Staging of Cancer, 4th edition (1992) published by Lippincott-Raven Publishers, Philadelphia.

rare with soft tissue sarcomas, but it is seen in selected subtypes such as epithelioid sarcoma, synovial sarcoma, and angiosarcoma.[15]

PRESENTING HISTORY AND PHYSICAL EXAMINATION

CLINICAL PRESENTATION

The clinical presentation of patients recently diagnosed with soft tissue sarcoma may vary because of the anatomically diverse nature of these tumors. Fifty percent of sarcomas arise in an extremity, most commonly in a lower extremity. The retroperitoneum is the second most common location (15%), followed by the trunk, head and neck, visceral organs, and breast.[9, 16] Tumor size at the time of presentation frequently depends on the area in which the tumor arises. For example, a superficial mass on a patient's forearm is usually noticed at a relatively small size, whereas a sarcoma located in the medial thigh may grow to a substantial size before it is discovered. Retroperitoneal sarcomas often are large at presentation because the abdomen and retroperitoneum can accommodate a large mass without significant symptoms.

The most common clinical presentation in a patient with a sarcoma of an extremity is a painless soft tissue mass that is often discovered by the patient or by a medical professional at physical examination. Symptoms often are not reported until the tumor grows large enough to place pressure on nearby nerves or vessels, causing pain, swelling, or numbness. Other symptoms from sarcomas of an extremity may include weakness or gait changes. Patients with intra-abdominal or retroperitoneal tumors most commonly present with vague abdominal pain or a palpable mass. Abdominal tumors can also produce symptoms of nausea, vomiting, abdominal distention, or early satiety. Visceral sarcomas often produce symptoms that affect the specific viscus involved. For example, patients with gastric leiomyosarcoma may present with symptoms related to gastrointestinal bleeding.

STAGING EVALUATION

The diagnostic evaluation for a patient suspected of having a soft tissue sarcoma should include a thorough medical history and physical examination. The medical history should include any past exposure to chemicals or radiation. A family history of genetic abnormalities is also important. A complete past medical history and physical examination are needed to evaluate any coexisting medical disease that may affect the implementation of multimodality treatment. The physical examination should include an accurate evaluation of the size and depth of the lesion relative to the investing fascia of the extremity and any attachment to superficial or deep structures. The functional status of the anatomic site is important to assess, along with an evaluation for any bone or neurovascular involvement. The status of regional lymph nodes should also be assessed, even though lymph node metastasis at presentation is uncommon.[15] A previous biopsy site should be examined for the orientation of the incision and overall wound healing, which may affect the timing and scope of subsequent surgical procedures.

The appropriate staging evaluation for a patient with a soft tissue sarcoma depends on the size and histologic grade of the primary tumor. The pertinent tests also depend on the site of the sarcoma and may include imaging studies and a biopsy, if these have not been performed. Imaging studies are critical for determining whether the tumor can be resected and for evaluating for the existence of metastatic disease.

Magnetic resonance imaging (MRI) is considered the most precise imaging modality for evaluation of a primary lesion in an extremity. A computed tomography (CT) scan of the abdomen and pelvis is recommended for the evaluation of a retroperitoneal sarcoma. Although CT is an accurate test for assessing the relation of the tumor to adjacent intra-abdominal structures, MRI is occasionally used to evaluate long-segment vascular involvement in the retroperitoneum, such as proximity of the tumor to the aorta or inferior vena cava. Under rare circumstances, if bone involvement is suspected, a plain radiograph or MRI scan is required to assess the extent of bony involvement. A bone scan is almost never required in the evaluation of the primary tumor.

To exclude pulmonary metastatic disease, a chest radiograph is required for almost all sarcoma patients. High-grade sarcomas larger than 5 cm in size require a CT scan of the chest because these patients are at increased risk of presenting with synchronous pulmonary metastases.[11] Intra-abdominal metastatic disease is more common with visceral or retroperitoneal sarcomas. In these cases, the abdominal CT scan of the primary lesion usually provides adequate imaging of the liver. Evaluation for brain or bone metastasis is not recommended unless the patient is symptomatic at the time of presentation.

BIOPSY

A soft tissue mass that has been growing, is larger than 5 cm, or has been present for more than 4 to 6 weeks requires a biopsy for pathologic diagnosis. Fine-needle aspiration may be an acceptable biopsy technique, provided that an experienced cytopathologist is available. A more common method used to diagnose soft tissue sarcoma is percutaneous core biopsy. A superficial lesion can commonly be biopsied with the use of direct palpation, but less accessible sarcomas often require an image-guided biopsy to safely sample the most heterogeneous component of the mass. For example, the majority of a large retroperitoneal tumor may be made up of a low-grade component, but cross-sectional imaging may reveal a radiographically more dense, possibly higher-grade component. This heterogeneous area should be biopsied to provide the greatest likelihood of detecting high-grade sarcoma. An incisional biopsy is rarely required but may be performed when a definite diagnosis cannot be achieved by less invasive means.

An excisional biopsy may be appropriate for a lesion smaller than 5 cm that is superficial and can be completely excised without damage to adjacent neurovascular structures. The proper orientation of the biopsy incision is important. For lesions of an extremity, the incision should be aligned parallel to the long axis of the extremity. Longitudinal orientation of the incision facilitates a future wide local excision to resect the mass completely while minimizing subsequent difficulties with primary wound closure. Adequate hemostasis at the time of biopsy is important to avoid local spread of viable tumor cells.

DIFFERENTIAL DIAGNOSIS

The differential diagnosis for a soft tissue mass includes both benign and malignant soft tissue tumors. Benign lesions most commonly mistaken for a sarcoma of an extremity or a superficial sarcoma of the trunk include a sebaceous cyst, lipoma, myxoma, neuroma, neurofibroma, hemangioma, and angioma. Biopsy of a suspicious soft tissue mass is the only means to conclusively exclude a malignant process.

Retroperitoneal masses such as lymphoma or primary or secondary germ-cell neoplasms may be mistaken for a retroperitoneal soft tissue sarcoma. Laboratory tests that show elevated levels of α-fetoprotein in serum support the diagnosis of a primary germ cell tumor, but a biopsy is required for a definitive diagnosis. Similarly, an increased level of lactic dehydrogenase may support the diagnosis of lymphoma. Patients with lymphoma may also present with constitutional symptoms of fever, night sweats, and weight loss in addition to peripheral adenopathy, but again a biopsy is required for a definitive diagnosis and for treatment planning.

TREATMENT

Soft tissue sarcomas usually are treated with a multimodality approach that combines surgery, chemotherapy, and radiation therapy (Fig. 15–1). Proper staging of a sarcoma is imperative to determine the appropriate components of the treatment plan.

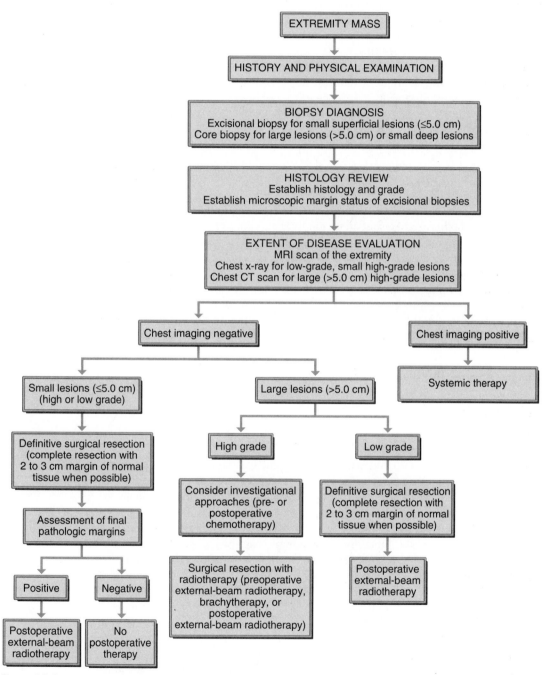

Figure 15–1. Treatment algorithm for primary soft-tissue sarcoma of an extremity.

SURGERY

Surgery is the primary therapy for all sarcoma patients with localized disease (AJCC stages I through III). Most patients with sarcoma of an extremity can be treated with a limb-sparing procedure rather than amputation. The objectives of limb-sparing surgery include removal of all gross tumor, attainment of negative microscopic surgical margins, and preservation of extremity function. Amputation is required only for a minority of patients with extremity sarcomas (<10%) and is avoided unless it is the only option for local control.

Wide local excision is recommended for surgical treatment of most sarcomas. This involves removal of the mass and a margin of normal tissue surrounding the tumor. The extent of resection depends on the size and location of the tumor in relation to nearby anatomic structures. Regional lymph node dissection is not performed because of the rare incidence of metastasis to the lymph nodes.

Patients with AJCC stage IIC or III tumors (G3 and 4, T2) are at an increased risk for distant metastasis. Multimodality treatment (chemotherapy, radiotherapy, and surgery) algorithms are often used for these patients. Adjuvant radiotherapy improves local control and is generally recommended for patients with tumors larger than 5 cm and for those with smaller lesions with positive microscopic surgical margins.

Hyperthermic isolated limb perfusion is an investigational treatment option for patients who have sarcoma of an extremity that is considered to be nonresectable without amputation. This procedure is available at selected institutions for patients for whom amputation is the only surgical option. Hyperthermic isolated limb perfusion involves infusing chemotherapeutic agents into an isolated extremity through an extra-anatomic heated perfusion circuit to treat the entire extremity directly without exposing the patient to the side effects of systemic chemotherapy. Clinical trials are ongoing to evaluate the efficacy of this therapy and to determine its role in the management of patients with sarcoma of an extremity.[17, 18]

RADIATION THERAPY

Radiation therapy is often used in addition to surgery to improve local control. When it is combined with surgery, three different treatment sequences can be used. Preoperative external beam irradiation is usually given at a dose of 50 Gy. A second approach is to give external beam irradiation after surgery, usually at doses between 60 and 65 Gy. Brachytherapy is a third option for patients who have a high-grade sarcoma and is usually given at a dose of 45 to 55 Gy. Brachytherapy is a type of interstitial radiotherapy that involves placing afterloading catheters into the tumor bed at the time of surgical resection. These catheters are then loaded with a radioactive material (usually iridium 192) and left within the body for 6 to 10 days during the postoperative period. Brachytherapy has the advantage of low cost and convenience for the patient but cannot be used for low-grade tumors.[13, 19, 20] Local control rates for all three radiation therapy approaches are comparable.[13, 21]

Intraoperative radiation therapy is a specialized technique that requires a dedicated operating room and therefore is not universally available. It usually is used to deliver a boost of 10 to 20 Gy in addition to conventional external beam irradiation, which is given to the patient before or after surgery. Intraoperative radiation therapy has the advantage of treating the tumor bed and tissues at greatest risk for local recurrence while minimizing the dose to adjacent viscera, thereby minimizing the risk of subsequent radiation-related local toxicity.

CHEMOTHERAPY

Chemotherapy is the primary treatment for patients who present with metastatic disease (AJCC stage IV). The role of chemotherapy in patients with localized sarcoma remains controversial.[22, 23] In many specialized centers in the United States, chemotherapy is provided to patients who have localized high-grade (stage IIIB) disease. This treatment can be given before surgery (neoadjuvant) or after surgery (adjuvant). The primary goal of systemic chemotherapy in patients who have localized disease is to minimize the risk of developing pulmonary metastases.

The two most common chemotherapeutic agents used for sarcoma are doxorubicin and ifosfamide. Cumulative administration of doxorubicin can lead to complications from cardiac toxicity, so these patients should be monitored closely. A patient who has received a cumulative dose of 400 to 500 mg/m^2 doxorubicin is considered to be at increased risk for cardiac toxicity. An echocardiogram, cardiac scan, and cardiac biopsy are recommended for the rare symptomatic patient to rule out doxorubicin-related cardiac toxicity. Ifosfamide can cause renal toxicity, so patients must be monitored closely while they receive this chemotherapeutic agent. Renal function tests are required to monitor for evidence of azotemia and renal dysfunction. Mesna, a urothelial protective agent, is often given in combination with ifosfamide to treat complications of hemorrhagic cystitis.

LOCALLY RECURRENT DISEASE

A patient with a primary soft tissue sarcoma must be monitored closely for local recurrence, which commonly appears within 3 years after completion of treatment. Treatment for a locally recurrent sarcoma is again dependent on the histologic subtype and grade. In addition, the scope and intensity of previous treatment, including prior surgery, radiation therapy, and chemotherapy, influence the treatment options available for patients who have locally recurrent disease. Further surgery with or without radiation therapy may be appropriate for low-grade sarcomas. Chemotherapy or radiation therapy (when feasible) may be recommended to treat locally recurrent disease in patients with a high-grade sarcoma, depending on the size and location of the recurrent tumor.

METASTATIC DISEASE

Patients who present with metastatic disease are considered to be candidates for systemic chemotherapy. Patients with resectable pulmonary metastases may be candidates for surgical excision. Pulmonary metastasectomy is associated with a defined long-term survival rate that ranges from 15% to 25%.[24, 25] Extrapulmonary metastatic disease is more difficult to treat. Patients who have extensive metastatic disease must be managed on an individual basis. Treatment often includes chemotherapy, surgery, radiation therapy, or a combination of these modalities.

MULTIDISCIPLINARY APPROACH TO DIAGNOSTIC WORKUP AND TREATMENT

The optimal approach to a patient with a diagnosis of soft tissue sarcoma involves multidisciplinary treatment planning. Pathology slides from previous biopsies and surgical procedures are reviewed by a pathologist who has experience with sarcomas before further staging evaluation is done and before the treatment plan is formulated. Outside imaging studies are reviewed by radiologists with expertise in soft tissue imaging to evaluate the primary tumor and its relation to adjacent structures and to assess any evidence of metastatic disease. In many specialized centers, each individual case is presented at a multidisciplinary conference that is attended by health care practitioners specializing in soft tissue sarcoma. Any further diagnostic studies are recommended at that time, and then a treatment plan is finalized and discussed with the patient.

POSTTREATMENT FOLLOW-UP

Long-term surveillance of a patient with soft tissue sarcoma consists of follow-up visits every 3 months for the first 3 years and includes appropriate imaging studies.[26] Most recurrences occur within the first 3 years[11]; therefore, frequent follow-up visits are recommended during that period. Afterward, the patient should be evaluated every 6 months for 2 years and then annually for 5 years. A medical history and physical examination should be performed at each follow-up visit, but routine laboratory tests are not necessary.

To detect local recurrence in a patient who had a sarcoma of an extremity requires both a baseline MRI scan and ultrasonography of the treated extremity 3 months after completion of treatment. These studies should be performed provided the patient has no local wound problems and the incision is well healed. High-quality ultrasonography can then be used at subsequent visits as a less expensive follow-up study to evaluate for recurrent disease. Any abnormality noted on subsequent follow-up physical examinations or ultrasound scans can be further investigated by a repeat MRI scan that can be compared with the baseline scan. A patient who had a retroperitoneal sarcoma requires a chest radiograph and a CT scan of the abdomen and pelvis every 3 months for the first 3 years to evaluate for recurrent or metastatic disease.

To detect distant metastases, a chest radiograph is required at each follow-up visit for patients who had high-grade sarcoma. Annual chest radiographs are sufficient for patients who had low-grade sarcoma. Any suspicious areas on a chest radiograph should be further evaluated with a CT scan of the chest to rule out metastatic disease.

CANCER PREVENTION

No specific steps have been recommended to prevent soft tissue sarcomas. Patients who have had these tumors should be encouraged to continue regular follow-up appointments to detect recurrent disease at an early stage. By closely monitoring these patients, evidence of recurrent disease can be detected early, when the tumor is small and is more easily treated with an appropriate multi-modality approach.

REFERENCES

1. Landis SH, Murray T, Bolden S, Wingo PA: Cancer statistics, 1998. CA Cancer J Clin 1998;48:6–29.
2. Pisters PWT, Fein DA, Somlo G: Soft-tissue sarcomas. In Pazdur R, Coia L, Hoskins W, et al (eds): Cancer Management: A Multidisciplinary Approach. Huntington, NY, PRR, 1996:491.
3. Hardell L, Eriksson M: The association between soft tissue sarcomas and exposure to phenoxyacetic acids: A new case-referent study. Cancer 1988;62:652.
4. Brady MS, Gaynor JJ, Brennan MF: Radiation-associated sarcoma of bone and soft tissue. Arch Surg 1992;127:1379.
5. Woodward AH, Ivins JC, Soule EH: Lymphangiosarcoma arising in chronic lymphedematous extremities. Cancer 1972;30:562.
6. Jones IT, Jagelman DG, Fazio VW, et al: Desmoid tumors in familial polyposis coli. Ann Surg 1986;204:94.
7. Sorensen SA, Mulvihill JJ, Nielsen A: Long-term follow-up of von Recklinghausen neurofibro-matosis: Survival and malignant neoplasms. N Engl J Med 1986;314:1010.
8. Malkin D, Li FP, Strong LC, et al: Germ line p53 mutations in a familial syndrome of breast cancer, sarcomas, and other neoplasms. Science 1990;250:123.
9. Pisters PWT, Brennan MF: Sarcomas of soft tissue. In Abeloff M, Armitage J, Lichter A, et al (eds): Clinical Oncology. New York, Churchill-Livingstone, 1995:1799.
10. Presant CA, Russell WO, Alexander RW, et al: Soft-tissue and bone sarcoma histopathology peer review: The frequency of disagreement in diagnosis and the need for second pathology opinions. The Southeastern Cancer Study Group experience. J Clin Oncol 1986;4:1658.
11. Pisters PWT, Leung DHY, Woodruff J, et al: Analysis of prognostic factors in 1041 patients with localized soft tissue sarcomas of the extremities. J Clin Oncol 1996;14:1679.
12. Hajdu SI, Shiu MH, Brennan MF: The role of the pathologist in the management of soft tissue sarcomas. World J Surg 1988;12:326.
13. Pisters PWT, Harrison LB, Leung DHY, et al: Long-term results of a prospective randomized trial of adjuvant brachytherapy in soft tissue sarcoma. J Clin Oncol 1996;14:859.
14. Sobin LH, Wittekind C, eds. TNM Classification of Malignant Tumours. New York, John Wiley & Sons, Inc., 1997:106–109.
15. Fong Y, Coit DG, Woodruff JM, et al: Lymph node metastasis from soft tissue sarcoma in adults: Analysis of data from a prospective database of 1772 sarcoma patients. Ann Surg 1993;217:72.
16. Brennan MF, Casper ES, Harrison LB, et al: The role of multimodality therapy in soft-tissue sarcoma. Ann Surg 1991;214:328.
17. Lienard D, Ewalenko P, Delmotte JJ, et al: High-dose recombinant tumor necrosis factor alpha in combination with interferon gamma and melphalan in isolation perfusion of the limbs for melanoma and sarcoma. J Clin Oncol 1992;10:52–60.
18. Eggermont AMM, Shraffordt-Koops H, Lienard D, et al: Isolated limb perfusion with high-dose tumor necrosis factor-α in combination with interferon-γ and melphalan for nonresectable extremity soft tissue sarcomas: A multicenter trial. J Clin Oncol 1996;14:2653.
19. Pisters PWT, Harrison LB, Woodruff JM, et al: A prospective randomized trial of adjuvant brachytherapy in the management of low grade soft tissue sarcomas of the extremity and superficial trunk. J Clin Oncol 1994;12:1150.
20. Janjan NA, Yasko AW, Reece GP, et al: Comparison of charges related to radiotherapy for soft tissue sarcomas treated by preoperative external beam irradiation versus interstitial implantation. Ann Surg Oncol 1994;1:415.
21. Harrison LB, Zelefsky MJ, Armstrong JG, et al: Brachytherapy and function preservation in the localized management of soft tissue sarcomas of the extremity. Semin Radiat Oncol 1993;3:260.
22. Bramwell V, Rouesse J, Steward W, et al: Adjuvant CYVADIC chemotherapy for adult soft tissue sarcoma: Reduced local recurrence but no improvement in survival. A study of the European Organization for Research and Treatment of Cancer Soft Tissue and Bone Sarcoma Group. J Clin Oncol 1994;12:1137.
23. Tierney JF: Adjuvant chemotherapy for localized resectable soft-tissue sarcoma of adults: Meta-analysis of individual data. Lancet 1997;350:1647–1654.
24. Gadd MA, Casper ES, Woodruff JM, et al: Development and treatment of pulmonary metastases in adult patients with extremity soft-tissue sarcoma. Ann Surg 1993;218:705.
25. Putnam JB Jr, Roth JA, Wesley MN, et al: Analysis of prognostic factors in patients undergoing resection of pulmonary metastases from soft tissue sarcomas. J Thorac Cardiovasc Surg 1984;87:260.
26. Pisters PWT: Combined modality treatment of extremity soft tissue sarcomas. Ann Surg Oncol 1998; in press.

Chapter 16

Melanoma

Carol Lacey, PA-C, and Paul Mansfield, MD

Melanoma was first described in the English literature by William Norris in 1820. Norris noted the association between moles and melanoma in patients who had fair hair color and complexions; he also noted that there was a family history in many cases.[1] He described the clinical features of his patients, who were predominantly male, and noted that they usually remained in good health until a very late stage of the disease. Norris wrote of pathologic features such as variation in pigmentation, presence of nodularity, satellite lesions around a primary growth, and widespread dissemination that could involve the lungs, liver, bone, and brain. He found that local recurrence occurred after minimal excision and recommended that wide excision be used. These observations hold true today. Although it was once uncommon, today melanoma is an increasingly important cause of disease and death in certain populations.[2]

INCIDENCE

The incidence of melanoma is increasing at a faster rate than that of any other cancer in the United States, and melanoma accounts for 2.5% of all cancers.[2] In 1935, a person had a risk of 1 in 1500 of developing melanoma in his or her lifetime. By 1980, the lifetime risk was 1 in 250. In less than half a century, the incidence of melanoma increased 600%.[2] Since 1980, the number of new cases of melanoma diagnosed annually has doubled, and it is estimated that melanoma will develop eventually in approximately 1 of every 95 whites.[2]

RISK FACTORS

SUN EXPOSURE AND PIGMENTARY TRAITS

Men or women who have light complexions and fair hair, especially red hair, and who have a tendency to sunburn after a relatively short exposure to bright sunlight have a twofold to threefold increased risk of developing melanoma compared with dark-haired persons, particularly when exposure results in a blistering sunburn, as often occurs during youth.[3] Melanoma is 80% more common in whites than in nonwhites.

Ultraviolet B radiation in the form of sunlight is thought to be an environmental carcinogen for melanoma because of its ability to initiate and promote growth of neoplastic cells, and it has been shown to induce melanoma in some laboratory animals. When photons in sunlight are absorbed by DNA, they can induce changes in the amino acid sequence or cause breaks in the DNA strand. Most cells are capable of repairing this damage but, for example, in patients with xeroderma pigmentosum, this capacity is lost, and the occurrence of skin cancer is frequent. Another area of interest and potential importance is how oncogenes that normally modulate cell division and differentiation, such as the *p53* tumor suppressor gene, can become damaged.[4]

FAMILY HISTORY

Between 5% and 10% of melanoma patients have a familial history of the disease.[5] Their risk of developing melanoma is increased by two to eight times and seems to be independent of other factors such as sun exposure.

DYSPLASTIC NEVI

Dysplastic nevi are melanocytic lesions that can be precursors of melanoma as well as markers of increased melanoma risk. The presence of dysplastic nevi, especially in a patient with a familial tendency for melanoma, results in a 7- to 70-fold increased risk for melanoma.[6, 7]

Dysplastic nevi are identified by certain clinical and histologic features. Clinically, dysplastic nevi tend to be larger than common acquired nevi and often measure more than 5 mm in the longest axis. The borders are fuzzy and irregular, unlike those of common acquired nevi, which are well demarcated. The pigmentation pattern is also irregular and variegated, with light, medium, and dark brown colors and components that are pink or tan. A so-called fried-egg shape may be created when the central nevus is a different shade of color from that of the peripheral component. Dysplastic nevi can occur anywhere on the skin surface but are more frequently seen on areas typically exposed to the sun, such as the back and chest (Fig. 16–1).

TYPES OF MELANOMA

Melanoma has several histologic types. The four most common types are discussed here. Each has unique clinical and histopathologic features that can have prognostic importance.

SUPERFICIAL SPREADING MELANOMA

Superficial spreading melanomas (Fig. 16–2) usually arise from a pre-existing pigmented lesion and constitute approximately 70% of all melanomas. The typical history is of slow change over several months or years, followed by a rapid growth phase. Superficial spreading melanomas are predominately flat because melanocytic growth occurs in a radial or horizontal pattern in the epidermal layer of the epithelium. The characteristic appearance is that of a

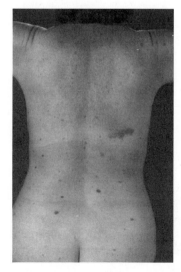

Figure 16–1. Dysplastic nevi.

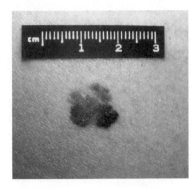

Figure 16–2. Superficial spreading melanoma.

pigmented lesion with multiple colors, including black, purple, brown, tan, and reddish pink, and irregular borders.

NODULAR MELANOMAS

Nodular melanomas (Fig. 16–3) commonly arise without evidence of a pre-existing nevus. They demonstrate a vertical growth pattern and are thicker than superficial spreading melanomas. Nodular melanoma is a more aggressive tumor and is seen in 15% to 30% of melanoma patients, typically those who are male. The elevation may be dark blue, or it may appear to be a pink or flesh-colored amelanotic lesion owing to a greater degree of atypia and a reduction of pigment synthesis.

LENTIGO MALIGNA MELANOMA

Lentigo maligna melanomas (Fig. 16–4) account for 4% to 10% of melanomas and usually are large (>3 cm), slow-growing, flat, notched, tan-colored lesions that occur on the face or arms of older persons. These lesions demonstrate a primarily radial growth pattern and a low propensity to metastasize. They almost always occur in skin areas of chronic severe sun damage (solar elastosis).

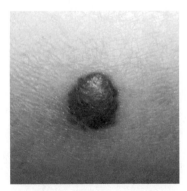

Figure 16–3. Nodular melanoma.

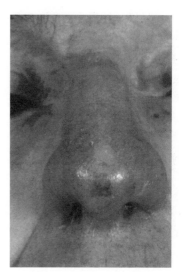

Figure 16–4. Lentigo maligna melanoma.

ACRAL LENTIGINOUS MELANOMA

The term acral lentiginous melanoma (Figs. 16–5 and 16–6) applies predominantly to a pattern of melanoma found on the palms, soles, and nailbeds (subungual). Although this growth pattern makes up only 2% to 8% of melanomas in whites, it accounts for 35% to 60% of melanomas in dark-skinned persons. Acral lentiginous melanomas resemble highly irregular tan or brown stains on the palmar or plantar surface. More than 75% of subungual lesions involve either the great toe or thumb and appear as brown or black discolorations in or under the nailbed. Acral lentiginous melanoma is often initially misdiagnosed as a fungal infection, ingrown nail, or trauma. However, the discoloration does not "grow out" with nail growth and will ulcerate if untreated. A lesion that does not respond readily to treatment, that does not grow out, or that is at all suspicious should be biopsied. Table 16–1 describes the features of benign pigmented lesions that are useful for differential diagnosis.

SIGNS AND SYMPTOMS

The cardinal feature of a skin lesion that proves to be a melanoma is change. This change may occur over weeks, months, or years. Lesions that grow so rapidly that they change in a matter of days are more likely to be inflammatory (e.g., pyogenic granuloma). Most, but not all, melanomas are noticed in an existing pigmented lesion. Early signs of malignancy include increase in size,

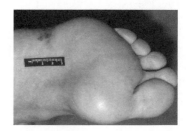

Figure 16–5. Acral lentiginous melanoma.

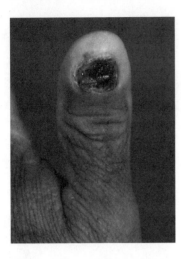

Figure 16–6. Acral lentiginous melanoma.

color change, increase in elevation (height), and itching. Late signs of malignancy include ulceration, bleeding, and tenderness. Pigmented lesions that change in any of these ways should be biopsied.

DIAGNOSIS

BIOPSY FOR HISTOPATHOLOGIC EVALUATION

Any lesion that has changed in size, shape, color, or contour or that has clinical features suggestive of melanoma should be biopsied. The biopsy may be either excisional or incisional (e.g., a punch biopsy of 3 to 6 mm), so long as it adequately represents the tumor's full thickness and level of invasion into the dermal layers; this information is vital to staging and determination of prognosis (Fig. 16–7). Shave biopsy or electrodesiccation of a suspected melanoma should be condemned.[8] The site of the excisional biopsy should be chosen carefully so as to sample the thickest area of the lesion and to orient the ellipse along the lines of skin tension and parallel to the direction of lymphatic drainage for consideration of definitive surgical therapy if necessary (Fig. 16–8). On extremities this is along the long axis of the limb, but near the joints the placement may vary. Punch biopsies are not generally recommended for lesions of the face because it is more difficult to achieve a cosmetically acceptable closure with a round, "cookie-cutter" defect.

Table 16–1. Differential Diagnosis of Pigmented Lesions

TYPE OF LESION	APPEARANCE
Seborrheic keratosis	Waxy, raised, "stuck on" lesion, dark brown; can be "scraped" off
Compound nevus	Well-demarcated, round to oval, ranging from flesh-colored to dark brown; sometimes has slightly irregular borders
Lentigo maligna	Flat, sharp bordered, medium to dark brown; solar variant on sun-exposed areas
Subungual hematoma	Red-brown area beneath nail; proximal clearing as nail grows out
Hemangioma	Purple nodule partially blanches to compression

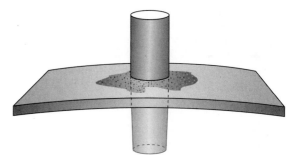

Figure 16–7. Skin punch biopsy.

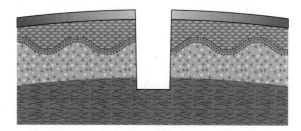

HISTOPATHOLOGIC CRITERIA

A lesion is diagnosed as melanoma if it demonstrates sufficient architectural and cytologic atypia.[9] In certain situations, particularly when evaluating metastatic lesions, immunohistochemical analysis using S-100 protein and HMB-45 antibodies is helpful. Primary lesions require an epidermal component. These

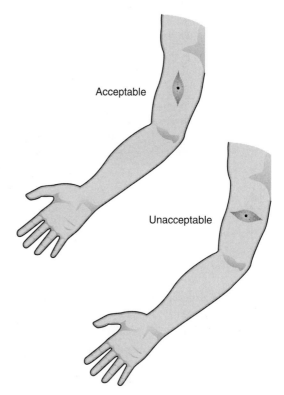

Figure 16–8. Orientation of excisional biopsy. Biopsy should be placed to minimize skin tension and parallel to the direction of lymphatic drainage.

markers can be found in paraffin-embedded tissue specimens. S-100 protein is expressed by virtually all melanomas, by other tumors, and by some normal cells, and its presence is highly sensitive for melanoma. HMB-45 is a monoclonal antibody that reacts to most types of melanoma and few other cells; it has a high specificity for melanoma.

STAGING

The most important information the pathologist provides is the melanoma's thickness (Breslow microstaging technique) and its level of invasion (Clark microstaging technique). Under the Breslow system (Fig. 16–9), an ocular micrometer is used to measure from the granular layer of the epidermis to the greatest depth of invasion. This provides a reproducible method for tumor staging and accurately correlates with the risk of metastatic disease, which is the single most powerful prognostic indicator.[10]

The Clark system categorizes five levels of invasion that reflect depth of penetration into the dermis or subcutaneous fat (see Fig. 16–9). The disadvantage of this system is that anatomic landmarks can be distorted and are not always clearly identified or reproduced.[10] The latest version of the staging system adopted by the American Joint Committee on Cancer (Table 16–2) is heavily based on microstaging of the primary tumor and the patterns of metastases. The most common first site of metastasis is the regional lymph node basin. Melanoma cells can also become entrapped in dermal lymphatics near the primary site (satellites) or between the primary tumor and regional lymph nodes (intransits). In stages I and II, the disease is localized and subdivided into A or B categories based on microstaging findings (thickness and level). Stage III represents nodal metastasis to the nodal basin or basins regional to the primary tumor. More than one basin may be affected by primary lesions on the trunk. Stage IV indicates either distant metastases or nodal metastases to basins other than the drainage sites of the primary tumor. The most common sites of metastasis are skin

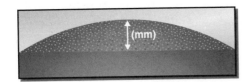

A

Figure 16–9. Melanoma tumor staging. *A*, Measurement of tumor thickness (Breslow). *B*, Levels of invasion (Clark).

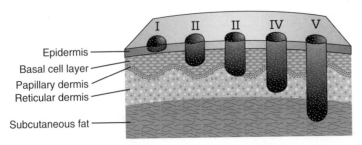

Epidermis
Basal cell layer
Papillary dermis
Reticular dermis

Subcutaneous fat

B

Table 16–2. Staging of Melanoma Using the TNM System

STAGE	TNM	CRITERIA° THICKNESS/METASTASIS	CLARK'S LEVEL
0	pTis	Melanoma in situ	I
I	pT1	≤0.75 mm	II
	pT2	>0.75 but < 1.5 mm	III
II	pT3a	>1.5 but <3 mm	IV
	pT3b	>3 but <4 mm	IV
III	pT4a	>4 mm or invades subcutaneous tissue	V
	pT4b	Satellite(s) within 2 cm of primary tumor	
	Any pT	N1 = Metastasis <3 cm in regional node(s)	
	Any pT	N2a = Metastasis >3 cm in regional node(s)	
	Any pT	N2b = In-transit metastasis >2 cm from primary tumor	
	Any pT	N2c = Both (N2a and N2b)	
IV	Any pT, any N	M1a = Metastasis in skin, subcutaneous tissue, or lymph node beyond regional nodes	
	Any pT, any N	M1b = Visceral metastasis	

Data from the American Joint Committee on Cancer: Manual of Staging of Cancer, 5th ed. Philadelphia, Lippincott-Raven, 1997.
°When pathologic thickness and level of invasion criteria (Clark) do not coincide with T classification, thickness of lesion should take precedence.
In-transit metastasis: >2 cm from primary tumor and limited to regional nodes.

(subcutaneous), lungs, brain, liver, and bone, but disease can metastasize anywhere. Unlike other malignancies, relatively few patients present with stage IV disease.

PRINCIPLES OF TREATMENT

PRIMARY MELANOMA

Primary melanomas are treated surgically with wide excision. Surgical margins are based on the thickness of the lesion, which correlates with the tumor's propensity for local recurrence. For lesions less than 1 mm thick, a minimum surgical margin of 1 cm (measured from each edge of the lesion or biopsy site) is adequate. For lesions more than 1 mm thick, a 2-cm margin of skin is required. For lesions more than 4 mm thick, a skin margin of 2 to 3 cm is required.

REGIONAL LYMPH NODES

Removal of lymph nodes is indicated if they are clinically palpable and suspected of having, or being positive for, metastases. In the clinically node-negative patient, the role of radical excision is less clear and must be based on parameters such as tumor thickness and other characteristics that indicate a propensity for spread. Tumors less than 1 mm thick affect the regional nodes in fewer than 5% of patients (and may not be evident for years), and node dissection is not usually indicated. For intermediate lesions that are 1 to 4 mm thick, occult nodal metastases are found in up to 20% of patients undergoing elective lymph node dissection.

A technique called intraoperative lymphatic mapping and sentinel node biopsy has been developed to identify for biopsy nodes that have the highest risk of containing tumor.[11] The sentinel node is found by intraoperatively injecting a radiolabeled sulfur colloid compound intradermally around the primary tumor site and finding the "hottest" lymph node with a handheld gamma probe. A blue dye is injected in a similar fashion to identify the sentinel lymph nodes visually at the time of surgical incision.[11] The node is removed and sent for pathologic evaluation. If no tumor is found, then a radical node dissection may be avoided. If tumor cells are present, there is a risk of additional nodal involvement and full dissection is warranted. This is a highly accurate test for detecting regional metastatic disease.[11]

METASTASES

As mentioned, the regional lymph nodes are the most common sites of tumor spread, followed by skin and subcutaneous tissue. Other potential sites include lung, liver, brain, and bone. Treatment with systemic chemotherapy alone has not resulted in significant improvement in survival, but clinical trials using combined immunologic, biologic, and chemotherapeutic agents have produced objective responses in a minority of patients, although the response frequently is short lived. Another area of investigation involves use of monoclonal antibodies directed to melanoma surface antigens to activate a host immune response to the melanoma, a so-called vaccine. Radiation therapy frequently is effective for local control and palliation. Surgery can benefit some selected patients who have distant metastatic disease.

SCREENING

In theory, early detection of thin tumors should reduce the morbidity and mortality rates of melanoma because thin lesions are associated with a high 5-year survival rate. However, the efficacy of early detection and screening programs remains untested by randomized trials because there is no good way to randomize this type of study.[12] Screening for primary melanoma consists of visual inspection of the skin of an asymptomatic person for suspicious lesions and, if such lesions are detected, referral of that person for biopsy. Screening practices vary and may range from a casual self-examination by someone at low risk to frequent, systematic, and total skin examinations by a skin specialist in patients identified as having risk factors. In general, the American Cancer Society recommends a cancer-related checkup in asymptomatic men and women every 3 years from age 20 to age 39 years and annually after 40 years of age. In addition, the American Academy of Dermatology provides free mass skin screenings by volunteer dermatologists every spring. Screening participants also complete a standardized form that asks about risk factors, changing conditions of moles, and family and personal history of skin cancer and melanoma.

Screening programs serve multiple purposes. They provide educational materials that help people identify personal risk factors, and they describe and stress the importance of skin self-examination. They also describe how to obtain definitive diagnosis, treatment, and follow-up, as well as risk-avoidance methods such as sun protection and avoidance of sun exposure during peak times.

PREVENTION

Cancer prevention for melanoma should identify high-risk individuals and populations at high risk and provide the following:

- Educational material at an early age regarding risk avoidance (reducing sun exposure, avoiding sunburn). This information could be disseminated through schools and by local media in the form of public service announcements.
- Instruction in the proper use of sunscreens and protective clothing.
- Impetus for changing cultural desires from sun worshipping to sun-exposure watching.
- Support of basic and clinical research studies.

CONCLUSION

Melanoma is a potentially preventable and curable disease if risk factors are identified and early detection is emphasized. With education and intervention, the morbidity and mortality rates associated with melanoma can be reduced.

REFERENCES

1. Silvers DN: On the subject of primary cutaneous melanoma: An historical perspective. In Fenoglio CM, Wolff M (eds): Progress in Surgical Pathology, vol 4. New York, Masson, 1982.
2. Kopf AW, Rigel DS, Friedman RJ: The rising incidence and mortality rate of malignant melanoma. J Dermatol Surg Oncol 8:760, 1982.
3. Gallagher RP, Elwood JM, Hill GB: Risk factors for cutaneous melanoma—the Western Canada Melanoma Study. Br J Cancer 51:543, 1985.
4. Matsui MS, Deleo VA: Photocarcinogenesis by ultraviolet A and B. In Mukhtar H (ed): Skin Cancer: Mechanisms and Human Relevance. Boca Raton, FL, CRC Press, 1995.
5. Holman CDJ, Armstrong BK: Pigmentary traits, ethnic origin, benign nevi, and family history as risk factors for cutaneous malignant melanoma. J Natl Cancer Inst 72:257, 1984.
6. Rigel DS, Rivers JK, Kopf AW, et al: Dysplastic nevi: Markers for increased risk of melanoma. Cancer 63:386, 1989.
7. Greene MH, Clark WH, Tucker MA: Acquired precursors of cutaneous malignant melanoma. Cancer 63:386, 1989.
8. Robinson JK: Fundamentals of Skin Biopsy. Chicago, Year Book Medical Publishers, 1986.
9. Barnhill RL, Mihm MC Jr: Histopathology of malignant melanoma and its precursor lesions. In Balch CM, Houghton AN, Milton GW, et al (eds): Cutaneous Melanoma, 2nd ed. Philadelphia, JB Lippincott, 1992:251–255.
10. Balch CM, Murad TM, Soong SJ, et al: A multifactorial analysis of melanoma: Prognostic histopathological features comparing Clark's and Breslow's staging methods. Ann Surg 188:732, 1978.
11. Ross MI, Reintgen D, Balch CM: Selective lymphadenectomy: Emerging role for lymphatic mapping and sentinel node biopsy in the management of early stage melanoma. Semin Surg Oncol 9:219, 1993.
12. Koh HK, Lew RA, Prout MN: Screening for melanoma and skin cancer: Theoretic and practical considerations. J Am Acad Dermatol 20:159, 1989.

Chapter 17

Hodgkin's Disease

Deborah E. Seigler, PA-C, and
Alejandro Preti, MD

Hodgkin's disease (HD) represents a therapeutic dilemma to even the skilled oncologist. The affected patients are usually young, in an active phase of life, and have a disease that is potentially curable yet life-threatening. The treatment modalities available (radiation therapy, chemotherapy, and combined therapy) have both short- and long-term complications. The challenge to the clinician is to design a treatment program that cures the patient of the disease but accomplishes that goal with the least amount of short- and long-term toxicity and, if possible, allows the patient to maintain an active lifestyle.

EPIDEMIOLOGY

HD is an uncommon disorder, representing 0.7% of all malignancies that occur annually in the United States.[1] However, it is one of the most common malignancies in young adults and has a 4:3 male-to-female ratio.[2] The incidence of HD follows a typical bimodal curve and has been stable over the last several years. In developed countries, the incidence is low in childhood, rapidly increases among teenagers (peaking at about age 25), and then declines through middle age, with a second peak in incidence at about age 60.[2] In underdeveloped countries, the initial peak incidence is in childhood and constantly increases with age.[2] The disease in young adults is more commonly seen in higher socioeconomic classes, whereas socioeconomic class does not appear to be a factor in older adults with the disease.[3]

ETIOLOGY

The cause of HD is unknown, although an infectious process has been suggested. The Epstein-Barr virus has been implicated in HD, and its role in the pathogenesis of the disease is currently being investigated.

The immunologic status of patients with HD is impaired, and the origin of this impairment has been closely scrutinized.[2] Impairment is exhibited in a variety of ways. A defect in cellular immunity is expressed by an unresponsiveness to skin testing with delayed-type antigens, even in patients with early-stage HD.[2] This inherent immunologic disregulation is further disrupted by treatment of the disease. Treatment with radiation and chemotherapy, as well as splenectomy if performed as part of staging, can all impair immunity further. This may provide a biologic explanation or rational basis for the increased incidence of infections and secondary malignancies in patients with HD in relation to their disease process and prior therapy.

CLINICAL PRESENTATION

Typically, patients with HD present with painless enlargement of a superficial central lymph node. The enlarged lymph node is usually supradiaphragmatic, and 60% to 80% first occur in the neck.[4] Axillary or mediastinal lymphadenopathy alone is less common. Most patients who present without peripheral lymphadenopathy have a mediastinal tumor that is detected on chest radiography. Subdiaphragmatic presentations alone are uncommon in young people but occur in approximately 25% of older patients.[4] HD spreads in a very predictable pattern from one lymph node chain to another.

About one third of patients with HD present with systemic symptoms at the time of diagnosis.[2] These systemic symptoms are known as "B" symptoms and include weight loss, night sweats, and fever. Fever is defined as body temperature higher than 38°C and is present in about 25% of patients at presentation.[2] The fever is usually low grade, initially occurs in the afternoon, and progresses as the disease progresses.[2] This cyclic fever is characteristic of HD and is known as Pel-Ebstein fever. Weight loss is defined as the unexplained loss of more than 10% of body weight during the preceding 6 months.[4] Itching is not considered to be a B symptom, but it is characteristic of HD and occurs in about one in eight patients.[2, 4]

A careful history and physical examination are the most important aspects of evaluating a patient who presents with enlarged lymph nodes. Careful attention to the presence of B symptoms is crucial. Infectious nodes are soft, tender, and usually less than 2 cm in diameter. Malignant nodes are generally firm, hard, rubbery, and nontender. They can be fixed to underlying tissue and are more than 2 cm in diameter. Peripheral (centrifugal) lymph nodes such as epitrochlear nodes usually are not involved by HD but rather by non-Hodgkin's lymphoma.

DIAGNOSIS

The diagnosis of HD is made under a microscope by a pathologist. Therefore it is mandatory that a large, intact lymph node, preferably the most central node in an involved group, be surgically resected and a specimen obtained.[4] The pathologic diagnosis depends on the presence of distinct, binucleated giant cells, termed Reed-Sternberg cells. Controversy about the origin of these cells is ongoing. Their identification in a lymph node specimen can be difficult, because Reed-Sternberg cells account for only a small fraction of the total cellular population. Finding Reed-Sternberg cells is only part of the diagnostic puzzle. The background cells and their ratios to Reed-Sternberg cells are also significant. Immunophenotyping may be helpful in distinguishing HD from other types of lymphoma.

CLASSIFICATION

The Rye Classification is a four-part histopathologic subclassification system used for HD (Table 17–1). Nodular sclerosis and mixed-cellularity subtypes account for 90% of all cases. Nodular sclerosis, the most common subtype, is usually found in younger patients. Patients with mixed-cellularity HD tend to be older. The lymphocyte-predominant subtype is thought to have a distinct biology and prognosis.[5] Patients with this subtype usually have localized disease, which is treated with local radiation therapy, and their prognosis is excellent. The lymphocyte-depletion subtype is the most uncommon, and most pathologists today would challenge its existence.

STAGING

The extent of disease (stage) at the time of diagnosis is the most important guide to prognosis and treatment in HD.[2] In 1971, the Ann Arbor symposium

Table 17-1. Histopathologic Classification of Hodgkin's Disease (Rye Classification)

HISTOLOGY	RELATIVE FREQUENCY (%)	ADDITIONAL CHARACTERISTICS	ESTIMATED 5-YEAR SURVIVAL RATE
Nodular sclerosis	30–60	Females > Males	>75%
Mixed cellularity	20–40	Males > Females	50–60%
Lymphocyte-predominant	5–10	Good response with radiation alone	90%
Lymphocyte-depleted	5–10	Elderly; may be HIV-associated	<50%

Data from Rosenthal DS, Eyre HJ: Hodgkin's Disease and Non-Hodgkin's Lymphomas. In Murphy GP, Lawrence W, Lenhard RE (eds): American Cancer Society Textbook of Clinical Oncology, 2nd ed. Atlanta, American Cancer Society, 1995:454.

on staging in HD recommended the four-part system that remains in general use today (Table 17–2). It is based on both clinical and pathologic staging. Important changes of the Ann Arbor system were made in 1989 at the Cotswalds conference. It was recognized that patients with bulky disease, including masses larger than 10 cm or mediastinal masses larger than one third of the chest wall diameter, had special circumstances requiring combined modality treatment and that the suffix "X" should be added to the stage in these patients.[1] Stages II and III should emphasize the number of nodal sites involved (e.g., stage II3).[3] Other changes were the subdivision of stage III into stages III1 and III2. Patients with stage III1 disease have splenic involvement or lymphadenopathy involving the splenic, celiac, or portal nodes; those with stage III2 disease have para-aortic, iliac, or mesenteric involvement.[1] Stage III was subdivided based on work done at the University of Chicago that showed a more favorable prognosis for patients with disease confined to the upper abdomen than for those with disease in the retroperitoneal, iliac, or mesenteric nodes.[3]

Clinical staging consists of the history, physical examination, radiographic studies (plain radiographs, computed tomography [CT] scans, lymphangiogram, and gallium scan), and bilateral bone marrow biopsies. Pathologic staging consists of information gained from histologic examination of tissue obtained in staging laparotomy with splenectomy.

Table 17-2. Ann Arbor Staging Classification for Hodgkin's Disease

Stage I
Involvement of a single lymph node region (I) or a single extralymphatic organ or site (IE)
Stage II
Involvement of two or more lymph node regions on the same side of the diaphragm (II) or localized involvement of an extralymphatic organ or site (IIE)
Stage III
Involvement of lymph node regions on both sides of the diaphragm (III) or localized involvement of an extralymphatic organ or site (IIIE), spleen (IIIs), or both (IIIsE)
Stage IV
Diffuse or disseminated involvement of one or more extralymphatic organs, with or without associated lymph node involvement; the organ(s) involved should be identified by a symbol: (P) pulmonary, (O) osseous, or (H) hepatic. In addition, (A) indicates an asymptomatic patient; (B) indicates the presence of fever, night sweats, or weight loss >10% of body weight.
Systemic Symptoms
Each stage is subdivided into A and B categories: B for those with defined systemic symptoms and A for those without. The B designation is given to those patients with (1) unexplained loss of >10% of body weight in the 6 months before admission, (2) unexplained fever with temperatures above 38°C, and (3) drenching night sweats. Pruritus alone does not qualify for B classification, nor does a short febrile illness associated with an infection.

From Rosen PJ, Lavey RS, Haskell CM: Hodgkin's disease. In Haskell CM, Berek JS (eds): Cancer Treatment, 4th ed. Philadelphia, WB Saunders Co., 1995:454.

The staging laparotomy with splenectomy was introduced in 1969. The procedure consists of splenectomy; biopsy of portal, hepatic, periaortic, iliac, celiac, and mesenteric lymph nodes; and a wedge and deep-needle biopsy of both lobes of the liver. It can uncover disease that is not appreciated with clinical staging. This is important because some patients who are assumed to have local disease, which is curable with localized treatment, may in fact have disseminated or extranodal disease, which requires systemic treatment as well. Some 30% of patients have their disease stage changed by laparotomy.[2] Splenic involvement is the most frequent cause of revision of disease stage. In the 1970s surgical staging was strongly recommended. In the late 1980s it became controversial given the consequences of splenectomy and abdominal surgery. Today laparotomy is being performed less and less often. Staging laparotomy should be performed only if the information obtained will change the patient's treatment, not the assigned stage of the disease.

Clinical staging procedures recommended for prognostic and therapeutic evaluation of HD are as follows:

Patient history with emphasis on identifying B symptoms and unexplained pruritus

Complete physical examination with attention to evaluation of lymphadenopathy, size of liver and spleen, and evaluation of bone tenderness

Laboratory studies (complete blood count with differential and platelet counts; erythrocyte sedimentation rate; biochemical profile including liver function studies, serum albumin, lactate dehydrogenase, and calcium measurements)

Measurement of β_2-microglobulin

Radiographic studies (chest radiograph; CT of chest, abdomen, and pelvis)

Bipedal lymphography (bilateral lower extremity lymphangiogram to detect gross defects in lymph node architecture)—it is sensitive for detecting clinical disease in para-aortic nodes and is superior and more sensitive than CT in evaluating abdominal disease if done by a skilled radiologist in a department with extensive experience.

Bilateral bone marrow biopsies—these should be done in all patients but are more likely to be positive in patients with B symptoms.

Procedures for use under special circumstances include the following:

Staging laparotomy (only if findings would change the treatment plan)

Magnetic resonance imaging (for evaluation of spinal cord compression or bone involvement but not brain, which is not involved by HD)

Gallium scan (for residual masses after treatment, which are very common in HD)—residual masses that are not gallium avid have been correlated with the absence of disease; hence, gallium scans have become a complementary study.

Technetium bone scan (when bone involvement is suspected).

PROGNOSTIC CRITERIA

In HD, stage at diagnosis is one of the most important prognostic indicators.[2] Patients who present with limited- or early-stage disease do better than those who present with advanced-stage disease. Other prognostic indicators that adversely affect outcome include advanced age, presence of B symptoms, tumor bulk or large mediastinal mass, pelvic or inguinal involvement, extensive splenic involvement, elevated erythrocyte sedimentation rate, and increased level of β_2-microglobulin. All these factors are taken into account for treatment decision making by the clinician. Several prognostic models that stratify patients into favorable and unfavorable categories have been proposed, but there is no consensus on which model to follow.

TREATMENT MODALITIES

The goals in HD are to cure the patient and to minimize the short- and long-term treatment complications. To formulate a treatment plan, the clinician must rely on the pathologic diagnosis, staging, and prognostic indicators. Once all the information has been gathered, therapy must be tailored specifically to each patient.

A variety of options are available to successfully treat HD. These include (1) radiation therapy alone, (2) chemotherapy alone, (3) combined-modality therapy—both radiation therapy and chemotherapy, and (4) autologous bone marrow transplantation.

Treatment design in HD is becoming more complex and controversial. In general, patients with early-stage HD (Ann Arbor stage I or II) receive radiation therapy. Patients with advanced disease (Ann Arbor stage III or IV) usually receive combination chemotherapy or combined-modality therapy. In patients with large mediastinal masses, combined-modality therapy is recommended regardless of stage. The role of chemotherapy for a subset of early-stage HD patients remains controversial.

Irradiation was the first effective treatment for patients with HD. The curative potential of radiation therapy is based on the predictable spread of the disease. The fundamental goal of treatment is to destroy all of the tumor cells in the known area of disease (involved-field radiation) and in the next suspected or contiguous lymph node chain (extended-field radiation). Radiation can be delivered to a variety of fields. Common fields used in treatment of HD include the involved field, the mantle field (cervical, supraclavicular, axillary, mediastinal, and hilar nodes), the inverted-Y field (para-aortic, iliac, and inguinal nodes), and the spade field (para-aortic and iliac nodes). If more than one field requires treatment, the region having the largest tumor bulk usually is treated first.

Several effective chemotherapy regimens are available for HD. They all require the use of combinations of drugs. The three major regimens used are MOPP (mechlorethamine, vincristine, procarbazine, and prednisone), ABVD (doxorubicin, bleomycin, vinblastine, and dacarbazine), and various combinations of MOPP and ABVD. Other less established but effective chemotherapy regimens are currently undergoing clinical trials. There is considerable debate about which regimen provides the maximum cure rate with the least iatrogenic complications.

In a landmark study conducted at the National Institutes of Health between 1964 and 1967, DeVita and colleagues[6] showed that combination chemotherapy with MOPP could potentially cure patients with advanced-stage HD. In 1986 the group published 20-year follow-up data for a number of patients with advanced HD who had received MOPP as their initial treatment. The data showed that a substantial number of these patients remained cured of their disease.[7] Despite the success of MOPP, not all patients given it are cured, and there is considerable associated toxicity. ABVD was developed initially as salvage therapy for those patients who failed to respond to MOPP. Early studies with ABVD showed that some patients who failed MOPP therapy achieved complete remission with ABVD. Later, ABVD was shown to produce rates of complete remission comparable to those achieved with MOPP.[2] Alternating cycles of

MOPP and ABVD (MOPP/ABVD regimen) have been shown to be effective for the primary treatment of advanced-stage HD. The main difference between MOPP, ABVD, and MOPP/ABVD does not appear to be in their effectiveness but rather in their toxicity profiles. There is more nausea, vomiting, neurotoxicity, sterility, and potential for secondary leukemia with MOPP; more cardiopulmonary complications are seen with ABVD.

Autologous bone marrow transplantation is offered to patients who experience relapse within the first year after chemotherapy and to patients who do not achieve a complete response after chemotherapy. It is considered curative treatment.

SURVEILLANCE

Patients who achieve a complete remission should be monitored at 3-month intervals during the first 2 years after therapy, at 4- to 6-month intervals during the next 3 years, and yearly after 5 years. A careful physical examination should be done at each visit. Patients who received radiation therapy should have careful skin examinations. Laboratory tests should include a complete blood count with differential, erythrocyte sedimentation rate, and measurements of alkaline phosphatase and liver transaminases. Thyroid function studies should be performed in patients who received radiation therapy, because the incidence of hypothyroidism in this group is significant. A chest radiograph should be obtained, and periodic CT scans are indicated.

LONG-TERM SIDE EFFECTS OF TREATMENT

The effectiveness of treatment in curing patients with HD has resulted in the recognition of associated long-term complications of treatment. Understanding the late complications of treatment plays a major role in the selection of a treatment program. If treatments are comparable in terms of curative potential, then the long-term side effects should guide the clinician in treatment selection. The clinician is obligated to inform the patient of potential complications before treatment.

The major complications associated with treatment of HD include secondary leukemia and solid tumors, sterility and loss of libido, cardiopulmonary toxicity, and hypothyroidism. A higher incidence of MOPP-related myelodysplastic syndrome and acute myelogenous leukemia is a well-recognized late complication of treatment.[3] The increased incidence is even higher in patients who received both radiation therapy and MOPP. The leukemogenic potential of MOPP seems to disappear 10 to 12 years after completion of therapy.[3] The incidence of solid tumors related to radiation therapy seems to increase 20 to 30 years after treatment; these tumors usually appear in the fields of previous irradiation. Lung cancer, particularly among smokers, is the most common secondary solid tumor, but breast, thyroid, stomach, skin, bladder, and head and neck cancers have all been reported.[8] Smoking cessation should be strongly encouraged in these patients.

Sterility related to both MOPP chemotherapy and radiation therapy is also a well-recognized complication of treatment.[3] Virtually all men are found to have an absence of spermatozoa after MOPP therapy, and women experience ovarian damage, as demonstrated by prolonged cessation of menses or by early menopause. Radiation therapy can result in sterility in men and ovarian failure and sterility in women. Men undergoing MOPP chemotherapy who still wish to conceive a child should have sperm cryopreserved before treatment. Surgical replacement of ovaries is sometimes offered to women who receive pelvic irradiation.

ABVD does not appear to be leukemogenic or to have the gonadal toxicity associated with MOPP,[3] but it does have significant cardiopulmonary toxicity.[3] This must be considered in patients who may undergo irradiation to the chest. Toxicity to the lungs and heart attributable to radiation therapy can be enhanced by ABVD chemotherapy.

Hypothyroidism is frequently observed in patients who received supradiaphragmatic irradiation. Because it can occur many years after treatment, diligent follow-up of long-term survivors is required.[3]

Radiation therapy given to young children can result in early closure of epiphyseal plates and can lead to growth defects.[8]

SUMMARY

HD is a potentially curable malignancy that usually occurs in persons of a relatively young age group. A wide range of therapeutic options are available, and treatment strategies for different stages of disease continue to be debated. Because of the potential for cure and long-term survival, the clinician is challenged to cure the patient while limiting the potential short- and long-term side effects of treatment.

REFERENCES

1. Engstrom GP, Sanford DB, Hagemeister FB: Hodgkin's disease. In Pazdur R (ed): Medical Oncology: A Comprehensive Review, 2nd ed. Huntington, NY, PRR, 1995:111–112.
2. Aisenberg AC: Hodgkin's disease. In Malignant Lymphoma: Biology, Natural History, and Treatment. Malvern, PA, Lea & Febiger, 1991:1–86.
3. Rosen PJ, Lavey RS, Haskell CM: Hodgkin's disease. In Haskell CM, Berek JS (eds): Cancer Treatment, 4th ed. Philadelphia, WB Saunders, 1995:952,958–960.
4. Rosenthal DS, Eyre HJ: Hodgkin's disease and non-Hodgkin's lymphomas. In Murphy GP, Lawrence W, Lenhard RE (eds): American Cancer Society Textbook of Clinical Oncology, 2nd ed. Atlanta, American Cancer Society, 1995:454.
5. Trudel MA, Krikorian JG, Neiman RS: Lymphocyte predominance in Hodgkin's disease: A clinicopathologic reassessment. Cancer 1987;59:99–106.
6. DeVita VT, Serpick A, Carbone PP: Combination chemotherapy in the treatment of advanced Hodgkin's disease. Ann Intern Med 1970;73:881–894.
7. Longo DL, Young RC, Wesley M, et al: Twenty years of MOPP therapy for Hodgkin's disease. J Clin Oncol 1986;4:1295–1306.
8. Kaufman D, Longo DL: Hodgkin's disease: Crit Rev Oncol Hematol 1992;13:157,177.

Chapter 18

Non-Hodgkin's Lymphoma

Amelia Ritty, PA-C, and Alejandro Preti, MD

INTRODUCTION

Non-Hodgkin's lymphomas (NHLs) are a heterogeneous group of lymphoproliferative disorders that have few common clinical features and many biologic differences. Each NHL represents the clonal expansion of a developmental compartment of a component of the lymphoid system, and each of these has a normal counterpart in the B-, or T-, or null cell systems. More than a dozen neoplasms of the lymphoid system are included in this category; they can originate in and spread to both lymph nodes and extranodal sites. For example, follicular lymphomas, which typically originate in the lymph nodes, may also involve the bone marrow. Mantle cell lymphomas have a predilection for the colon, and mucosa-associated lymphoid tissue (MALT) lymphomas have a predilection for the stomach. Burkitt's lymphoma, which generally begins in the lymphoid system, tends to spread early to the central nervous system (CNS).

EPIDEMIOLOGY

NHL occurs roughly three times as frequently as Hodgkin's disease. The American Cancer Society estimates that, in 1995 alone, 50,000 persons in the United States were diagnosed with NHL and almost 23,000 died of this disease.[1] Among malignant neoplasms, NHL ranks sixth in both incidence and mortality.[2] Treatment has improved, and many patients today are cured.[2] The incidence of NHL is increasing at a rate of 3% to 4% annually, second only to the increasing incidence of malignant melanoma.[2] The incidence of NHL has increased by more than 65% since the 1970s and by almost 150% since 1950.[2] The reason for this increase is not clear. Lymphomas associated with the acquired immunodeficiency syndrome (AIDS) account for some of the new NHLs seen within the last decade in young and middle-aged men from urban areas, but these cases account for only a small percentage of the overall increase in incidence.[2] The incidence of disease in elderly white men, extranodal presentations, and high-grade malignancies are all increasing progressively with age and at various rates.[1]

ETIOLOGY

The cause of most types of NHLs is unknown, but great progress has been made in understanding the pathogenesis of these diseases. Abnormal immune regulation and viral and bacterial factors have all been implicated in the development of NHLs. Molecular genetic events, cytogenetic abnormalities, oncogenes, and regulators of gene transcription and the cell cycle have also been implicated as etiologic agents. At least one specific chromosomal abnormality (translocation, deletion, or duplication) is involved with each NHL subtype.[2] Research is now being done to identify the detailed mechanisms that begin with a primary oncogenic event and lead to dysregulated cell division and the development of the abnormal cells in each NHL subtype. Recent evidence shows that each neoplastic transformation is a multistep process. Changing the paths that normally regulate mitosis requires several events. The usual sequence begins with dysplasia, followed by hyperplasia, metaplasia, and finally, neoplasia.[2]

The incidence of NHL is higher in patients who have both primary and secondary immune deficiencies. Acquired immunodeficiency states (AIDS and organ or bone marrow transplantation), congenital immunodeficiency syndromes, and certain autoimmune disorders (Sjögren's syndrome, rheumatoid disease, lupus erythematosus, and Hashimoto's thyroiditis) are also associated with the development of NHL. The mechanism is thought to be related to chronic deficiencies in immune surveillance and antigenic stimulation.[2]

Viruses may cause specific NHLs. For instance, the Epstein-Barr virus, a DNA virus, is associated with Burkitt's lymphoma, and human T-cell lymphotrophic virus type I (HTLV-1), an RNA virus, is associated with adult T-cell leukemia/lymphoma. Similarly, the etiopathogenesis of MALT lymphomas has been associated with the presence of *Helicobacter pylori*.

The development of NHLs may also be treatment related or associated with exposure to chemical or physical agents. Previous treatment of Hodgkin's disease or polycythemia vera with alkylating agents with or without radiation therapy predisposes a patient to the development of high-grade B-cell lymphomas. Some combination chemotherapy regimens and drugs such as alkylating agents, cyclosporine, and azathioprine have also been associated with the development of NHL. In addition, hydantoin anticonvulsants and herbicides have been implicated in the development of NHL.[2, 4, 5]

Cytogenetic abnormalities are commonly found among NHL subtypes. Burkitt's lymphoma is usually associated with oncogene translocations at t(8;14), t(8;22), or t(8;2). Marker chromosomes at 14q+ and 6q+ are seen in about 60% of all NHLs,[1] but their significance is unknown. Follicular lymphomas show genetic translocation at t(14;18), and t(11;14) is often found in patients with mantle cell lymphomas.[6]

Today, immunophenotypic studies are done to aid in establishing the diagnosis of NHL. Cell surface antigens in lymphoma tissue are detected by immunoperoxidase staining or flow cytometry. The surface marker characteristics are not totally lineage specific but distinguish lymphomas from myeloid and epithelial neoplasms. A diagnosis of NHL is based on morphology, immunophenotype (to determine lineage and monoclonality), cytogenetics (karyotype), and gene rearrangement studies.

CLINICAL PRESENTATION

Although most patients with NHL are asymptomatic, approximately 20% give a history of nonspecific constitutional or B symptoms (fevers, drenching night sweats, weight loss). Signs and symptoms are extremely variable depending on the site, extent, and type of disease present.[1–3]

Follicular lymphomas are usually slow-growing, and patients present with a long-standing history of "waxing and waning" lymphadenopathy (cervical and supraclavicular). Diffuse large cell lymphoma can appear as a mass that grows rapidly (over a period of days) and usually is localized to lymph node chain areas (e.g., neck, supraclavicular, axillary, groin, mesenteric). Such lymphomas can result in a large mediastinal mass that may produce superior vena cava syndrome, dysphagia, dysphonia, or spinal cord compression, either extrinsically from an involved lymph node chain or intrinsically from leptomeningeal disease. Typically, MALT lymphoma can present as a gastric ulcer, and mantle cell lymphomas as multiple lymphomatoid polyps.

Painless lymphadenopathy of superficial lymph nodes is the most common complaint of both patients with Hodgkin's disease and those with NHL. Involvement of Waldeyer's ring and the gastrointestinal tract is common in patients with

MALT lymphomas. Patients who have Hodgkin's disease or NHL with mediastinal lymphadenopathy may present with cough, dyspnea, or dysphagia.

Systemic symptoms such as fevers and night sweats may be seen in patients with NHL. Weight loss is common, and overwhelming fatigue and generalized weakness are reported by approximately 10% to 15% of patients at presentation.[3] Patients may also describe pain, which can be (1) in bone, as a result of localized areas of bony destruction or diffuse marrow infiltration; (2) neurogenic, caused by spinal cord compression, nerve root infiltration, meningeal involvement, or varicella zoster virus; (3) retroperitoneal, usually referred to the back, suggestive of massive retroperitoneal node involvement; or (4) visceral, because of gastrointestinal, liver, or splenic involvement by disease.[3, 5]

A thorough physical examination should be performed and should include a careful evaluation of all lymph node chains, including the submental, infraclavicular, iliac, popliteal, epitrochlear, and femoral chains. The size, number, consistency, tenderness, and location of all nodes should be documented. If nodal consistency is rock hard, carcinoma should be suspected; if the consistency is rubbery, infection or lymphoma should be suspected.[4] The patient's head and neck, especially the tonsils and oropharynx, should be examined thoroughly. Cervical nodes are most commonly involved in follicular lymphoma, and rapid progression to abdominal nodes, liver, and spleen may produce bulky asymptomatic disease. Hepatosplenomegaly and abdominal masses must be ruled out on physical examination and imaging studies.

Signs of obstruction resulting from visceral compression by enlarged lymph nodes (e.g., superior vena cava syndrome, edema of an extremity) may be present. Symptoms of bowel, urinary tract, and respiratory tract obstructions are often present. A complete and detailed neurologic examination is necessary to determine the presence of neuropathy and nerve root or spinal cord compression.

The most common extranodal sites of NHL are the gastrointestinal tract, Waldeyer's ring, skin, orbit, paranasal sinuses, testes, thyroid, salivary glands, and the CNS.[2, 4] Presenting symptoms and measurements of surrounding nodes should be documented in the patient's medical record to facilitate future evaluations. Such measurements allow determinations of response to therapy, recurrence, and the indolence or aggressiveness of the disease.

DIAGNOSIS

Whenever peripheral lymphadenopathy is present, excisional biopsy of one of the largest accessible lymph nodes is recommended.[5] Smaller lymph nodes may be more easily excised but often are not involved pathologically. When planning a diagnostic biopsy, it should be remembered that the inguinal and axillary lymph nodes are frequently enlarged because of chronic inflammation or infection and may not provide optimal specimens. Pathologists with expertise in interpreting fine-needle aspirates may perform this type of biopsy on tissue for staging, but an excisional lymph node biopsy is essential for primary diagnosis. If there are no accessible involved lymph nodes, open biopsy of suspicious organs is necessary for diagnosis. If disease is shown by computed tomography (CT) scanning to be restricted to the abdomen and tissue is needed to make a diagnosis, a laparotomy may be necessary.[3, 4] If cytopenia or abnormal circulating cells are found on hematology studies, bone marrow biopsy and aspiration are imperative for diagnosis.

A history of "waxing and waning" adenopathy is usually described by the patient before a diagnosis of lymphoma is made. However, lymphadenopathy does not always signal lymphoma. Many other reasons for nodal enlargement include viral or other infections (especially in children and young adults) and systemic immune disorders such as rheumatoid arthritis, Sjögren's syndrome, systemic lupus erythematosus, and infection by the human immunodeficiency virus (HIV), which may be undocumented. If any lymphadenopathy in these nodes does not resolve with treatment of the underlying infection or illness, or if it is progressive or asymmetric, a biopsy must be done.[4] Similarly, other conditions may be responsible for the described symptoms or enlargement of lymph nodes. For example, findings in the occipital and posterior auricular nodes are frequently benign; enlargement may be caused by scalp infection. Likewise, infection in the lower extremities may produce shotty inguinal nodes, which is not typical of NHL. Isolated high or middle cervical nodes may indicate occult primary carcinomas of the head and neck and not NHL. Finally, the supraclavicular areas should be carefully palpated to reveal any abnormal lymph nodes and to avoid unnecessary biopsies of the mediastinal and hilar lymph nodes. Further details on the workup for lymphadenopathy are given in Figure 18–1.

CLASSIFICATION

For prognostic and management purposes, NHLs are subdivided according to the Working Formulation as being of low, intermediate, or high grade. These clinicopathologic subdivisions are based on the presence or absence of follicular structure, cell size, and details of the nuclear and cytoplasmic characteristics.[2] In general, low-grade lymphomas are considered to be indolent or nonaggressive, whereas intermediate- and high-grade lymphomas are considered to be aggressive and to have a short natural course if untreated. Extensive morphologic studies, immunophenotyping, cytogenetic analyses, and gene rearrangement studies may be performed, but they may not be necessary for determining either the diagnosis or the prognosis.

Although multiple classification schemes have been used in the past and are used currently in Europe, the Working Formulation and the Rappaport Classification system are most often used in the United States.[1, 2, 4, 5] As stated, the Working Formulation divides NHLs according to clinicopathologic classification (biologic aggressiveness). However, this scheme does not address T- or B-cell origin and excludes lymphomas such as cutaneous T-cell lymphomas. The Rappaport Classification divides all lymphomas into nodular and diffuse types but does not accommodate NHL subtypes such as lymphoblastic lymphoma. These two classification systems are shown in Table 18–1. Because of advances in the characterization of NHLs, a new classification system is being developed in the United States[2, 6]; it will include the NHL subtypes currently excluded by the Working Formulation and Rappaport Classification.

LOW-GRADE LYMPHOMAS

Low-grade lymphomas include small cell lymphocytic and follicular lymphomas. Approximately two thirds of low-grade NHLs are clinical stage III or IV at diagnosis because of bone marrow involvement (>50% of all cases), mesenteric

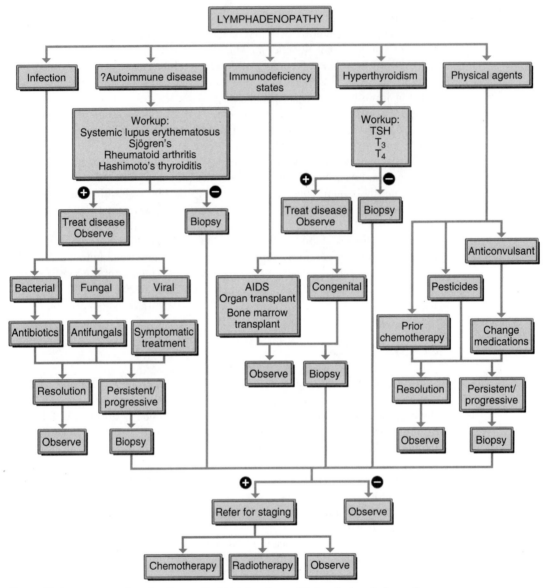

Figure 18–1. Diagnostic algorithm for non-Hodgkin's lymphoma. Workup for lymphadenopathy.

nodes, or liver involvement. However, because of their indolent nature, low-grade lymphomas may not require therapy for years and can be managed by close observation only.[4, 5]

SMALL CELL LYMPHOCYTIC LYMPHOMA

This is a low-grade neoplasm of an uncommon small B-cell lymphocyte. The cellular morphology is indistinguishable from that seen in chronic lymphocytic leukemia. This type of NHL should be considered a disseminated disease even though dissemination may not be proved during the clinical workup. Small cell

Table 18–1. Histologic Groups in Non-Hodgkin's Lymphoma

WORKING FORMULATION	RAPPAPORT CLASSIFICATION
Low grade	
Small lymphocytic	Well-differentiated lymphocytic lymphoma (WDL)
Follicular small cleaved lymphocytic	Nodular, poorly differentiated lymphocytic lymphoma (NPDL)
Mixed follicular small cleaved cell and large cell	Nodular mixed lymphoma (NM)
Intermediate grade	
Follicular, predominantly large cell	Nodular histiocytic lymphoma (NHL)
Diffuse small cleaved cell	Diffuse, poorly differentiated lymphocytic lymphoma (DPDL)
Diffuse large cell (cleaved or uncleaved)	Diffuse histiocytic lymphoma (DHL)
Mantle cell lymphoma	
High grade	
Diffuse large cell or immunoblastic	Diffuse histiocytic lymphoma (DHL)
B-cell	
T-cell	
Polymorphic	
Lymphoblastic	Lymphoblastic lymphoma
Small noncleaved	Diffuse undifferentiated lymphoma (DUL)
Burkitt's or non-Burkitt's	

Data from Rosenthal DS, Eyre HJ: Hodgkin's disease and Non-Hodgkin's lymphomas. In Murphy GP, Lawrence W, Lenhardt RE (eds): American Cancer Society Textbook of Clinical Oncology, 2nd ed. American Cancer Society, 1995:456–469.

lymphocytic lymphoma is rarely seen in patients younger than 20 years of age, and it occurs more often in men than in women (ratio of 2:1).[2] Five percent of small cell lymphocytic lymphomas evolve into aggressive and fatal diffuse large cell or immunoblastic lymphoma.[2]

FOLLICULAR LYMPHOMAS

These NHLs exhibit follicular or nodular structures. In the United States, 30% to 40% of all nodal NHLs are follicular. Follicular lymphomas are further subdivided into small cell, mixed small and large cell, and large cell types. Follicular lymphomas with small cleaved lymphocytes have the most favorable prognosis; however, because it is typically found to have disseminated beyond the primary site at diagnosis, the disease may be resistant to treatment. Follicular lymphoma has a recurrence rate of 15% to 20% per year. Approximately 50% of follicular lymphomas evolve into aggressive and unresponsive disorders that show histologic transformation and clinical disease progression to other sites.

INTERMEDIATE-GRADE LYMPHOMAS

Intermediate-grade NHLs include follicular and diffuse large cell lymphomas and mantle cell lymphomas. Follicular large cell lymphomas are the least common subtype, accounting for only 3% to 4% of all NHLs.[1] Mantle cell (centrocytic) lymphoma accounts for approximately 8% of all NHLs. The peak incidence is seen in patients in the eighth decade of life, with two thirds of these diagnoses being made in patients older than 50 years of age.[2] Mantle cell lymphoma has a male-to-female ratio of 2:1.[2] The mantle cell is a medium-sized lymphocyte that is irregularly shaped, as opposed to being round and cleaved. Disease of this subtype is typically categorized as stage III or IV at diagnosis because of bone marrow involvement. Of all classified lymphomas, mantle cell lymphomas are the most resistant to therapy; they carry a poor prognosis. The last type of intermediate-grade lymphoma, diffuse large cell lymphoma, constitutes between 25% and 30% of the total annual incidence of NHL. Its incidence increases through the years of middle age and peaks in the eighth decade of life. If it is left untreated, the expected survival time is only about 1.5 years; with combination chemotherapy, the cure rate is 30% to 50%.[2] If it is localized, diffuse large cell lymphoma is curable with radiation therapy, which today is most commonly combined with chemotherapy.[2]

HIGH-GRADE LYMPHOMAS

High-grade NHLs are classified as large cell, immunoblastic (T-cell), and small noncleaved cell lymphomas. Immunoblastic lymphomas of B-cell origin are considered as large cell lymphomas and are not classified separately. AIDS-related lymphomas, also of B-cell origin, are high-grade, aggressive, and highly fatal. Another high-grade lymphoma that may complicate AIDS is Burkitt's lymphoma. A small noncleaved cell tumor, Burkitt's lymphoma divides rapidly, with a potential cell doubling time of 12 to 24 hours. The Epstein-Barr virus has been implicated as a causative agent. Prominent and early involvement of the jaw bone is characteristic of Burkitt's lymphoma, which is endemic in regions of central Africa. Its increased incidence in other areas of the world has been related to the increase in patients with AIDS, a population in which Burkitt's lymphoma is often found. If detected in an early stage, Burkitt's lymphoma is treated as lymphoma and has a 50% to 70% cure rate. When in an advanced stage, Burkitt's lymphoma is treated as leukemia and the cure rate drops significantly.

T-CELL LYMPHOMAS

T-cell lymphomas are a heterogeneous group of lymphoid tumors characterized by malignant transformation of the T lymphocytes. This group includes convoluted T-cell lymphoma, a lymphoblastic lymphoma with markedly convoluted nuclei; cutaneous T-cell lymphoma, which exhibits clonal expansion of malignant T lymphocytes in various stages of differentiation and malignant infiltration of the skin; and adult T-cell leukemia, which is believed to be caused by human T-cell lymphotrophic virus type 1 (HTLV-1). Some T-cell lymphomas have a 50% rate of complete remission when treated with the conventional CHOP chemotherapeutic regimen (cyclophosphamide, doxorubicin, vincristine, and prednisone). However, T-cell lymphomas also have a tendency for later recurrences. The poor survival rate seen in patients with localized disease is often the result of extensive tumor burden.[5]

Lymphoblastic Lymphoma

High-grade, lymphoblastic lymphoma usually has a precursor T-cell origin. Although it accounts for only 3% to 4% of all NHLs, its incidence rises to 50% of all NHLs found in children.[2] A common presentation of this tumor is a rapidly growing anterior mediastinal mass in a male younger than 20 years old. Because meningeal involvement is common, aggressive chemotherapy should include CNS prophylaxis.[4] Microscopically, lymphoblastic lymphoma is identical to T-cell acute lymphoblastic leukemia, which is arbitrarily distinguished from lymphoblastic lymphoma by the presence of more than 30% blasts in the bone marrow.[2, 4] Without aggressive chemotherapy, the prognosis is poor.

Peripheral T-Cell Lymphomas

These are mature T-cell neoplasms. In the United States, the incidence of this tumor in adults with NHL is less than 15%.[1] Diagnosis is extremely difficult without T-cell receptor gene studies. Several types of peripheral T-cell lymphomas have been identified. Those that occur rarely but are highly aggressive include angioimmunoblastic lymphoma (also called immunoblastic lymphoma), anaplastic large cell lymphoma, midline granuloma, and lymphomatoid granulomatosis.

Cutaneous T-Cell Lymphomas

Mycosis fungoides and Sézary syndrome are the most common cutaneous T-cell lymphomas. All are malignant cutaneous lymphoproliferative disorders of helper (CD4-positive) T cells. Patients usually have a long history of undiagnosed skin disease before a specific diagnosis is made. The malignant infiltration to the skin may be the only initial manifestation of the disease.

Adult T-Cell Leukemia/Lymphoma

This T-cell lymphoma was identified in 1977 in southwestern Japan. Since its identification, it has also been seen in the Caribbean, in Brazil, and in the southeastern coastal United States. It is characterized by lymphadenopathy, hepatosplenomegaly, skin involvement, absence of a mediastinal mass, and subacute or chronic leukemia. Antibodies to HTLV-1 are found in more than 90% of patients with this disease. Adult T-cell leukemia/lymphoma is found equally in men and women, who usually are between the ages of 30 and 60 years. Recent studies suggest that this disease has a smoldering, indolent, and chronic pattern.[6]

EXTRANODAL LYMPHOMA

In the United States, 25% of NHLs are primarily extranodal, and each extranodal site has specific characteristics and treatment requirements.[2, 4–6] Approximately 50% of all extranodal lymphomas arise in the gastrointestinal tract and are of B-cell origin.[1, 3-5] The most favorable extranodal sites for localized lymphomas are the lungs, skin, orbit, salivary gland, and uterine cervix, because these lymphomas tend to have an indolent course.[5] Lymphomas that occur in the brain, especially those that also involve the retina, tend to have a rapidly progressive course and are associated with the Epstein-Barr virus. Between these two extremes are lymphomas of the stomach, large and small intestines, Waldeyer's ring, thyroid, bone, breast, and testes. Prognosis for these lymphomas depends on the extent of disease; disease spread beyond the primary site organ usually results in rapid progression. When the brain is the extranodal site, dissemination to viscera is often absent. Treatment of lymphoma localized to the brain includes intrathecal chemotherapy and radiation therapy. Within the brain, this is a rapidly progressive disease. Prognosis is poor, and patients have a short survival time. NHLs that occur in the gastrointestinal tract may be treated with irradiation and chemotherapy, and sometimes also with surgery. MALT lymphomas are more prone to occur in the gastrointestinal tract and, if they are progressive, may result in bowel and ureteral obstruction, biliary obstruction, hepatosplenomegaly, and perforation. When bone is the extranodal site, disease that is localized may be treated with irradiation and chemotherapy. Any malignant cells still present in the bony region after treatment usually remain dormant for a prolonged period; therefore, the prognosis for NHLs localized to bone is very good.[3]

STAGING

The patient's history and results of physical examination; laboratory studies that include a complete blood count, erythrocyte sedimentation rate, and liver function studies; CT scans of the abdomen, chest, and pelvis; and bilateral bone marrow biopsies are combined to determine the extent of disease at presentation and constitute the standard clinical staging workup. A gallium scan is commonly done to complement CT scans of suspected intermediate-grade NHLs. A bone scan should be performed only if bone involvement is suspected. A diagnostic lumbar puncture is indicated in lymphoblastic, AIDS-related, and Burkitt's lymphomas and in intermediate- and high-grade lymphomas that involve the bone marrow, a sinus, or the testes. Lymphangiography is used for staging only if the finding of retroperitoneal adenopathy is equivocal on CT scans or if its presence will change the treatment plan. Upper gastrointestinal tract and small bowel series should be performed if the patient is symptomatic or mesenteric adenopathy is suspected. Upper gastrointestinal endoscopy is also recommended for patients in whom disease involves Waldeyer's ring.

TREATMENT

The determination of appropriate treatment of an NHL is based primarily on the histology and the extent of disease (stage); in addition, treatment of an extranodal NHL also depends on the site. Many treatment planning options are available, but several factors must be considered. Advanced age of the patient and large tumor bulk are important comorbidity factors. Other factors that affect treatment recommendations include systemic symptoms, multiples sites of disease, an increased level of lactate dehydrogenase, disease dissemination to extranodal sites, and poor performance status (i.e., prognostic variables). These factors may be related to tumor burden. Most NHLs disseminate early and widely by a hematogenous route and not by contiguous node extension. For this reason, chemotherapy is the primary treatment modality, with irradiation as an adjunct therapy.[3]

Observation is a reasonable approach in the asymptomatic elderly patient who has indolent disease.[2, 4] Radiation therapy may be used for localized disease or palliative care. Single or combination chemotherapy of various intensities can be used, with special regimens for Burkitt's, lymphoblastic, and pediatric lymphomas.[1] High-dose chemotherapy with bone marrow transplantation or stem cell rescue and clinical trials that include monoclonal antibodies are additional options for patients with recurrent lymphoma.

As stated previously, AIDS-related lymphomas are high-grade, aggressive, and highly fatal B-cell tumors. Treatment of these lymphomas is a highly specialized area of expertise. A long-term study by the National Cancer Institute on antiretroviral therapy has been in progress for 2 years. Results to date have shown that NHL developed in 19% of patients with severe HIV infection. There was also a close correlation between a low CD4 count (<50 cells/μL) and NHL occurrence.[2] Seventy-five percent of NHLs originate in an extranodal site in AIDS patients. By frequency, these sites include the gastrointestinal tract (25%), the CNS (25%), and bone. Rapid dissemination to bone marrow and meninges is characteristic. Treatment is limited by the CD4 count, despite the use of granulocyte colony-stimulating factor, and is a critical prognostic variable. HIV/RNA load testing may be even more accurate for prognosis in these patients.[7] Rapid response to treatment and early recurrence after treatment are typical of NHLs in AIDS patients.

CHEMOTHERAPY

A discussion of all chemotherapeutic agents and regimens is not necessary for the primary care provider. Patients should be referred to a medical oncologist or hematologist for treatment (see Referral Criteria). Follow-up coordination and communication between the advanced clinical practitioner and the oncologist/hematologist is vital to the patient's care.

In 1955, when it was discovered that alkylating agents, particularly chlorambucil (Leukeran), were effective in the management of NHL, treatment of these tumors has changed dramatically.[5] Today combination chemotherapy with regimens such as CHOP are commonly used with curative intent to treat NHL.

RADIATION THERAPY

Radiation therapy is a local treatment, affecting only those areas in the selected radiation field.[3] Irradiation is currently used to treat localized and regional (stage I to III) low-grade NHLs and bulky, higher-grade NHLs. Irradiation may also be used for palliative treatment of symptoms in patients with advanced NHL of any histology. For instance, it is used to alleviate obstruction of superior vena cava syndrome, spinal cord compression, ureteral obstruction, and intractable pain caused by the tumor mass.

SURGERY

Surgery is used primarily to establish the diagnosis of NHL. It does not have a role in the treatment or management of NHL except in some instances of gastrointestinal involvement. Because irradiation and chemotherapy in patients whose disease involves the gastrointestinal tract puts them at risk for perforation, surgical resection of involved gastric and small bowel lymphomas is a treatment consideration.[1-5]

BIOLOGIC THERAPY

Interferon therapy has resulted in a response rate of approximately 40% for low-grade NHL and is currently used as part of their management. Monoclonal antibodies conjugated with radionuclides or toxins are currently in phase I and II clinical trials and have shown encouraging results. Patients with NHL that is refractory to conventional therapies may be considered for such studies.

PROGNOSTIC FACTORS

Prognostic factors are tumor or host variables that have been correlated with patient outcome or disease status, or both. For instance, early (stages I and II) versus late (stages III and IV) disease is a major prognostic factor. In general, host variables of prognostic significance include advanced age (>65 years) and poor performance status (Zubrod scale >1). Tumor variables associated with poor prognosis are bulky disease (>7 to 10 cm), presence of systemic (B) symptoms, more than one involved extranodal site, and elevated levels of lactate dehydrogenase and β_2-microglobulin.[1]

Today, NHLs are stratified into favorable and unfavorable categories on the basis of systems or scores that include most of the variables mentioned. Concomitant medical problems, such as a history of cardiac disease, renal and hepatic insufficiency, or respiratory disease, also limit the outcome.

REFERRAL CRITERIA

Clinical presentation and baseline studies are used to guide the decision of whether to refer a patient to an oncologist/hematologist. Lymphadenopathy that does not resolve after treatment for an underlying infection or disease requires investigation. Progression of lymphadenopathy in an asymmetric pattern, multiple sites of involvement, or an increase in extent or size of lymph nodes also requires investigation. Mediastinal and hilar adenopathy seen on routine chest radiographs should be further evaluated with a CT scan of the chest. CT scans of the abdomen should be done in cases of frank jaundice because they may reveal liver involvement or extrahepatic biliary obstruction caused by NHL.

Hematologic abnormalities identified by the complete blood count may include lymphocytosis, autoimmune hemolytic anemia, or thrombocytopenia. These findings may be caused by bone marrow involvement, and referral to an oncologist/hematologist is necessary for the performance of bone marrow biopsy and aspiration. Blood chemistry abnormalities may include elevations in markers of liver function, elevated creatinine and blood urea nitrogen, hypercalcemia, hyperuricemia (caused by the rapid cell turnover rate in aggressive NHLs), and hypergammaglobulinemia (on protein electrophoresis analysis). In case of these findings, the patient should promptly be referred to an oncologist/hematologist for appropriate further evaluation.

SURVEILLANCE POLICY

Patients whose disease has completely or partially remitted after treatment should be monitored carefully. Regularly scheduled follow-up appointments with the attending oncologist/hematologist should be encouraged. Most patients are seen every 3 months for the first 1 to 2 years after treatment, then every 6 months for 3 years, and then once annually. The follow-up schedule may vary with the individual practitioner and by disease status. Alternating visits between the specialist and the primary care provider may be an option if both medical providers agree with the patient's plan of care. Radiology and laboratory studies are best performed by the oncologist/hematologist during follow-up and restaging to ensure consistent results, views, and techniques for comparison. Elderly patients who exhibit signs of "failure to thrive," depression, or dementia should also be monitored. These vague complaints may be caused by NHL.

EFFECTS OF THERAPY

All treatments have both short- and long-term effects, and these effects depend on factors such as the chemotherapeutic agents used, the dose intensity and frequency, the amount of radiation given, and the extent of radiation fields. Patients who undergo any type of chemotherapy are at risk for anemia, neutropenia, and thrombocytopenia. Depending on the dosage and duration of treatment, these conditions may be slow to resolve on completion of therapy. Anemia that occurs during treatment or within the immediate follow-up period may be alleviated by erythropoietin, which may be given during and after treatment. However, anemia that does not resolve or that occurs (as shown by changes in the complete blood count) after a reasonable posttreatment period may have a different cause and should be investigated before any type of growth factor is given.

Some of the more common sequelae of chemotherapy agents include congestive heart failure (doxorubicin), pulmonary fibrosis or restrictive disease (bleomycin), hematuria (cyclophosphamide), and peripheral neuropathies (vincristine). All agents can cause anemia, neutropenia, and thrombocytopenia. Finally, patients who have undergone allogeneic bone marrow transplantation are at risk for graft-versus-host disease and should be monitored by the oncologist/hematologist.[1, 4]

Radiation therapy may cause local fibrosis and hyperpigmentation to the irradiated site. If a therapeutic field includes bony regions that are bone-marrow dense (i.e., the sternum, pelvis, or spine), myelosuppression may be prolonged or permanent. Radiation therapy to visceral organs can cause pulmonary fibrosis and scarring, esophagitis or stricture, or permanent alopecia if the whole brain has been irradiated. Improved technology and accurate, precise irradiation of selected fields have lessened the long-term effects of radiation therapy.[3]

CONCLUSION

NHL is a disease that affects people of all ages and lifestyles. As a primary care provider, the advanced clinical practitioner must be aware of the wide array of symptoms and presentations of NHL to provide a timely and accurate diagnosis. Coordination and communication with the attending oncologist/hematologist facilitates quality and continuity of care.

REFERENCES

1. Rosenthal DS, Eyre HJ: Hodgkin's disease and non-Hodgkin's lymphomas. In Murphy GP, Lawrence W, Lenhardt RE (eds): American Cancer Society Textbook of Clinical Oncology, 2nd ed. Atlanta, American Cancer Society, 1995:456–469.
2. Aisenberg A: Coherent view of non-Hodgkin's lymphoma. J Clin Oncol 1995;13:2656–2675.
3. Wasserman TH, Glatstein E: Non-Hodgkin's lymphomas. In Perez CA, Brady LW (eds): Principles and Practice of Radiation Oncology, 2nd ed. Philadelphia, JB Lippincott, 1992, pp 1329–1344.
4. Casciato D, Lowitz B: Manual of Clinical Oncology, 2nd ed. Boston, Little, Brown, 1988.
5. Aisenberg A: Malignant Lymphoma. Malvern, PA, Lea & Febiger, 1991.
6. Chappuis PO, Sappino AP: Update: Lymphoid neoplasms. Molecular characterizations of non-Hodgkin's lymphomas: Impact on patient management. Semin Hematol 1995;32:237–241.
7. Adair M, Burian P, Jones S, et al: Caring for the HIV-positive patient: Exciting changes in treatment. J Am Acad Physician Assts 1996; 9(90):52–61.

Chapter 19

Acute and Chronic Leukemias—A Concise Review

Kathryn L. Boyer, MS, PA-C, and Hagop Kantarjian, MD

Leukemias are malignant neoplasms of the blood-forming (hematopoietic) tissues.[1] Hematopoiesis is the formation and development of blood cells. The bone marrow is the primary organ that produces red blood cells, white blood cells (WBCs), and platelets—the final products of proliferation and differentiation of primitive cells, called stem cells. Stem cells mature into blood cells of all hematopoietic lineages in a process that continues throughout life. The process is disrupted, however, by leukemia, a malignant disorder caused by defects of the stem cells at different stages of maturation, with subsequent clonal expansion of the myeloid (red cell, granulocyte, platelet) or lymphoid (lymphocyte) lineages. Leukemia often manifests itself when suppression of normal hematopoiesis results in anemia, infections, or hemorrhage. Leukemia was first documented in 1827 by Velpean, but it was ignored until Virchow, credited with recognizing "weisses Blut" (white blood), mentioned it in 1847.[2] The first substance used to treat leukemia (chronic myeloid leukemia) was arsenic oxide, which produced a complete, although transient, remission. Radiation therapy was used later. Until the 1940s, leukemia was considered virtually incurable.[2] Today we have an arsenal of chemotherapy drugs, but current therapies still are not completely effective in treating the various leukemias.

Leukemias are classified into four major types: acute myeloid (AML), acute lymphocytic (ALL), chronic myeloid (CML), and chronic lymphocytic (CLL) leukemia, depending on which cell lines are involved. Acute versus chronic is a distinction determined by the observed duration of the patient's survival, although the two conditions involve different pathophysiologic processes. Paradoxically, acute leukemias to date have had better potential for cure than the chronic types. Acute leukemias are characterized by arrest in the maturation of stem cells that results in massive accumulation of immature nonfunctional cells, or blasts.[3] This process is potentially curable if the neoplastic clone is eliminated, which will allow reestablishment of normal hematopoiesis. Chronic leukemias, in contrast, result from a defect in cell reproduction that leads to unregulated proliferation and hence overexpansion of a spectrum of differentiated cells.[3] Programmed cell death, called apoptosis, may also be defective, leading to an abnormal accumulation of mature cells. Therapy is directed at reducing the tumor burden, suppressing the defective clonal element, and returning the patient's life to normal for as long as possible. In the future, a better understanding of the different mechanisms that cause each type of leukemia will lead to the development of more specific and effective therapies.

ACUTE LEUKEMIAS

GENERAL INFORMATION

MEDICAL EMERGENCY

At the initial diagnosis, acute leukemia should be considered a medical emergency. Any person with pancytopenia, a deficiency of all elements in the blood, is at an increased risk of infection, bleeding, and problems related to severe anemia, such as high-output cardiac failure. If immediate treatment is not available at the time the acute leukemia is diagnosed, the patient should be transfused with blood products to raise the values of deficient blood elements to acceptable levels. The neutropenic patient should be given oral antibiotics to prevent infection. At this point, rapid and efficient referral to a major cancer center is imperative. If the patient is in stable condition before the initiation of chemotherapy, this treatment has a greater chance of success.[4] Patients with AML who are not treated have a median survival time of approximately 2 months. When the blast count in the peripheral circulation exceeds 50,000 to 100,000/μL of blood, leukostasis (the accumulation of blasts or other WBCs in blood vessels) can cause altered mental status, retinal hemorrhage, cerebrovascular accidents, priapism, local perivascular tissue infiltration, and organ failure, especially of the pulmonary and renal systems. Emergency therapy for leukostasis includes hydration, hydroxyurea (a cytolytic drug), and/or leukapheresis, in which leukocytes are removed from withdrawn blood and the remainder is returned to the patient.[3] Rapid destruction of large numbers of leukemic cells (tumor lysis syndrome) by hydroxyurea or chemotherapy can cause life-threatening acute metabolic derangements. These can be avoided by vigorous hydration, alkalinization, the use of allopurinol, close observation, and early initiation of hemodialysis when necessary.

CHEMOTHERAPY CONSIDERATIONS

During chemotherapy, patients with acute leukemia must be monitored closely with frequent blood counts, transfusions of blood products to prevent severe anemia and hemorrhage, and administration of prophylactic antimicrobial drugs during times of severe neutropenia. Sulfamethoxazole-trimethoprim or ciprofloxacin is commonly used for broad-spectrum antibacterial coverage, fluconazole for prevention of candidiasis. Despite prophylaxis, patients are still at high risk of life-threatening infections throughout the duration of chemotherapy; attention to any temperature elevation is therefore imperative. Electrolyte imbalances occur during chemotherapy cycles and should be corrected whenever possible to avoid cardiac arrhythmias and other physiologic disturbances.

ACUTE MYELOID LEUKEMIA

AML is a rare malignancy. It is characterized by infiltration of bone marrow by abnormal hematopoietic precursors that disrupt normal production of several cell lines. It can be subdivided by the FAB (French-American-British Cooperative Group) system into specific types, depending on which cell lines are involved (Table 19–1).[1–6]

EPIDEMIOLOGY

The overall incidence of AML is approximately 4 per 100,000 persons in the United States and England,[4] and it increases with age, from 1 in 100,000 in people younger than 35 years to 15 in 100,000 for those older than 75.[3] Rates are slightly higher among men and Anglo-Saxons. Although in general the cause of AML is unknown, it is the type of leukemia most strongly linked to radiation exposure, chemical exposure (benzene), or previous use of alkylating agents.[1] Japanese atomic bomb survivors experienced a 20-fold increase of AML,[5] and the incidence of the disease is 10 times higher than normal among manufacturing

Table 19–1. French-American-British Cooperative Group (FAB) Classification of Acute Myeloid Leukemia by Morphology and Cytogenetics

FAB	INCIDENCE (%)	CELL MORPHOLOGY	CHARACTERISTICS	CYTOGENETICS	CONSIDERATIONS
M0	2–3	Undifferentiated	Large granular blasts	Diploid (normal)	May be confused with ALL
M1	20	Acute myeloblastic	Auer rods	trisomy 8, -5, -7	
M2	30	Acute myeloblastic with differentiation	Auer rods	trisomy 8, -5, -7, t(8;21)	
M3	10	Acute promyelocytic (APL)		t(15;17)	>30% promyelocytes
					Associated with DIC
					Treat with idarubicin and all-*trans*-retinoic acid (an oral differentiating agent)
M4	25–30	Myelomonocytic	Myelomonocytic blasts	inversion 16	Tissue infiltration
M4Eo		(Subtype of M4)	>5% eosinophils		
M5	10	Monocytic	Monoblasts	t(9;11), t(8;16), 11q-	Monocytic infiltration of skin, gingiva; hemorrhage common, especially of lung
M6	4	Erythroleukemia	Dysplastic erythrocytes	-5, -7, trisomy 8	
M7	1–3	Megakaryocytic	Megakaryocytes with shaggy borders	trisomy 21, inversion 3	Myelofibrosis in 20% to 30%

Blast, immature, undifferentiated cell; Auer rods, granular, lamellar bodies in cytoplasm of some abnormal granulocyte precursors; t(15;17), genetic translation of chromosomes 15 and 17; -5, monosomy 5; -7, monosomy 7; 11q-, deletion of long arm of chromosome 11; t(8;21): genetic translocation of material of chromosomes 8 and 21; t(9;11): genetic translocation of material of chromosomes 9 and 11; t(8;16): genetic translocation of material of chromosomes 8 and 16.

workers exposed to benzene.[2] Children who have received epipodophyllotoxins (highly toxic compounds with antineoplastic and cathartic properties) for ALL are at increased risk of developing AML in later years.[3] Secondary AML, which may occur 1 to 7 years after treatment with alkylating agents or other chemotherapeutic drugs, has a poorer prognosis than newly occurring leukemia. In addition, 25% of AML patients have a history of myelodysplastic syndrome (MDS).[6] Several congenital disorders—Down syndrome (20 times the risk), Fanconi's anemia, Klinefelter's syndrome, Turner's syndrome, and Wiskott-Aldrich syndrome—may terminate in AML.[3] The overall prognosis for AML remains guarded, with the cure rate ranging from 10% to 60%, depending on the patient's age, performance status, and organ function; the leukemia cell characteristics including chromosomal abnormalities; and the presence or absence of an antecedent hematologic disorder.

PRESENTATION

Occasionally, AML is discovered on a routine blood test of an asymptomatic patient, but most patients have physical complaints arising from disruption of normal blood component production. These include fatigue and shortness of breath (anemia), bleeding and bruising (thrombocytopenia), and fever with or without infection (neutropenia). Most common are upper respiratory infections, although occasionally a patient presents with pneumonia. Bone pain or infiltration of skin (leukemia cutis), gingiva, or other soft tissues usually suggests monocytic variants.[3] Less often, patients have collections of myeloblasts/chloromas or granulocytic sarcomas in any soft tissue. These may be isolated findings initially; however, bone marrow infiltration is inevitable, and treatment is warranted.

LABORATORY FINDINGS

Laboratory studies usually reveal pancytopenia, although patients may have any combination of anemia, thrombocytopenia, and leukopenia. Blasts and other immature WBCs may be present in the peripheral blood, and because of rapid cell turnover lactate dehydrogenase and uric acid may be elevated. In acute promyelocytic leukemia, coagulation profiles should be evaluated carefully, because disseminated intravascular coagulation (DIC) may occur when these cells disintegrate and release procoagulants. Leukocytosis, an increase of leukocytes, may also be present and is a medical emergency, because leukostasis in perivascular tissues can cause headaches, altered mental status, dyspnea, and ultimately fatal pulmonary or intracranial hemorrhages. Acute leukemias usually can be diagnosed from the peripheral smear, but bone marrow aspiration and biopsy should always be performed to determine the proper classification. In AML, the bone marrow aspirate has more than 30% blasts (<5% blasts is normal), of which more than 3% are positive for myeloperoxidase stain. Patients with M4 or M5 morphology are positive for monocytic stains (peroxidase and esterase). Patients with M6 disease have diffuse cytoplasmic positivity for PAS stain (see Table 19–1).[1–6] Histochemical stains of bone marrow blasts are crucial for diagnosis of AML type, but cell immunophenotyping and electron microscopy are helpful in difficult cases. Most patients for whom all stains are negative (acute undifferentiated leukemia) are treated as having AML, because immunopheno-typing usually demonstrates positive myeloid markers, which are also indicators of AML type.

Immunophenotyping (the determination of malignant cells in the immune system) of AML blood or marrow should show positivity for myeloid markers such as CD11b, CD13, CD14, CD15, and CD33.[3] Auer rods may be present. They are granular, lamellar bodies in cytoplasm of some cells; their presence is virtually diagnostic of leukemia. In acute promyelocytic leukemia, the M3 sub-type, the bone marrow may have less than 30% blasts but usually more than 70% progranulocytes. Cytogenetic studies, preferably done on bone marrow, result in abnormal findings in 50% to 60% of patients.[4]

TREATMENT

Although AML was an almost universally fatal disease 30 years ago, 25% of patients are now being cured with improved therapy regimens and supportive care. Initial treatment for AML is aimed at eradicating the leukemic clone and allowing normal hematopoiesis to be re-established. Treatment usually has two components: induction of remission and postremission therapy. Patients with most AML subsets are treated similarly, with a combination of cytarabine (ara-C) given by continuous infusion for 7 days and anthracyclines (daunorubicin, doxorubicin, idarubicin) given for 3 days as bolus injection. This is the 3 + 7 regimen that produces a 70% rate of complete remission (CR).[4] CR is defined as more than 1500 circulating neutrophils per microliter, more than 100,000 platelets per microliter, less than 5% bone marrow blasts with more than 20% cellularity, and normal maturation in all cell lines.[7] High-dose ara-C has improved prognosis overall, but particularly among younger patients and those with favor-able chromosomes. Idarubicin seems to be superior to other anthracyclines. In acute promyelocytic leukemia, the use of all-*trans*-retinoic acid, an oral agent that fosters maturation of cells, with chemotherapy frequently results in CR after one course. Allogeneic bone marrow transplantation (BMT) during first remission is reserved for patients who have a poor prognosis with chemotherapy, and it is offered to all patients who experience relapse after front-line induction chemotherapies. Other combinations of chemotherapeutic agents are currently being investigated, but the overall prognosis for patients with AML, especially those with some cytogenetic abnormalities, remains poor (Table 19–2).[3, 4, 7]

Table 19–2. Cytogenetics, Complete Remission Rates, and Cure Rates of Acute Myelogenous Leukemia

CYTOGENETICS	FAB CLASSIFICATION	OVERALL INCIDENCE (%)	COMPLETE REMISSION RATE (%)[*]	CURE RATE (%)[†]
Diploid (normal)	Any	50	70	25
t(8;21)	M2	5–10	90	40–50
Inversion 16	M4	5–10	90	40–50
t(15;17)	M3	10	80	60
-5, -7, trisomy 8	Any	20–30	50–60	<10
11q23, others	M5	10–20	50–70	10–15

[*]Circulating neutrophils >1500/μL, platelets >100,000/μL, bone marrow blasts <5%, and normal maturation of other bone marrow cells as seen in aspiration differential.
[†]One-year event-free survival.

MYELODYSPLASTIC SYNDROMES

The MDS are clonal proliferative disorders in which ineffective blood formation results in progressive deficiencies in the peripheral circulation.[1] The MDS include refractory anemia (RA), refractory anemia with ringed sideroblasts (RARS; a sideroblast is a red blood cell containing iron), refractory anemia with excess blasts (RAEB), refractory anemia with excess blasts in transformation to AML (RAEB-T), and chronic myelomonocytic leukemia (CMML) (Table 19–3).[4, 5, 8] Disease progression can be slow, but it often results in fatal pancytopenia or progression to AML.

EPIDEMIOLOGY

The reported incidence of MDS is 1 in 100,000, and it occurs more commonly in persons older than 60 years of age.[1] The cause in most cases is unknown, but some cases arise 3 to 7 years after exposure to chemotherapy with alkylating agents.[8] Other cases have been seen in patients with a history of irradiation or benzene exposure.[8] Chromosomal abnormalities are found in up to 75% of patients, the most common being -5, -7, $+8$, -17, similar to those found in AML.[8]

PRESENTATION

Patients may complain of fatigue, pallor, bruising, bleeding, or infection, which are direct consequences of bone marrow failure. Positive physical findings are unusual; 15% to 20% of patients have splenomegaly. Laboratory studies reveal peripheral pancytopenias, especially anemia, usually macrocytic (with abnormally large red blood cells). The bone marrow is hypercellular and shows dysplasia in at least one cell line.

TREATMENT

The prognosis and the course of disease progression are variable; patients with RA or RARS have the best prognosis and are treated with supportive care

Table 19–3. Myelodysplastic Syndromes

DISEASE	MARROW BLASTS (%)	BLOOD BLASTS (%)	RINGED SIDEROBLASTS 15% IN MARROW	ABSOLUTE MONOCYTES IN BLOOD PER MICROLITER	UNTREATED MEDIAN SURVIVAL (YR)
RA	<5	≤1	—	<1000	3
RARS	<5	≤1	⊕	—	3
RAEB	5–20	<5	±	—	1½
RAEB-T	21–30	≥5	±	<1000	1½
CMML	≤20	<5	±	>1000	1½

CMML, chronic myelomonocytic leukemia; RA, refractory anemia; RARS, refractory anemia with ringed sideroblasts; RAEB, refractory anemia with excess blasts; RAEB-T, refractory anemia with excess blasts in transformation; ringed sideroblasts, nucleated red cells containing iron granules in cytoplasm around the nucleus.

(erythropoietin, growth factors, transfusions). Intensive combination chemotherapy is investigational and is reserved for patients with RAEB and RAEB-T. With therapy like that for AML, the CR rate is 70% to 80% for patients with favorable chromosomes, and the projected 3-year event-free survival (EFS) rate is about 50%. In MDS patients with unfavorable chromosomal types, the CR rate is still 50%, but most patients relapse and the projected 3-year EFS rate is 10% or less. Allogeneic BMT may offer a potential cure for eligible patients, with reported long-term EFS rates of 20% to 40%. Other investigational agents include growth factors (granulocyte colony-stimulating factor [G-CSF], granulocyte-macrophage colony-stimulating factor [GM-CSF], erythropoietin), particularly for patients with low blast counts (<10%) and without monocytosis; combinations of growth factors and chemotherapy (e.g., ara-C); and new agents (e.g., decitabine, topotecan), some of which have promising results.

ACUTE LYMPHOCYTIC LEUKEMIA

ALL is a malignant clonal proliferation of lymphoid precursors whose maturation is arrested. It is one of the first malignancies that responded to chemotherapy and one of the first to be cured in a large percentage of affected children.

EPIDEMIOLOGY

ALL is the most common malignant disease of childhood, accounting for about 80% of all childhood leukemias but only about 20% of leukemias in adults.[9] A slight male predominance exists in the United States, and more whites and Hispanics are afflicted than people of any other ethnic group. ALL represents approximately 1% to 2% of all cancers,[9] with 3000 to 5000 new cases diagnosed each year in the United States. Its incidence has a bimodal age distribution, with the first peak occurring at about 3 to 5 years of age[1] and the second at about 50 years of age; the incidence then increases up to 2 cases per 100,000 in persons older than age 65. The incidence ratio of AML to ALL is 6:1.[4]

The cause of ALL is unknown, and risk factors, although studied extensively, have not been determined conclusively. Genetic and environmental correlations continue to present themselves. ALL risk is significantly increased among identical twins of ALL patients. In addition, siblings of patients with ALL have a fourfold greater risk of developing the disease than do members of the general population.[9] Certain congenital disorders have been associated with an increased risk of leukemia. Exposure to high-dose radiation is a definite risk factor in ALL, especially if the exposure is in utero.[9] As is true for AML, Japanese atomic bomb survivors have had a 20-fold increased risk of ALL.[9] Chemical exposure, especially to benzene, has been associated with an increased risk of acute leukemia, but only one third of such cases are ALL. Clusters of increased incidence suggest an infectious cause of the disease, but this has been difficult to substantiate. Viruses are considered mutagens capable of inducing the clonal malignancy associated with leukemia. Human T-cell lymphotropic virus type 1 (HTLV-1) is a known viral cause of human T-cell leukemia, and this suggests that other viruses, specifically Epstein-Barr virus, may contribute to the onset of ALL.[1, 10]

PRESENTATION

As the leukemic clone multiplies abnormally in the bone marrow and impairs normal hematopoiesis, the signs and symptoms of ALL appear abruptly. Most common are malaise, fatigue, bone pain, bleeding/bruising, weight loss, and fever without an obvious infectious cause.[9] These symptoms are often mistakenly attributed to an infectious rather than a malignant process. About 10% of patients feel well and are asymptomatic.[4] Twenty percent to 60% of patients with ALL have lymphadenopathy with painless, mobile nodes. About 75% of patients present with hepatomegaly with or without splenomegaly, although liver function usually is preserved.[9] The degree of lymphadenopathy and hepato-splenomegaly correlates with the tumor burden, so that their presence portends a worse prognosis. Occasionally, other organs may be involved, including the kidneys, lungs, heart, eyes, gastrointestinal tract, and skin. Central nervous system (CNS) involvement, although present initially in only 10% of patients, eventually occurs in 50% to 75% if prophylaxis for CNS disease is not given as part of therapy.[3] CNS leukemia manifests itself with signs and symptoms of increased intracranial pressure, such as headaches that are worse when the patient is lying down, papilledema, nausea, vomiting, irritability, and lethargy. Meningismus is common and usually affects cranial nerves III, IV, VI, and VII.[9] Testicular involvement occurs in 25% of children but is rare in adults. Mediastinal masses are noted with the leukemic stage of lymphoblastic lymphoma, or T-cell ALL, whereas bulky abdominal nodes, CNS involvement, and facial neuropathies suggest Burkitt lymphoma or other forms of mature B-cell ALL.[9]

LABORATORY FINDINGS

The WBC count usually is high, perhaps more than 100,000 cells/μL, frequently with a large number of circulating lymphoblasts. These blasts may be difficult to distinguish morphologically from myeloblasts in 20% to 30% of cases; histochemical staining for terminal deoxynucleotidyl transferase (TdT) activity is imperative for diagnosis. The absolute neutrophil count is frequently low despite the high total WBC count. Symptoms of leukocytosis are seldom seen, because lymphoblasts are small and do not readily sludge in blood vessels. Normochromic, normocytic anemia is almost universal, and thrombocytopenia is the rule, with two thirds of patients presenting with platelet counts lower than 50,000/μL. As with other leukemias, uric acid and lactic dehydrogenase may be elevated and reflect the large tumor burden. Clinical coagulopathies are uncommon, but chemical disseminated intravascular coagulation is frequently seen. A bone marrow that contains more than 30% blasts, of which at least 30% stain positive for TdT and fewer than 3% stain positive for myeloperoxidase, is diagnostic of ALL.[11] Because the defect represents a maturation arrest and accumulation of immature cells, the bone marrow biopsy is most often hypercellular.

Immunophenotyping has become important not only for distinguishing B-versus T-cell lineage but also for determining the level of differentiation present, which may be important for making therapeutic decisions. In ALL of B-cell origin (85%), immunophenotyping is positive for B-cell markers CD19 and CD20; when the CD10 marker (common acute lymphoblastic leukemia antigen, or CALLA) is found, the disease is referred to as CALLA+ ALL. T-cell ALL (15% of cases) is positive for at least two of the T-cell markers, CD1 and

CD8. Immunophenotyping is essential for diagnosis and for tailoring of therapy, which is influenced by prognosis. Patients with T-cell ALL, for example, have had improved success with combined therapy with cyclophosphamide and ara-C, whereas patients with mature B-cell ALL require short-term, dose-intensive therapy but no maintenance with mercaptopurine or methotrexate (Table 19–4).[1, 3, 5, 9–11, 18]

DIFFERENTIAL DIAGNOSIS

ALL may be confused initially with infectious causes or other malignancies that cause lymphocytosis and lymphadenopathy. Infectious causes that must be ruled out include toxoplasmosis, cytomegalovirus infection, and mononucleosis.[6] The bone marrow is normal in infection but not in ALL. Other malignancies that must be ruled out are AML, CLL, CML in lymphoid blast phase, non-Hodgkin's lymphoma in leukemic phase, small cell lung cancer, and Ewing's sarcoma.[6] The diagnosis is fairly straightforward once a bone marrow analysis is performed.

TREATMENT

Treatment in adults is modeled after childhood ALL regimens because of favorable results. About 75% of treated adults achieve a CR, although only 30% to 40% are cured. Practitioners at the M. D. Anderson Cancer Center use a combination of drugs in an alternating regimen in which vincristine, doxorubicin, hyperfractionated cyclophosphamide, and dexamethasone are alternated with high doses of methotrexate and cytarabine for eight courses, ideally spanning a 6-month period. Dexamethasone is used rather than prednisone because of its greater CNS penetration. Depending on the patient's predicted CNS relapse risk, 4, 8, or 16 intrathecal injections are given, with methotrexate alternating with cytarabine. CNS prophylaxis reduces the risk of CNS relapse to less than 5%.[10] The duration of neutropenia is shortened with the use of growth factors such as G-CSF or GM-CSF. Prophylactic antibiotic use may prevent opportunistic infections during neutropenic periods.

Maintenance therapy consists of 2 years of vincristine, methotrexate, mercaptopurine, and prednisone and is not necessary for patients with mature B-cell ALL. Allogeneic BMT during first remission remains controversial, but it should be pursued in patients with a poor prognosis, such as those with Philadelphia chromosome-positive ALL (see later discussion). In these patients with a human leukocyte antigen (HLA)-identical sibling, the best time for BMT is during the first remission; in other patients the optimal time for BMT is if relapse occurs during chemotherapy.[9] Autologous BMT is not recommended because of high relapse rates.

CHRONIC LEUKEMIAS

CHRONIC MYELOGENOUS LEUKEMIA

CML, or chronic myeloid or granulocytic leukemia, was described by Craigie in 1845 as "listlessness . . . swelling and hardness in the left epigastric region

Table 19-4. Acute Lymphocytic Leukemia Types as Determined by Cell Type and Cytogenetics

CELL TYPE	INCIDENCE OF ALL PATIENTS (%)	CYTOGENETICS	POSITIVE MARKERS	MISCELLANEOUS
T cell	15–20	Diploid (normal)	CD_2, CD_5, CD_6, CD_7	Mediastinal mass common
B cell	75–80	Nonspecific abnormalities or diploid	CD_{19}, CD_{20}, CD_{10}	
Mature B cell	2–7	t(8;14)	CD_{19}, CD_{20}	Burkitt's lymphoma is this type
		t(8;21)		
		t(8;22)		
Philadelphia chromosome-positive*	15–20	t(9;22)	Usually B-cell markers are positive	Very poor prognosis

*Philadelphia chromosome = translocation of genetic material between chromosomes 9 and 22 t(9;22).

. . . perspiration at night . . . blood vessels filled with grumus and clots containing lymph or purulent matter."[12] CML is a clonal myeloproliferative disorder caused by a malignant transformation of the primitive hematopoietic stem cell and characterized by extreme granulocytosis, with a high number of immature forms and splenomegaly.[1, 13] CML has historical significance as the first human malignant condition associated with a consistent cytogenetic abnormality—the Philadelphia (Ph) chromosome, t(9;22)—which made the disease a model for molecular oncogenesis.[3] CML also has therapeutic significance; it was one of the first malignant diseases in which the use of a biologic agent (interferon-α [IFN-α]) was successful in suppressing the neoplastic clone and improving survival.[13] CML has three distinct phases: chronic or benign, with an estimated survival time of 3 to 7 years; accelerated, with median survival time of 6 to 18 months; and acute or blastic, in which death is imminent in approximately 3 months.

EPIDEMIOLOGY

CML accounts for 0.3% of all cancers and 20% of all leukemias in the United States.[11] The annual incidence of 1.3 per 100,000 persons increases with age[3]; the median age at presentation is 45 years.[1] Men have a rate 1.7 times higher than women.[3] The cause of CML is unknown. Although the clonal malignancy (Ph) is a reciprocal translocation of genetic material between chromosomes 9 and 22, there is no proven familial tendency for the disease. No correlation exists among monozygotic twins, and no genetic factors have been linked to CML.[13] Exposure to radiation may promote evolution of CML in 7 to 10 years, and there is an increased incidence among atomic bomb survivors.[14] CML comprises one fifth of the leukemias that occur in patients treated with radiation for cervical cancer or ankylosing spondylitis, a degenerative disease of the vertebrae.[13] No association with chemicals or infectious agents has been demonstrated.[3]

In CML the presence of the chromosomal abnormality portends a better prognosis than its absence. The Ph chromosome is present in 95% of CML patients; the remaining 5% are Ph-negative, which makes treatment progress difficult to monitor.

PRESENTATION

About 40% of cases of chronic phase CML are detected in asymptomatic patients when a routine blood count is done for unrelated problems. Clinical characteristics vary according to stage of disease. In the early chronic phase, symptoms may be absent or mild, but patients may experience an insidious onset of nonspecific problems such as malaise, fatigue, fever, weight loss, night sweats, or decreased exercise tolerance. Symptoms of splenomegaly, such as early satiety, left upper-quadrant fullness or pain, and referred left-shoulder discomfort, may be present. Splenomegaly can range from absent to massive, and hepatomegaly is present in up to 40% of patients.[13] Symptoms of hyperviscosity in patients with leukocytosis include tinnitus, stupor, visual changes from retinal hemorrhages, Roth spots, and even cerebral vascular accidents. Symptoms and laboratory abnormalities worsen as the disease progresses. In 20% of patients, the ill-defined accelerated phase goes clinically undetected, and the patient progresses rapidly from the chronic to the blastic phase.[13] The acute, or blastic, phase is often heralded by fever, bone pain secondary to marrow expansion, weight loss, night sweats, and increasing splenomegaly.[14] Symptoms of anemia and infectious processes are also common secondary to progressive pancytopenia (Table 19–5).[3, 11, 16, 17]

LABORATORY DATA

In the chronic phase, leukocytosis with increased eosinophils, basophils, large platelets, and sometimes thrombocytosis, possibly to 1,000,000/μL, may occur. Hemoglobin and hematocrit are usually normal. The WBC count may be cyclic, fluctuating in 30- to 60-day cycles, which should be remembered during therapy. A low leukocyte alkaline phosphatase score is seen in chronic-phase CML. An elevated score in a patient with a high WBC count suggests a leukemoid ("resembling leukemia") reaction or infection, which must be distinguished from true leukemia before treatment. Increased numbers of blasts and basophils (>20%) in the peripheral blood, platelets fewer than 100×10^9/L, and additional chromosomal abnormalities signify the accelerated phase.[13] In the blastic phase, abnormal laboratory findings include a rapidly increasing WBC count with circulating blasts, immature cells, and basophils.[15] Lactic dehydrogenase and uric acid levels may be increased, reflecting the increased tumor burden. Increased blasts (30%) in bone marrow or blood, extramedullary masses, or clonal evolution (development of additional chromosomal abnormalities) may identify blastic transformation. Clonal evolution often includes the addition of Ph^2 (a double Philadelphia chromosome), trisomy 8, or iso17.[13] Leukostasis may occur if the peripheral blast count exceeds 50,000 to 100,000 per microliter, with tissue

Table 19–5. Characteristics of Chronic Myelogeneous Leukemia, with Laboratory Values by Stage

CHARACTERISTIC	CHRONIC PHASE	ACCELERATED PHASE	BLAST/ACUTE PHASE
Symptoms	None to minimal	Moderate	Pronounced
Splenomegaly	Mild to massive	May increase	May be massive
White blood cell count	↑ ↑	Erratic	↑ or ↓
Peripheral blood differential	<1–2% blasts	↑ basophils, occasional blasts, ↑ immature cells	Circulating blasts >25%
Hemogloblin	Usually normal	Normal to ↓	↓
Platelets	↑ or normal	Erratic	↓
Leukocyte alkaline phosphatase score	Low	↑ or normal	Normal
Bone marrow	<5% blasts	Basophils, ↑ immature cells, ↑ ± ↑ blasts	>30% blasts
Cytogenetics (chromosomes)	85% Ph⁺ (t(9;22))	Ph⁺ ± clonal evolution	Ph⁺ ± clonal evolution
Expected survival	5–7 yr	12–18 mo	3–6 mo
Therapy	IFN-α every day; late: homoharringtonine + cytarabine	Decitabine chemotherapy (DAC)	Myeloid → AML-like Lymphoid → ALL-like Undifferentiated → AML-like

Clonal evolution, development of additional chromosomal abnormalities.

infiltration affecting the lymph nodes, skin, subcutaneous tissue, bone, and, rarely, the cerebral spinal fluid.

In the chronic phase, the bone marrow differential is normal. It is hypercellular, up to 90%, with an increased myeloid-to-erythroid ratio of 10:1 to 30:1 (normal is 2:1 to 4:1).[13] Blasts are fewer than 5% (which is normal), and the percentage of basophils is normal or low. As the disease progresses, the number of blasts, immature cells, and basophils increases. Blast crisis is identified when a bone marrow aspirate or peripheral blood shows more than 30% blasts that are myeloid (50%), lymphoid (25%), or undifferentiated (25%) in phenotype. Histochemical stains and immunophenotyping can assist with this distinction, which is important for therapeutic decisions. Lymphoid blast transformation has a better prognosis than the others; the patient usually reverts to the chronic phase after ALL-like chemotherapy.

DIFFERENTIAL DIAGNOSIS

Until the presence of the Philadelphia chromosome is identified in cytogenetic studies, CML may be confused with either a leukemoid reaction or CMML, one of the MDS.[15] Among the hematologic features that distinguish CML from other entities is a low leukocyte alkaline phosphatase score, which is elevated in other disease processes.[14]

TREATMENT

The goal of treatment is to achieve a complete hematologic remission (complete normalization of peripheral counts and absence of splenomegaly)[16] and a complete cytogenetic remission with elimination of the Philadelphia clone. Busulfan has been used, but its toxicity to lungs, marrow, and myocardium can be severe.[15] Hydroxyurea (Hydrea) is an inexpensive, nontoxic oral medication that controls the WBC count in 70% of patients in chronic phase but does not suppress the chromosomal abnormality. It has no value in the acute phase of the disease. IFN-α, used clinically since the mid-1980s, established complete hematologic remission in about 80% of CML patients treated with IFN alone and produced a major cytogenetic response in 30% to 40% of patients in the chronic phase of CML.[13, 17] Average time to a complete cytogenetic response in a patient with chronic-phase CML who is sensitive to IFN is 22 to 24 months. Several groups have documented a survival advantage with IFN use and shown that median survival is longer in patients receiving IFN treatment than in patients treated with hydroxyurea or busulfan.[17] In addition, the interval between chronic and accelerated or blast phases was prolonged in patients treated with IFN. As a result of this well-documented survival benefit, IFN has become the standard of care for Ph-positive CML patients. The recommended dosage is 5,000,000 U/m^2 (or the maximum tolerated dose) administered subcutaneously daily for a minimum of 3 years.[13] Early side effects are usually limited to flu-like symptoms such as fever, headache, chills, and decreased appetite; chronic side effects include fatigue, depression, insomnia, CNS changes, and immune complications such as hypothyroidism and collagen vascular disorders. These may be severe in 10% of patients and require dose reduction in 30% to 50% of patients.[16] One method used at the M. D. Anderson Cancer Center is to combine IFN with low-dose ara-C for a synergistic effect. Results thus far are promising and show an increased cytogenetic response after 4 years of study.[16] Homoharringtonine, a plant alkaloid, has had favorable responses in chronic-phase patients who are resistant or intolerant to IFN. New agents, including chemotherapeutic agents (decitabine, topotecan), differentiating agents (retinoic acid), and immunomodulators, are currently being investigated.

Patients in the accelerated phase present more of a treatment challenge. They are currently treated with decitabine with the goal of controlling blood counts, palliating symptoms of splenomegaly, and slowing progression to the blastic phase. Chemotherapy regimens for patients in the blastic phase are similar to those used for patients with acute leukemia, but they have shown little success in myeloid or undifferentiated blast crisis.

Allogeneic BMT from a matched sibling is curative in 40% to 60% of patients; the outcome is better if transplantation is performed during the chronic phase.[13] BMT has the best outcome in younger patients because the incidence and severity of complications and of graft-versus-host disease (GVHD) increase with advancing age. Overall results depend on the patient's age at the time of transplantation, stage of disease, and preparative regimens. The relapse rate is consistently 20% after allogeneic BMT.[15] Prior treatment with IFN does not adversely affect overall survival, disease-free survival, time to engraftment, incidence of GVHD, or 100-day BMT-related mortality.[13] T-cell-depleted marrow decreases GVHD incidence but increases relapse rate and graft failure.[15] Many of the patients with no histocompatible relative who have received matched, unrelated donor transplants have had discouraging results: 80% experience acute GVHD, more than 50% experience chronic GVHD, and the 2-year mortality rate is higher than 50%.[16] Still, BMT is curative in selected subsets of patients, more often in those younger than 30 years of age.

CHRONIC LYMPHOCYTIC LEUKEMIA

CLL, an indolent lymphoproliferative disorder, is the most common leukemia in the Western hemisphere in people older than 50 years of age.[18] Ninety-five percent of CLL cases result from accumulation of slowly proliferating, long-lived B lymphocytes derived from a single clone. The remaining 5% have an aggressive T-cell leukemia that is usually refractory to therapy.[19] Dysplastic lymphocytes accumulate in blood, marrow, lymph nodes, and spleen, disrupting normal organ function. More extensive involvement indicates more aggressive disease.

EPIDEMIOLOGY

The incidence varies according to geographical area. In the United States, CLL comprises 30% of all adult leukemias,[11] in Asia only 2.5%.[20] CLL constitutes about 0.9% of all cancers, with an annual incidence of 5.2 per 100,000 in people older than 50 years of age and 30.4 per 100,000 in those more than 80 years old.[3, 14] Ninety percent of patients are older than 50 years.[18] The male-to-female ratio is 2 to 3:1.[1, 14] In CLL patients, the incidence of nonlymphoid neoplasms is twice that of the general population, possibly because of decreased immune surveillance.[20] One third of these cancers are pulmonary neoplasms, with colorectal cancer, melanoma, other skin cancers, and soft tissue sarcomas, especially fibrous histiocytomas, occurring more often than in the general population.[14, 20]

The cause of CLL is unknown, and B-cell CLL is the only leukemia not associated with radiation, chemicals, or drug exposure. However, a twofold to sevenfold increase in familial tendency for CLL has been identified.[3] CLL evolves in the setting of immunodeficient states, suggesting that altered immune function may be of pathophysiologic importance in the development of the disease.[3] No infectious cause or association of CLL and viruses—specifically, Epstein-Barr virus, cytomegalovirus, and herpes simplex virus—has been identified.[19] Between 10% and 25% of patients with CLL experience some type of autoimmune disorder during the course of the disease.[6]

PRESENTATION

Clinically, patients with CLL are extremely variable. Unexplained lymphocytosis on a routine blood test is the single initial abnormality in about 25% of patients. Some patients present with autoimmune disorders, such as autoimmune hemolytic anemia or idiopathic thromobocytopenic purpura, a hemorrhagic disease that is often accompanied by the presence of immunoglobulin G.[20] Other presenting symptoms include shortness of breath, bleeding, and B symptoms (fatigue, fever with drenching night sweats, weight loss), usually secondary to the hypermetabolic state that accompanies leukocytosis. Some patients complain of early satiety or left upper-quadrant discomfort secondary to splenomegaly.[19] More often, patients present with bothersome lymphadenopathy or recurrent bacterial, viral, or fungal infections caused by defective humoral immune function.[20] Most of the clinical features arise from an accumulation of neoplastic lymphocytes in lymphoid organs and decreased activity of lymphoid and myeloid systems because normal-functioning cells are crowded out.[14] Some patients experience an unexplained exaggerated response to insect bites. In advanced disease states, anemia and thrombocytopenia occur secondary to bone marrow failure. Despite high WBC counts (often $>300 \times 10^9$/L), signs and symptoms of leukostasis are rare.[3, 19] The Rai classification, presented in Table 19–6, represents clinical staging of CLL.[3, 14, 19, 20]

Not surprisingly, the most common physical finding is lymphadenopathy, usually cervical, with small, discrete, nontender, mobile nodes.[19] Any or all of the lymph node-bearing areas may be affected. Occasionally, localized masses of nodes may be present.[18] Splenomegaly and hepatomegaly are common. Petechiae and ecchymotic lesions may be present with thrombocytopenia. Despite widespread and sometimes massive lymphadenopathy, lymphedema is uncommon.[19]

LABORATORY DATA

Small, mature-appearing lymphocytes with occasional variation and damage observed as "smudge cells" are characteristic of CLL.[3] At diagnosis, a patient with CLL must have an absolute lymphocyte count higher than 5000 cells/μL with at least 30% involvement of the marrow and demonstrable clonality.[20] Anemia is present in 35% of patients at diagnosis, and thrombocytopenia in 25%; both of these conditions result from bone marrow infiltration or autoimmune destruction.[3] Persistent thrombocytopenia may be caused solely by hypersplen-

Table 19–6. Chronic Lymphocytic Leukemia Staging According to the Rai System

RAI STAGE	CLINICAL CHARACTERISTICS	MEDIAN SURVIVAL (YR)°	TREATMENT
0	Lymphocytosis with BM involvement	>10	Observation
I	Lymphocytosis + lymphadenopathy (LAD)	8	Observation
II°	Lymphocytosis + LAD + hepatomegaly or splenomegaly	5–6	Usually observe; if symptomatic, treat as in stage III or IV
III°	Lymphocytosis + hemoglobin <11 gm%	<2	Fludarabine (chlorambucil ± prednisone in past)
IV°	Lymphocytosis + anemia + thrombocytopenia platelets <100 × 10⁹/L	<2	Fludarabine ± splenectomy; steroids if immune-mediated thrombocytopenia

°The variability within stages results in widely diverse outcomes. Stages II, III, IV may include lymphadenopathy and/or hepatomegaly and/or splenomegaly. BM, bone marrow.

ism, in which case splenectomy is recommended and usually results in normalization of the platelet count.[20] When thrombocytopenia is associated with the presence of antiplatelet antibodies or idiopathic thrombocytopenic purpura (ITP), corticosteroids are of benefit. Hypogammaglobulinemia is common and may be profound. β_2-Microglobulin may be elevated; it is an important prognostic indicator of disease activity.

The degree of bone marrow infiltration ranges between 30% and 99%. The pattern of the bone marrow biopsy may be nodular (more local disease), interstitial, mixed nodular and interstitial, or diffuse (more extensive disease). Bone marrow biopsy helps initially to determine the extent of disease and during follow-up to document the patient's response to treatment. Cytogenetic abnormalities are present in 20% to 40% of patients, the most common ones involving chromosomes 12, 13, and 14, with trisomy 12 occurring in 20% to 60%.[20] Any chromosomal abnormality indicates an unfavorable prognosis.

Imaging studies, such as chest radiographs and chest and abdominal computed tomography scans, may be necessary to determine subclinical hepatosplenomegaly and the true extent of lymphadenopathy. Patients often have significant hilar, para-aortic, retroperitoneal, or pelvic lymphadenopathy that cannot be detected on physical examination.

PATHOLOGY AND IMMUNOLOGY

Lymphocyte accumulation probably begins in lymph nodes and then spreads to other lymphoid tissue, including the bone marrow. Crowding of the normal hematopoietic precursors may result in anemia, thrombocytopenia, agranulocytosis, and abnormal immunoglobulin production, leading to decreased immunity and increased susceptibility to infections. Immunophenotyping of blood and marrow in B-cell CLL shows positivity for B-cell markers CD5, CD19, CD20, CD23, CD25, and coexpression of CD5+CD19.[11, 20] Surface immunoglobulin measurement is important for establishing clonality of the lymphoid population.[20] In addition, the CD4 to CD8 ratio may be reversed at diagnosis.[19] T-cell CLL accounts for 5% of all CLL cases. T cells arise from post-thymic tissue and have an immunophenotype positive for T-cell markers CD2, CD3, CD4, and CD7.[21] T-cell CLL has a poor prognosis and a poor response to chemotherapy.

Most patients with CLL die of infection, bleeding as a result of progressive disease, or other illness unrelated to leukemia. In 10% of patients, CLL is transformed into aggressive, diffuse large cell lymphoma (Richter's transformation)[14]; this usually is heralded by the abrupt onset of fever, hepatosplenomegaly, and an enlarged group of lymph nodes. Other features of transformation include elevated lactic dehydrogenase, progressive lymphadenopathy, B symptoms, monoclonal gammopathy (disturbed immunoglobulin synthesis), and extranodal involvement.[14] As a result of this aggressive transformation, the patient usually dies within 5 months, regardless of therapy.[20] Another type of CLL transformation is to prolymphocytic leukemia (PLL), which is marked by 11% to 55% prolymphocytes (large cells with prominent nucleoli) in blood and splenomegaly disproportionately large compared with lymphadenopathy.[19, 20]

DIFFERENTIAL DIAGNOSIS

CLL is distinguished from other causes of lymphocytosis and lymphadenopathy by bone marrow aspirate analysis with immunophenotyping and bone marrow biopsy. Infectious causes of lymphadenopathy and lymphocytosis (pertussis, infectious mononucleosis, cytomegalovirus infection, toxoplasmosis) produce large activated T lymphocytes, but the bone marrow should be normal.[11] CLL must be distinguished from other malignancies, such as hairy cell leukemia, PLL, non-Hodgkin's lymphoma in the leukemic phase, and Waldenström's macroglobulinemia.[19] Lymphocytic infiltration of the gastrointestinal tract, salivary glands, lungs, or ocular area raises the possibility of mucosa-associated lymphoid tissue (MALT) lymphoma.[19] Clinical features, complete blood count, immunophenotyping, analysis of bone marrow aspirate and biopsy, and possibly tissue biopsy may be necessary to diagnose CLL or one of its variants correctly.

TREATMENT

Not all CLL patients require treatment, nor would they benefit from it. Moreover, the best time to institute treatment is not completely clear. Indications for intervention are advanced CLL phase (Rai stage 3 or 4), severe lymphocytosis, lymphocyte doubling in less than 1 year, diffuse infiltration of bone marrow, and presence of systemic symptoms such as fevers, weight loss, night sweats, bulky lymphadenopathy, splenomegaly, recurrent infections, or refractory autoimmune events. The front-line therapy for patients at M. D. Anderson Cancer Center is fludarabine, a purine nucleotide analog, combined with cyclophosphamide, an alkylating agent, both given intravenously. Up to six courses of this combination may be given. An earlier study showed a complete response rate of 60% and a partial response rate of 80% when fludarabine was given alone.[20] Drugs that have been used most commonly in CLL are chlorambucil (a nitrogen mustard) and prednisone, both given orally. Response rates have varied among studies, ranging from 38% to 75%.[19] Often patients become resistant to this therapy, at which point they should be referred to a comprehensive cancer center for further therapy. Fludarabine may soon become the standard of care for CLL. Other modalities of treatment, such as intravenous immunoglobulin

G, recombinant interleukin-2, monoclonal antibodies, and other cytokines, are currently being investigated.

VARIANTS OF CHRONIC LYMPHOCYTIC LEUKEMIA

Hairy cell leukemia (HCL) is an indolent disorder characterized by the infiltration of bone marrow and spleen by lymphocytes with unusual "hairy" cytoplasmic projections, leading to pancytopenia and splenomegaly. HCL represents 2% of all leukemias in the United States.[20] The median age of onset is 50 years, and it affects men four times more often than women. Its cause is unknown, and no associations with radiation, chemical exposure, or genetic predisposition have been proven, although 15 cases of familial HCL have been documented.[20] No specific cytogenetic abnormality has been associated with HCL.

Patients with HCL seek medical attention for recurrent infections, abdominal discomfort secondary to splenomegaly, weight loss, or symptoms of anemia. They seem to have a propensity for opportunistic infections, probably because of neutropenia, and vasculitis.[3] Splenomegaly, present in 90% of patients at diagnosis, can be massive. Lymphadenopathy is uncommon. Anemia and thrombocytopenia are found in 80% of patients at diagnosis; leukopenia, especially neutropenia, is present in more than 50%.[20] Bone marrow aspiration often yields a "dry tap," but if it is successful the leukemia cells stain positive for the tartrate-resistant isoenzyme of acid phosphatase (TRAP), which is characteristic of HCL.[22] The biopsy of hypercellular bone marrow reveals the histologic "fried egg" pattern that is also pathognomonic of HCL.[3] Immunophenotyping of HCL shows positivity for monoclonal surface immunoglobulin and markers CD11c, CD19, CD20, CD22, and CD25 and is usually negative for CD5.[20] HCL may be confused with malignant lymphomas, splenic lymphoma with villous lymphocytes, CLL, and MDS.[20] The positive TRAP stain of blood and marrow, combined with marker results, can differentiate HCL from these other malignancies. Splenectomy was the treatment of choice until 1984, when IFN-α treatment replaced surgery.[20] About 80% of patients responded to IFN for 12 to 18 months, but they required long-term subcutaneous injections. The nucleoside analog 2-chlorodeoxyadenosine (2-CDA), given by 7-day continuous infusion, has been shown to eliminate neoplastic lymphocytes in more than 90% of patients and is now the treatment of choice.[19] Toxicity is mild (leukopenia for about 2 months after chemotherapy), and the potential for cure is high. Rare relapses can be treated with another course of the same drug. Follow-up should be annual, with complete blood count, bone marrow aspiration with TRAP stain, and biopsy.

Prolymphocytic Leukemia

PLL is one tenth as common as CLL, usually occurs later in life, and is more common in men.[3] PLL is characterized by splenomegaly with minimal lymphadenopathy, increased lymphocytes, and increased prolymphocytes; it is usually B cell in origin.[20] Immunophenotyping shows CD5 negativity and strong FMC-7 positivity, distinguishing PLL from CLL.[3] Karyotypes include chromosomal transformations t(11;14) and t(6;12) and abnormalities involving chromosome 14.[20] Chemotherapy similar to that used for CLL has been used with some response, but median survival ranges from 17 weeks to 3 years.[20]

Large Granular Lymphoma/Leukemia

This is a T-cell malignancy; the median age at occurrence is 57 years. Symptoms may include recurrent bacterial infections and autoimmune phenomena including rheumatoid arthritis. Splenomegaly is common, lymphadenopathy rare.[20] Patients are usually neutropenic and anemic but not thrombocytopenic. Markers expressed are CD2, CD3, CD8, CD56, and CD57.[19, 21] Often this disease runs an indolent course, making observation the best approach until progression occurs.[20] If treatment becomes necessary, some of the therapies are splenectomy, IFN-α, G-CSF, and nucleoside analogues.

FOLLOW-UP AND SURVEILLANCE

More patients are surviving leukemia now, and some are cured, probably as a direct result of improved treatments. Physician assistants and nurse practitioners who monitor leukemia patients must be aware of the increased incidence of infections, greater risk of bleeding, and potential for second malignancies. A relapse is always possible. Complete blood counts, which must be done regularly for these patients, are the best method of detecting a relapse early. Any change in WBC count, hemoglobin, or platelets must be followed up faster than in a nonleukemic patient. Bone marrow aspiration may be required to rule out relapse before a patient is referred to a comprehensive cancer center.

Because leukemia patients may be taking medication for years, advanced care practitioners and family physicians must be aware of side effects and toxicities of these medications. Influenza vaccines should be given to patients with chronic leukemia, and to those with acute leukemia provided their WBC count is

Normal Hematopoiesis			
BONE MARROW		**PERIPHERAL BLOOD**	
NORMAL %	**CELL TYPE**	**CELL TYPE**	**NORMAL %**
0.3–5.0	Blast	Blast	0
1.8–8.0	Promyelocyte	Promyelocyte	0
5.0–20.0	Myelocyte	Myelocyte	0
13.0–32.0	Metamyelocyte	Metamyelocyte	0
7.0–30.0	Neutrophil	Neutrophil	42–66
0.5–4.0	Eosinophil	Eosinophil	1.0–4.0
0.0–0.7	Basophil	Basophil	0.0–1.0
3.0–17.0	Lymphocyte	Lymphocyte	24–44
0.0–2.0	Plasma cell	Plasma cell	0
0.5–5.0	Monocyte	Monocyte	1.0–6.0
0.1–2.0	Reticulocyte	Reticulocyte	0.0–1.0
1.0–8.0	Pronormoblast	Mature red blood cell	
7.0–32.0	Normoblast	Mature red blood cell	
	Megakaryocyte	Platelet	140–144 $\times$ 10^9/L

Data from Hoffbrand AV, Pettit JE: Essential Haematology, 3rd ed. London, Blackwell Scientific Publications, 1993:1–11, 244.

within normal limits. Any persistent infection should be watched closely and investigated rapidly.

REFERENCES

1. Mauer AM: The Leukemias. In Berkow R, Fletcher AJ, Bondy PK, et al (eds): The Merck Manual, 16th ed. Rahway, NJ, Merck Research Laboratories, 1992:1233–1245.
2. Goasguen JE, Bennett JM, Henderson ES: Biologic diagnosis of leukemias. In Henderson ES, Lister TA, Greaves MF (eds): Leukemia, 6th ed. Philadelphia, WB Saunders, 1996:8–33.
3. Mitus AJ, Rosenthal DS: The adult leukemias. In Murphy GP, Lawrence W Jr, Lenhard RE Jr (eds): American Cancer Society Textbook of Clinical Oncology, 2nd ed. Atlanta, American Cancer Society, 1995:486.
4. Ghaddar HM, Estey EH: Acute myelogenous leukemia. In Pazdur R (ed): Medical Oncology: A Comprehensive Review, 2nd ed. New York, PRR, 1995:27.
5. Wiernik PH: Acute leukemias. In DeVita VT Jr, Hellman S, Rosenberg SA (eds): Cancer Principles and Practice of Oncology, 3rd ed. Philadelphia, JB Lippincott, 1989:1809
6. Hoffman R, Williams DA: Molecular and cellular biology of hematopoiesis. In Stein JH, Hutton JJ, Kohler PO, et al (eds): Internal Medicine, 4th ed. St. Louis, CV Mosby, 1994:684.
7. Cheson BD, Casselith PA, Head DR, et al: Report of the National Cancer Institute-sponsored Workshop on Definitions of Diagnosis and Response in Acute Myeloid Leukemia. J Clin Oncol 1990;8:813.
8. Appelbaum FR: Bone marrow failure. In Stein JH, Hutton JJ, Kohler PO, et al (eds): Internal Medicine, 4th ed. St. Louis, Mosby, 1994:873.
9. Cortes JE, Kantarjian HM: Acute lymphocytic leukemia. In Pazdur R (ed): Medical Oncology: A Comprehensive Review, 2nd ed. New York, PRR, 1995:3.
10. Preti HA, Kantarjian HM: Acute lymphocytic leukemia in adults: An update. Tex Med 1994;90:52.
11. Wallach J: Hematologic diseases. In Interpretation of Diagnostic Tests, 5th ed. Boston, Little, Brown, 1992:330.
12. Craigie D. A case of disease of the spleen in which death took place in consequence of purulent matter in the blood. Edinburgh Medical Surgeon 1845;64:400.
13. Cortes JE, Talpaz M, Kantarjian HM: Chronic myelogenous leukemia. In Pazdur R (ed): Medical Oncology: A Comprehensive Review, 2nd ed. New York, PRR, 1995:57.
14. Fialkow PJ, Singer JW: Chronic leukemias. In DeVita VT Jr, Hellman S, Rosenberg SA (eds): Cancer Principles and Practice of Oncology, 3rd ed. Philadelphia, JB Lippincott, 1989:1836.
15. Barnett MJ, Eaves CJ: Chronic myeloid leukemia. In Henderson ES, Lister TA, Greaves MF (eds): Leukemia, 6th ed. Philadelphia, WB Saunders, 1996:535.
16. Kantarjian HM, O'Brien S, Anderlini P, et al: Treatment of CML: Current status and investigational options. Blood 1996;87:8.
17. Talpaz M: Use of interferon in the treatment of chronic myelogenous leukemia. Semin Oncol 1994;21(suppl 14):3.
18. Hutton JJ: The leukemias and polycythemia vera. In Stein JH, Hutton JJ, Kohler PO, et al (eds): Internal Medicine, 4th ed. St. Louis, CV Mosby, 1994:887.
19. Keating MJ: Chronic lymphocytic leukemia. In Henderson ES, Lister TA, Greaves MF (eds): Leukemia, 6th ed. Philadelphia, WB Saunders, 1996:554.
20. Fayad L, O'Brien S: Chronic lymphocytic leukemia and associated disorders. In Pazdur R (ed): Medical Oncology: A Comprehensive Review, 2nd ed. New York, PRR, 1995:37.
21. Van Dongen JJM, Adriaansen HJ: Immunobiology of leukemia. In Henderson ES, Lister TA, Greaves MF (eds): Leukemia, 6th ed. Philadelphia, WB Saunders, 1996:95.
22. Hoffbrand AV, Pettit JE: Essential Haematology, 3rd ed. London, Blackwell Scientific Publications, 1993:244.

Chapter 20

Multiple Myeloma and Other Plasma Cell Dyscrasias

Elizabeth S. Waxman, RN, MSN, OCB, CNS, and Donna M. Weber, MD

INTRODUCTION

Multiple myeloma is a plasma cell dyscrasia, a disorder characterized by the abnormal growth of a clonal population of plasma cells resulting in the production of monoclonal immunoglobulin.[1] Other plasma cell dyscrasias include monoclonal gammopathy of unknown significance (MGUS), solitary plasmacytoma of bone (SPB), asymptomatic myeloma, Waldenström's macroglobulinemia, and amyloidosis.

The monoclonal immunoglobulin produced in multiple myeloma is commonly referred to as the monoclonal or M protein.[1] Although an excessive amount of the M protein is produced, it is often functionally ineffective, and uninvolved immunoglobulins are often suppressed, resulting in a defective humoral immune response.[1] Complications of myeloma include anemia, fractures, pain, renal failure, infection, nerve compression, and hypercalcemia.[2] This chapter focuses primarily on multiple myeloma and briefly reviews other plasma cell dyscrasias.

MULTIPLE MYELOMA

EPIDEMIOLOGY

Multiple myeloma represents 1% of all the malignancies in the United States.[3] The annual incidence of this disease per 100,000 people is 4.7 among white males and 3.2 among white females; among African Americans, the frequency doubles to 10.2 in males and 6.7 in females.[2] The onset of multiple myeloma is late, with the peak occurrence between the fifth and seventh decades of life.[4] Multiple myeloma is the most common lymphoid malignancy in African Americans and the second most common in whites, for whom non-Hodgkin's lymphoma ranks first.[5] The incidence of myeloma increases with age. The median age at onset is 68 years for men and 70 years for women.[5] The median age at death from myeloma is 70 years for men and 71 years for women.[6]

No predisposing events appear to be important in the origin of multiple myeloma.[2] Some events that have been suggested include radiation exposure (in radiologists and radium dial workers) and occupational exposure (in agricultural, chemical, metallurgic, rubber, pulp, paper, and leather tanning industries).[2] Another suggested risk factor is chemical exposure to benzene, formaldehyde, hair dyes, paint sprays, or asbestos.[7] Most of these associations have been countered by studies that found negative correlations.[7]

It was initially reported that survivors of the atomic bombing of Hiroshima had a greater risk of developing multiple myeloma, but longer follow-up data now refute any evidence of increased risk among survivors.[8] Some reports do suggest that a lower level of prolonged radiation exposure may have caused some cases of multiple myeloma among radiologists and radium dial painters.[9, 10] No relation has been shown between the incidence of multiple myeloma and exposure to diagnostic x-rays or therapeutic irradiation.[7, 11]

Another risk factor associated with multiple myeloma may be intense, prolonged exposure to benzene.[12] This association remains unproved and may never be demonstrated because of current industrial safeguards.[2]

GENETICS

Multiple myeloma is not generally considered to be an inherited disease, although there have been numerous reports of multiple cases in the same family.[7] A specific chromosomal abnormality has not been detected in patients with multiple myeloma, although chromosomal abnormalities frequently have been observed.[3, 4]

Multidrug resistance is a phenomenon often observed in late-stage multiple myeloma, especially after prolonged treatment. P-glycoprotein, the product of the multidrug resistance gene, serves as a pump, preventing antineoplastic agents from being retained in malignant cells and thus allowing those cells to proliferate. The level of p-glycoprotein expression in previously untreated myeloma patients is low. The level increases in patients with refractory or relapsing disease after cumulative exposure to certain chemotherapeutic agents such as vincristine and doxorubicin.[13]

CLINICAL MANIFESTATIONS

Twenty percent of patients with multiple myeloma are completely asymptomatic and are diagnosed by chance. The majority, however, present with symptoms, which can vary significantly. The most common symptom is bone pain, especially from fractures of vertebral bodies or lytic rib lesions.[2] Other findings include anemia, hypercalcemia, azotemia, and recurrent infections.[2]

Bone disease is a common feature: 70% of patients have lytic lesions at initial presentation.[14] These lesions, which are visible on plain skeletal radiographs, are the result of accelerated osteoclast formation and bone destruction.[14]

Anemia in patients with multiple myeloma is primarily caused by replacement of the bone marrow space by myeloma cells. A normocytic, normochromic anemia is present in 60% of patients at the time of diagnosis.[5] Patients with or without renal failure may also have decreased levels of erythropoietin, which can worsen the degree of anemia.[15]

Hypercalcemia, defined as a corrected serum calcium level higher than 11.5 mg/dL, is present in 20% of newly diagnosed patients.[2] The high level of calcium is secondary to progressive bone destruction.[2] Prolonged immobility may exacerbate the hypercalcemia.[2] One should suspect the clinical manifestation of hypercalcemia in patients with myeloma who complain of nausea, fatigue, confusion, polyuria, or constipation.

Renal failure is noted in 20% of patients at diagnosis.[1] Another 20% of patients with multiple myeloma develop this complication in later stages of the disease.[16] Casts of Bence Jones proteins in the renal tubules are the most common cause of renal insufficiency, but hypercalcemia, dehydration, and infection may also contribute.[17]

The principal type of lesion associated with renal failure is "myeloma kidney," in which the renal tubules are filled with damaging, dense casts surrounded by nucleated giant cells.[1] These large, dense casts lead to the formation in the tubules of precipitates that can obstruct and rupture the tubular epithelium.[1] Interstitial inflammation, fibrosis, and tubular degeneration may occur, resulting in renal failure.[3, 18] The tubular casts have been shown to contain light-chain immunoglobulins (the Bence Jones proteins), which may be directly toxic to the renal tubular epithelium.[4]

Amyloidosis complicates multiple myeloma in 10% to 20% of patients.[3, 18] Kidneys with plasma cell-produced amyloid deposits are generally large, and amyloid is deposited in the arterial walls, interstitial tissue, and glomeruli.[14] Renal failure usually results from arterial and tubular damage.[14]

Patients with multiple myeloma have an increased susceptibility to bacterial infections because of impaired host defense mechanisms.[4, 19] Common infectious organisms include *Staphylococcus aureus, Streptococcus pneumoniae, Escherichia coli, Haemophilus influenzae, Pseudomonas*, and *Klebsiella*.[1] Mechanisms responsible for the immunosuppression and infection include hypogammaglobulinemia; neutropenia and qualitative defects in neutrophil and complement systems; and immobility secondary to bone disease.[1] Steroids, which are often used in the treatment of multiple myeloma, render the patient susceptible to bacterial, viral (herpes zoster), and fungal infections.

INITIAL WORKUP AND DIAGNOSIS

The initial evaluation of the myeloma patient should include a bone marrow aspiration; complete blood count with differential and platelet count; chemical survey, including determinations of blood urea nitrogen, creatinine, calcium, total protein, albumin, lactate dehydrogenase (LDH), and uric acid; serum protein electrophoresis and immunofixation; quantitative assay of immunoglobulins; 24-hour urine collection for urine protein electrophoresis and immunofixation; and a skeletal survey. β_2-microglobulin (B2M) and LDH are often helpful prognostic factors. Examination of the bone marrow aspirate should reveal the presence of plasmacytosis. The complete blood count with differential and platelet count may reveal cytopenias resulting from extensive bone marrow replacement by plasma cells.

Serum protein electrophoresis usually indicates the presence of the abnormal M protein in the blood, and immunofixation identifies the type of immunoglobulin involved. Quantitative assay of immunoglobulins can demonstrate which immunoglobulin is overproduced and often reveals reduction of uninvolved immunoglobulins. The light chains (Bence Jones proteins) are excreted in the urine and may be quantitated by 24-hour urine collection and electrophoresis. The presence of bone marrow plasmacytosis greater than 20% and of monoclonal protein in the serum or urine is usually required for the diagnosis of multiple myeloma.[2] Rarely, patients present with bone marrow plasmacytosis and multiple lytic lesions without monoclonal protein detected in the serum or urine.[2] Bone lesions should be evaluated using plain radiographs. Nuclear bone scans generally detect blastic bone disease (bone growth) and are usually negative because of the purely lytic nature of the bone lesions in myeloma. These scans can be positive when fractures complicate lytic bone lesions.

Serum prognostic factors include B2M and LDH. B2M is one of the most important prognostic indicators of multiple myeloma, because it reflects the extent of disease in a single measurement.[2] Because B2M is excreted in the urine, impaired renal function elevates the serum level. If renal insufficiency is present when the B2M level is determined, the result must be corrected using nomograms before it is used for prognostic purposes. An elevated B2M (>6 μg/mL) is considered to be a poor prognostic feature.[14] High serum levels of LDH have been associated with shortened survival time (median, 9 months) and with drug resistance in both treated and untreated patients.[20, 21] The Durie-Salmon and M. D. Anderson staging systems for multiple myeloma are presented in Tables 20–1 and 20–2, respectively.

The differential diagnosis of multiple myeloma includes MGUS, SPB, asymptomatic myeloma, Waldenström's macroglobulinemia, and amyloidosis. These are discussed in a later section.

Table 20-1. Durie-Salmon Staging System for Multiple Myeloma

STAGE	CRITERIA	MYELOMA CELL MASS

I	Hemoglobin >10 g/dL
	Serum calcium ≤12 mg/dL (normal)
	Normal bone or solitary plasmacytoma on radiography
	Low M-component production rate
	  IgG <5 g/dL
	  IgA <3 g/dL
	  Urine light-chain
	  M component <4 g/day
		<0.6 (low)

II	Not fitting stage I or III	0.6–1.20 (intermediate)

III	Hemoglobin <8.5 g/dL
	Serum calcium >12 mg/dL
	Multiple lytic bone lesions on radiography
	High M-component production rate
	  IgG >7 g/dL
	  IgA >5 g/dL
	  Urine light-chain
	  M component >12 g/day
		>1.20 (high)

SUBCLASSIFICATION		
A	Normal renal function (serum creatinine level <2.0 mg/dL)	—
B	Abnormal renal function (serum creatinine level ≥2.0 mg/dL)	—

Data from Durie BGM, Salmon SE: A clinical staging system for multiple myeloma. Cancer 1975;36:842–854.

PATHOLOGY

On examination of the peripheral blood smears, a normocytic, normochromic anemia may be present.[5] The markers for plasma cells are CD38, plasma cell antigen 1,[5] and cytoplasmic immunoglobulin (κ or λ). Usually normal B-cell markers such as CD19 and CD20 are not present. On occasion, in immature, advanced disease, cells positive for CD10, also known as common acute lymphoblastic leukemia antigen (CALLA), are noted. Cells are often positive for CD10 in other hematologic malignancies, including leukemias and non-Hodgkin's lymphomas.

As previously stated, in multiple myeloma there is an overproduction of a monoclonal immunoglobulin and suppression of the uninvolved immunoglobulins. In a healthy person, during normal cellular differentiation and division, the B lymphocytes mature into plasma cells that manufacture and secrete large quantities of immunoglobulins, which normally contribute to humoral immunity.[1] Five classes of immunoglobulins are secreted: IgM, IgA, IgD, IgE, and IgG. IgM is the initial immunoglobulin produced during a primary immune response.

Table 20-2. M. D. Anderson Staging System for Multiple Myeloma

STAGE	CRITERIA	MYELOMA CELL MASS
I	Hemoglobin >10.5 g/dL Corrected serum calcium ≤11.0 mg/L Serum myeloma protein <4.5 g/dL	Low
II	Not fitting stage I or III	Intermediate
III	Hemoglobin <8.5 g/dL Coreceted serum calcium >11.5 mg/dL	High

From Papadimitrakopoulou V, Weber DM: Multiple myeloma and other plasma cell dyscrasias. In Pazdur R (ed): Medical Oncology: A Comprehensive Review, 2nd ed. Huntington, New York, PRR Inc., 1995:130.

IgG is the primary immunoglobulin, is more specific than IgM, and can cross the placenta, thereby conferring passive immunity to newborns.[1] IgA is the immunoglobulin in saliva, tears, and secretions of the gastrointestinal and respiratory tracts and plays a primary role in protecting mucous membranes and vital organ systems by maintaining the first line of defense.[4] IgD and IgE are found in lesser amounts in the plasma and are involved in lymphocytic differentiation and allergic response, respectively.[1]

In order of frequency, the types of M protein produced and found in the serum or urine or both are: IgG (60%), IgA (20%), IgD (2%), and IgE (<0.1%).[2] IgM is usually elevated in Waldenström's macroglobulinemia. In most cases of multiple myeloma, only one class of immunoglobulin is overproduced. However, there are cases in which two immunoglobulins are overexpressed; in these situations, the patient is said to have a biclonal elevation.[2]

TREATMENT OVERVIEW

Treatment decisions are determined by the initial patient presentation and the stage of disease. Patients with indolent disease and asymptomatic patients can be observed without treatment. When signs and symptoms of disease progression occur, including an increase in the M protein level, anemia, fatigue, compression fractures, hypercalcemia, and renal failure, then systemic chemotherapy is the treatment of choice and must be started immediately. Although therapy can often induce prolonged remissions and overall survival measured in years, myeloma is not considered curable.

Newly diagnosed patients with low- or intermediate-mass multiple myeloma may be treated with melphalan and prednisone (Table 20–3). Despite multiple therapeutic trials, combination chemotherapy has not proved to be superior to melphalan and prednisone alone.[22] Although this regimen is effective, the response time is short, the median remission is 2 years, and the median survival time for all patients is 3 years.[2] Patients with low-tumor-mass disease usually have improved survival compared with patients with high-tumor-mass disease.

If the myeloma does not respond to the first course of melphalan and prednisone and significant myelosuppression is not noted, then the same agents are given a second time, with a 20% increase in the dose of melphalan and the same dose of prednisone.[23] The patient should have a complete blood count, differential, and platelet count done at least weekly during the first course to assess myelosuppression. The melphalan dose is increased with each course of treatment until adequate myelosuppression occurs.[23]

Systemic chemotherapy is also indicated for use with relapsing disease. VAD (vincristine, doxorubicin, and dexamethasone) is the treatment of choice for patients with disease that relapses despite treatment with melphalan and prednisone and may produce responses in 35% of such patients (see Table 20–3).[2] VAD is also an appropriate regimen for patients presenting with renal failure and hypercalcemia, since these drugs are hepatically metabolized and further dose adjustments for reduced kidney function are unnecessary.[2] VAD also provides rapid normalization of renal function and calcium levels in patients who respond to treatment.[2] Patients with plasma cell leukemia also benefit from therapy with VAD rather than melphalan and prednisone alone. In patients whose myeloma does not respond to initial therapy with melphalan and predni-sone, pulse dexamethasone alone provides response rates similar to those pro-

Table 20–3. Proposed Standard Treatment of Multiple Myeloma

DISEASE/PATIENT STATUS	TREATMENT APPROACH
Untreated Myeloma	
Low-risk disease, age ≥70 yr, or major medical problems	Melphalan/prednisone: melphalan 8 mg/m²/day PO and prednisone 100 mg/d PO on days 1–4
High-risk disease, renal failure, or hypercalcemia	VAD: vincristine 0.4 mg/day IV and doxorubicin 9 mg/m²/day IV (both drugs continuous infusion) on days 1–4; dexamethasone 40 mg/day PO on days 1–4, 9–12, and 17–20
With spine radiotherapy	Dexamethasone 40 mg/day PO on days 1–4, 9–12, and 17–20
Maintenance Therapy	Interferon-α 3,000,000 U SC TIW
Resistant Myeloma	
Resistant to melphalan/prednisone	
Unresponsive	Dexamethasone or VAD as above
Relapsing	VAD as above
Resistant to VAD or dexamethasone	Cyclophosphamide 300 mg/m² q 12 h × 6 doses on days 1–3; vincristine 2 mg IV and doxorubicin 50 mg/m² IV (both drugs by continuous infusion over 48 hr) days 4 & 5; dexamethasone 40 mg/day PO on days 1–4, 9–12, and 17–20; granulocyte colony-stimulating factor (G-CSF) 5 μg/kg starting day 10.
Primary refractory disease ≤1 yr (high or intermediate tumor mass)	Myeloablative therapy and blood stem cell transplantation

From Papadimitrakopoulou V, Weber DM: Multiple myeloma and other plasma cell dyscrasias. In Pazdur R (ed): Medical Oncology: A Comprehensive Review, 2nd ed. Huntington, New York, PRR Inc., 1995:129.

duced by VAD (25%) and should be considered the treatment of choice for patients with primary refractory disease (see Table 20–3).

Radiation therapy also plays a large role in the treatment of multiple myeloma, which is usually radiosensitive. Approximately 70% of patients with multiple myeloma eventually require and potentially benefit from irradiation.[24] Treatment of painful, disabling bony sites is usually rapid and successful, leading to decreased requirements for narcotics or analgesics and increased functional capacity, thereby enabling the patient to carry on with activities of daily living.[14] The addition of pulse dexamethasone during treatment with radiation may also provide pain relief and additional response.

Patients who present with back pain, lower extremity weakness, or numbness and are diagnosed with spinal cord compression must start treatment with steroids and radiation therapy immediately, because cord compression is an oncologic emergency. The steroids should be given in a pulse fashion: the same dose, 4 days on and 4 days off steroids, for 3 weeks, regardless of radiation therapy. The steroids usually are given on days 1 through 4, 9 through 12, and 17 through 20.[2] This approach avoids severe myelosuppression, which often occurs when chemotherapy is combined with radiation in these patients.[2]

Myeloablative therapy with stem cell support is currently being investigated as a treatment for multiple myeloma. Both allogeneic and autologous approaches have been studied.[14] Allogeneic bone marrow transplantation requires a human leukocyte antigen (HLA)-typed and -matched donor and requires that the patient have good cardiac, pulmonary, hepatic, and renal function. Potential advantages of allogeneic bone marrow transplantation include the fact that the patient is not required to have minimal bone marrow involvement by disease and a theoretical graft-versus-myeloma effect.[14] This approach is generally reserved for patients with relapsing or late refractory disease because there is a high rate of early mortality and morbidity.

Myeloablative therapy with autologous stem cell support is associated with less mortality and morbidity than allogeneic transplantation, particularly with regard to graft-versus-host disease.[14] An acceptable matched donor is not required, because the stem cells are collected from the patient. Stem cells may be collected either by harvesting the bone marrow or by peripheral blood stem cell collection (the most common method). Recent studies suggest a survival advantage for patients who receive a transplant early in the course of their disease.[25] Others have reported that patients whose disease has not responded to pulse dexamethasone and a more intensive alkylating agent treatment and are still within the first year of therapy are most likely to benefit, whereas those with late primary refractory disease, those with disease in refractory relapse, and those in remission are less likely to benefit.[26] At The University of Texas M. D. Anderson Cancer Center, we generally reserve transplantation for patients with primary refractory disease within the first year of therapy (see Table 20–3), but this approach varies among different centers.

REMISSION CRITERIA

Complete remission is defined as complete disappearance of serum M protein and urine Bence Jones protein by the most sensitive technique (immunofixation) and no monoclonal plasma cells in the bone marrow.[5] At M. D. Anderson Cancer Center, partial remission is defined as a 75% reduction in the serum M protein level, at least a 95% reduction in the urine Bence Jones protein excretion, and fewer than 5% bone marrow plasma cells as determined by two consecutive laboratory evaluations at least 1 month apart.[5] Patients in remission often have an increase in previously suppressed levels of uninvolved immunoglobulins.

REMISSION MAINTENANCE THERAPY

Patients in complete or partial remission may be given maintenance therapy. Interferon-α administered by subcutaneous injection, compared with no therapy, prolongs the first remission by approximately 6 months but confers no survival advantage.[27] Treatment with interferon should continue until relapse of myeloma (see Table 20–3). Maintenance therapy with melphalan and prednisone may also prolong remissions but is generally more myelosuppressive and is associated with a slight risk of a secondary leukemia or myelodysplasia.[2]

SURVEILLANCE

Ambulatory patients whose myeloma is in complete or partial remission should have monthly follow-up visits. Before each appointment, laboratory evaluation usually includes a complete blood count with differential and platelet count; measurement of blood urea nitrogen, creatinine, calcium, total protein, and albumin; serum protein electrophoresis; quantitative assay of immunoglobulins (at least at the first outpatient visit); and a 24-hour urine collection for urine protein electrophoresis. Periodic measurement of LDH and B2M is often helpful because these are measures of drug resistance, short survival, and tumor mass.[2] At the first sign of relapse, as determined by a rising serum or urine M protein (25% increase), hypercalcemia, renal failure due to myeloma, or new or enlarging lytic lesions, maintenance therapy should be discontinued and appropriate treatment initiated (see Table 20–3).

OTHER PLASMA CELL DYSCRASIAS

Multiple myeloma is one of a group of plasma cell disorders that also includes MGUS, SPB, asymptomatic myeloma, Waldenström's macroglobulinemia, and amyloidosis.

MONOCLONAL GAMMOPATHY OF UNKNOWN SIGNIFICANCE

MGUS occurs in 1% of normal persons older than 40 years, and the frequency increases with increasing age.[5] There is an overlap between the findings for patients with MGUS and those for patients with stage I myeloma (or macroglobulinemia) that can often be recognized by serial follow-up of the patient for at least 1 year without any form of treatment.[6] In MGUS, the M-component level remains at a low over many years, but in malignant plasma cell disorders, the M-component level gradually rises, and other signs and symptoms of the disease develop.[6] Patients usually have low levels of monoclonal protein (<2.5 g/dL), preserved uninvolved immunoglobulins, minimal marrow plasmacytosis, and no evidence of lytic bone lesions.[2] Patients with elevated M protein are observed periodically without treatment, because most will not require treatment.[6] During the first year, the patient should be reevaluated by laboratory tests and clinical examination every 3 to 4 months. If after 1 year the level of M protein remains stable and the patient remains asymptomatic, follow-up may continue at intervals of 6 months or longer. Of patients diagnosed with MGUS, 1.5% have disease progression to a malignant B-cell neoplasm (multiple myeloma, lymphoma, amyloidosis).[28]

SOLITARY PLASMACYTOMA OF BONE

Patients with SPB present with a solitary lytic bone lesion that, when biopsied, reveals malignant plasma cells.[29] Approximately 5% of patients with myeloma have SPB with no identifiable disease elsewhere, and approximately 50% of patients with SPB have evidence of a monoclonal protein in the serum or urine (see Table 20–3).[30] If careful evaluation including a negative magnetic resonance imaging study reveals no evidence of systemic disease, it is common practice to treat the solitary lesion with local radiation therapy.[14] The dose of radiation usually is 45 Gy.[2] Multiple myeloma becomes evident in most patients with time, and only 20% to 30% remain free of disease for more than 10 years.[31–33] The rapid development of myeloma is inevitable for patients with SPB in whom a monoclonal protein is present in serum or urine (or both) before treatment and persists after treatment.[32] The median time to disease progression is 2 years.[29] Treatment with subcutaneous interferon-α is currently being evaluated in an attempt to inhibit disease evolution.[2] When progression to generalized disease occurs, the median survival from that point is identical to that of other patients with multiple myeloma.[14]

ASYMPTOMATIC MYELOMA

Twenty percent of patients with multiple myeloma are diagnosed by chance during screening evaluations that reveal an elevated serum protein level.[2] Because these patients have no symptoms of disease, their disease is described as asymptomatic myeloma. The characteristics of asymptomatic myeloma include median monoclonal immunoglobulin levels higher than 3 g/dL and plasma cells accounting for more than 10% of bone marrow cells.[14] Features absent in the patient with asymptomatic myeloma include renal insufficiency, hypercalcemia, significant anemia (hemoglobin >10.5 g/dL), and lytic bone lesions. These patients should have close monitoring, including serial measurements of B2M, serum protein electrophoresis, 24-hour urine protein electrophoresis, and periodic bone surveys, because these indicators may reflect disease progression. Systemic chemotherapy should not be initiated until there is evidence of disease progression, because many patients may remain stable for many years.[2]

Recent studies have helped define prognostic criteria for groups at high risk for disease progression. These include serum M protein higher than 3 g/dL, Bence Jones proteinuria greater than 50 mg/dL, and IgA type.[2] Patients with two or more of these characteristics have short times to progression (median, 18 months); the absence of any of these features has been associated with much later disease progression (median, >5 years).[2] One study found that 40% of asymptomatic patients had marrow involvement on magnetic resonance imaging despite normal skeletal surveys; this type of presentation also predicted early disease progression.[34] Asymptomatic patients with a lytic bone lesion should probably be treated at presentation, because the time to progression is short (median of 8 months).[2]

WALDENSTRÖM'S MACROGLOBULINEMIA

Another disease entity that must be considered in the differential diagnosis of multiple myeloma is Waldenström's macroglobulinemia, a rare low-grade lymphoid malignancy composed of mature plasmacytoid lymphocytes with monoclonal IgM production.[2] Waldenström's macroglobulinemia usually affects older persons and can cause symptoms as a result of tumor infiltration of the marrow, lymph nodes, or spleen; circulating IgM (hyperviscosity, cryoglobulinemia, or cold agglutinin anemia); and tissue deposition (neuropathy, glomerular disease, or amyloidosis). Some other clinical features include hemorrhage, cutaneous lesions, and bone disease.[35]

Tumor infiltration of Waldenström's macroglobulinemia can cause the pancytopenia seen in other malignancies when the marrow is replaced by disease. In Waldenström's macroglobulinemia, malignant plasmacytic lymphocytes often infiltrate lymph nodes and the spleen, accounting for the enlargement of these organs in about 40% of patients.[14] Usually, the adenopathy is generalized and modest in presentation, with nodes between 2 and 5 cm; usually splenomegaly also is not severe, with the spleen palpated 3 to 5 cm below the left costal margin.[14]

Hyperviscosity is the condition in which a patient's serum is thicker, or more viscous, than normal. Research studies have shown that IgM immunoglobulins are particularly prone to cause hyperviscosity because of their larger size.[14] When IgM concentrations reach 3 g/dL, the viscosity rises more rapidly. Symptoms of hyperviscosity are often seen when the serum viscosity is four times normal. It is important to determine the symptom threshold for each patient and to keep the IgM concentration below that level.[14]

Patients with hyperviscosity often complain of vision problems and can have neurologic syndromes. Visual problems include decreased visual acuity, blurred vision, and diplopia.[14] On funduscopic examination, there may be distended, tortuous retinal veins, commonly referred to as sausage-like vessels.[14] Neurologic syndromes in macroglobulinemia are caused either by hyperviscosity or by involvement of the peripheral nerves by the monoclonal protein.[14] Symptoms caused by hyperviscosity include headache, confusion, lethargy, coma, dizziness, and vertigo.[36] These symptoms are usually gradual in onset; however, if untreated, they progress over time secondary to increasing IgM concentrations.[14] Reversibility of the symptoms depends on recognition of hyperviscosity and initiation of treatment with plasmapheresis followed by chemotherapy.[14] Peripheral neuropathies, usually mixed motor and sensory, are seen in 5% of patients with macroglobulinemia and are often associated with a myelin-associated glycoprotein.[14] Reversal of the peripheral neuropathy may be possible when the IgM level is reduced.[14]

Other manifestations of circulating IgM are cryoglobulinemia and cold agglutinin disease. In the former, cryoglobulins can be formed when the monoclonal IgM reacts with IgG to form a complex, or they may be associated with the monoclonal IgM alone.[37] This occurs in 5% to 10% of patients with macroglobulinemia.[14] Typical symptoms associated with cryoglobulins are usually caused by precipitation of these proteins on exposure to cold and commonly include Raynaud's phenomenon and digital ischemia.[14] In approximately 33% of patients with Waldenström's macroglobulinemia, the IgM immunoglobulins have cold-reactive properties.[14] Hemolytic anemia may occur if a cold agglutinin is present. This is usually caused by an antibody associated with the Ia antigen on the red blood cell. Treatment should be aimed at lowering the IgM level to alleviate symptoms.

Renal dysfunction and amyloidosis are rare manifestations found in patients with Waldenström's macroglobulinemia.[14] Hemorrhagic complications are common presenting signs of macroglobulinemia.[14] The actual mechanisms that cause hemorrhage are complicated and unclear. IgM interacts with several coagulation proteins, including factors V, VII, and VIII and the prothrombin complex.[37] In some cases, IgM binds to fibrinogen, causing poor fibrin formation, clot retraction, and prolonged prothrombin time. Platelets can become coated with the monoclonal immunoglobulin, causing abnormal platelet aggregation and adhesion.[38] The clinical manifestations are epistaxis, retinal hemorrhage, and other mucous membrane bleeding.[14] These complications can be reversed by lowering the circulating IgM level through plasmapheresis or chemotherapy.

Cutaneous manifestations of Waldenström's macroglobulinemia are rare, but occasionally they are the first sign of the disease.[14] Two types of skin lesions occur.[39] One is a violaceous plaque or tumor composed of an infiltrate of malignant lymphocytes; the other is a shiny pink papule composed of hyaline deposits of the IgM monoclonal protein.[14] Patients may have one or both types of lesions.[39] Both tend to regress with successful chemotherapy.[16] A small percentage of patients with Waldenström's macroglobulinemia develop overt lytic or osteopenic bone disease. The malignant plasmalymphocytic lymphoma cells do not generally produce osteoclast activity factors as do the malignant plasma cells in myeloma, and therefore lytic bone lesions are noted in only 10% of patients.[14]

Oral alkylating agents (e.g., chlorambucil, melphalan, cyclophosphamide) alone or in combination with prednisone generally produce response rates of 50%.[40] Plasmapheresis is often used initially to treat hyperviscosity and to decrease the level of circulating immunoglobulins.[6] Systemic treatment is continued until the IgM level plateaus, at which point treatment can be discontinued until there is evidence of rising serum M protein, hyperviscosity, or other evidence of relapse.[5] Remission criteria are similar to those for myeloma, and more than 50% reduction in adenopathy is required. Complete remission is rarely achieved; patients who respond to treatment have a reported median survival time of 50 months, and nonresponders, 25 months.[41]

A new chemotherapeutic agent, cladribine (2-CdA), is being used in the treatment of Waldenström's macroglobulinemia. Cladribine has induced remissions of long duration (median of 18 months) in more than 80% of previously untreated patients with only two courses of therapy.[2] Patients are monitored in unmaintained remission and generally respond to reinitiation of cladribine at relapse.[2] Cladribine has induced responses in 54% of patients with primary resistant disease and in 70% of patients who have had a relapse off treatment.[2] Patients with relapsing disease resistant to alkylating agents (refractory relapse) are less likely to benefit from cladribine (response rate 18%) and should be considered for more intensive therapies.[2]

AMYLOIDOSIS

Primary amyloidosis is another plasma cell disorder that must be differentiated from multiple myeloma. Ten percent to 15% of patients with multiple myeloma also have amyloidosis; however, people with amyloidosis do not necessarily have myeloma. The presenting symptoms of amyloidosis (with or without myeloma) include weakness, weight loss, ankle edema, dyspnea, paresthesias, lightheadedness, and syncope secondary to orthostatic hypotension.[42] Nocturnal aching of the hands can be symptomatic of median nerve compression associated with carpal tunnel syndrome caused by amyloid infiltration of the transverse carpal ligament.[5] Physical findings include enlargement of the tongue, hepatomegaly, purpura, and ankle edema, which usually is caused by congestive heart failure or nephrotic syndrome.[5] The tongue frequently shows indentations from the teeth and may prevent closure of the mouth.[5] The tissues most subject to amyloid deposition in myeloma include the tongue, gastrointestinal tract, heart, skin, nerves, and skeletal muscle.[5] Purpura of the eyelids is characteristic of amyloidosis, and unilateral or bilateral periorbital purpura may appear suddenly after the head is placed in a dependent position.[5] Skin manifestations include plaques, papules, or nodules.[5] An electrocardiogram of a patient with amyloidosis may demonstrate low voltage.[5] A two-dimensional echocardiogram may reveal thickening of the ventricular walls, septum, or papillary muscles and pericardial effusion.[43]

The classic method of diagnosing amyloidosis has been rectal biopsy, which is positive in more than 60% of patients.[5] Another method of establishing the diagnosis of amyloidosis is to aspirate abdominal fat and stain the specimen with Congo red. This latter method has been positive in more than 70% of patients.[5]

Treatment for amyloidosis with myeloma is the same as treatment for multiple myeloma: systemic chemotherapy with melphalan and prednisone continued for at least 1 to 2 years.[5] The treatment may stop or slow further amyloid deposition, but it does not affect the amyloid deposits already present.[5] Congestive heart failure secondary to amyloidosis is considered to be a poor prognostic feature of amyloidosis and usually does not respond to cardiac glycosides.[44] Symptom management and relief of edema may be achieved through the use of diuretics.[5]

CONCLUSION

The patient with a plasma cell dyscrasia has a chronic disease that can often be controlled so that long periods of remission occur. However, no cure is available at this time. Multiple myeloma and other plasma cell dyscrasias usually respond to similar treatments. One exception is Waldenström's macroglobulinemia, which responds to nucleoside analogs like cladribine, which in many cases induces long remissions of excellent quality. Therapy for these disorders is aimed at achieving remission or, in later stages of the disease, at palliation and pain control. One of the most important goals of patient care is to keep the patient mobile and ambulatory so that he or she can continue participating in activities of daily living.

REFERENCES

1. Sheridan CA: Multiple myeloma. In Groewald SL, Frogge MH, Goodman M, Yarbro CH (eds): Cancer Nursing Principles and Practice, 3rd ed. Boston, Jones & Bartlett, 1993:1230–1237.
2. Papadimitrakopoulou V, Weber DM: Multiple myeloma and other plasma-cell dyscrasias. In Pazdur R (ed): Medical Oncology: A Comprehensive Review, 2nd ed. Huntington, NY, PRR, 1995:127–138.
3. Bubley GJ, Schnipper LE: Multiple myeloma. In Holleb AI (ed): American Cancer Society Textbook of Clinical Oncology. Atlanta, American Cancer Society, 1991:397–409.
4. Oken MM: Multiple myeloma. Med Clin North Am 1984;68:757–787.
5. Salmon SE, Cassady JR: Plasma cell neoplasms. In DeVita VT, Hellman S, Rosenberg SA (eds): Cancer: Principles and Practice of Oncology, 4th ed. Philadelphia, JB Lippincott, 1993:1984–2025.
6. Mellstedt A, Aahre A, Bjorkholm M, et al: Interferon therapy in myelomatosis. Lancet 1979;1:245–247.
7. Riedel DA, Pottern LM: The epidemiology of multiple myeloma. Hematol Oncol Clin North Am 1992;6:225–247.
8. Preston DL, Kusumi S, Tomonaga M, et al: Cancer incidence in atomic bomb survivors. Part III: Leukemia, lymphoma, and multiple myeloma, 1950–1987. Radiat Res 1994;137:568–597.
9. Lewis EB: Leukemia, multiple myeloma, and aplastic anemia in American radiologists. Science 1963;142:1492–1494.
10. Stebbings JH, Lucas HF, Stehney AF: Mortality from cancers of major sites in female radium dial workers. Am J Intern Med 1984;5:435–439.
11. Bofetta P, Stellman SD, Gardinkle L: A case control study of multiple myeloma nested in the American Cancer Society prospective study. Int J Cancer 1989;43:554–559.
12. Rinsky RA, Smith AB, Hornung R, et al: Benzene and leukemia. N Engl J Med 1987;316:1044–1050.
13. Grogan TM, Spier CM, Salmon SE, et al: P-glycoprotein expression in human plasma cell myeloma: Correlation with prior chemotherapy. Blood 1994;81:490–495.
14. Shulman LN: Plasma cell diseases and related disorders. In Handin RJ, Lux SE, Stossel TP (eds): Blood: Principles and Practice of Hematology. Philadelphia, JB Lippincott, 1995:885–913.
15. Ludwig H, Fritz E, Kotzmann H, et al: Erythropoietin treatment of anemia associated with multiple myeloma. N Engl J Med 1993;322:1693–1699.

16. Johnson WJ, Kyle RA, Pineda AA, et al: Treatment of renal failure associated with multiple myeloma: Plasmapheresis, hemodialysis, and chemotherapy. Arch Intern Med 1990;150:863–869.
17. Cohen DJ, Sherman WH, Osserman EF, et al: Acute renal failure in patients with multiple myeloma. Am J Med 1984;76:247–256.
18. Ellison DH, Johnson BM: Renal fluid and electrolyte disorders in the critically ill immunosuppressed patient. In Parrillo JE (ed): The Critically Ill Immunosuppressed Patient: Diagnosis and Management. Rockville, MD, Aspen, 1987:81–118.
19. Jacobson DR, Zolla-Pazner S: Immunosuppression and infection in multiple myeloma. In Wiernik PH (ed): Neoplastic Disease of the Blood. New York, Churchill Livingstone, 1991:415–426.
20. Barlogie B, Smallwood L, Smith TL, et al: High serum levels of lactate dehydrogenase identify a high-grade lymphoma-like myeloma. Ann Intern Med 1989;110:521–525.
21. Dimopoulos MA, Barlogie B, Smith TL, et al: High serum lactate dehydrogenase level as a marker for drug resistance and short survival in multiple myeloma. Ann Intern Med 1991;115:931–935.
22. Alexanian R, Haut A, Khan AU, et al: Treatment for multiple myeloma: Combination chemotherapy with different melphalan dose regimen. JAMA 1969;208:1680.
23. Boccadoro M, Pileri A: Standard chemotherapy for myelomatosis: An area of great controversy. Hematol Oncol Clin North Am 1992;6:371–382.
24. Bosch A, Frias Z: Radiotherapy in the treatment of multiple myeloma. Int J Radiat Oncol Biol Phys 1988;15:1363–1369.
25. Harousseau JL, Attal M, Divine M, et al: Autologous stem cell transplantation after first remission induction treatment in multiple myeloma: A report of the French registry on autologous transplantation in multiple myeloma. Blood 1985;85:3077–3085.
26. Alexanian R, Dimopoulos M, Smith T, et al: Limited value of myeloablative therapy for late multiple myeloma. Blood 1994;83:512–516.
27. Alexanian R, Weber DM: Whither interferon for myeloma and other hematologic malignancies. Ann Intern Med 1996;124:264–265.
28. Kyle RA: Monoclonal gammopathy of undetermined significance (MGUS): A review. In Hoffbrand AB, Lasch HG, Nathan DE, Salmon SE (eds): Clinics in Hematology. Eastbourne, MI, WB Saunders, 1982:123–150.
29. Knowling MA, Harwood AR, Bergsagel DE: Comparison of extramedullary plasmacytomas with solitary and multiple plasma cell tumors of bone. J Clin Oncol 1983;1:255.
30. Dimopoulos MA, Goldstein J, Fuller L: Curability of solitary bone plasmacytoma. J Clin Oncol 1992;10:587–590.
31. Dimopoulos MA, Moulopoulos A, Delasalle K, et al: Solitary plasmacytoma of bone and asymptomatic multiple myeloma. Hematol Oncol Clin North Am 1992;6:359–369.
32. Chak LY, Cox RS, Bostwick DG, et al: Solitary plasmacytoma of bone: Treatment, progression, and survival. J Clin Oncol 1987;5:1811–1815.
33. Bataille R, Sany J: Solitary myeloma: Clinical and prognostic features of a review of 114 cases. Cancer 1981;48:845.
34. Moulopoulos L, Dimopoulos MA, Smith TL, et al: Prognostic significance of magnetic resonance imaging in patients with asymptomatic multiple myeloma. J Clin Oncol 1995;13:251–256.
35. Dimopoulos MA, Alexanian R: Waldenström's macroglobulinemia. Blood 1994;83:1452–1459.
36. Somer T: Rheology of paraproteinaemias and the plasma hyperviscosity syndrome. Baillieres Clin Haemotol 1987;1:695.
37. Patterson WP, Caldwell CW, Doll DC: Hyperviscosity syndromes and coagulopathies. Semin Oncol 1990;17:210.
38. Godal HC, Borchgrevink CF: The effect of plasmapheresis of the hemostatic function in patients with macroglobulinemia Waldenström and multiple myeloma. Scand J Clin Lab Invest 1965;17(suppl 84):133.
39. Mascaro JM, Montserrat E, Estrach T, et al: Specific cutaneous manifestations of Waldenström's macroglobulinemia: A report of two cases. Br J Dermatol 1982;106:217.
40. Carter P, Koval JJ, Hobbs JR: The relation of clinical and laboratory findings to the survival of patients with macroglobulinemia. Clin Exp Immunol 1977;28:241–249.
41. MacKenzie MR, Fudenberg HH: Macroglobulinemia: An analysis for forty patients. Blood 1972;39:874.
42. Kyle RA: Amyloidosis. In Hoffbrand AV, Lasch HG, Nathan DG, Salmon SE (eds): Clinics in Hematology. Eastbourne, MI, WB Saunders, 1982:151–180.
43. Siqueira-Filho AS, Cunha CLP, Tajik AJ, et al: M-Mode and two dimensional echocardiographic features in cardiac amyloidosis. Circulation 1981;63:188–196.
44. Kyle RA, Greipp PR, O'Fallon WM: Primary systemic amyloidosis: Multivariate analysis for prognostic factors in 168 cases. Blood 1986;68:220–224.

Chapter 21

Complications of Cancer Treatment

Paula Trahan Rieger, MSN, RN, ANP, CS, OCN, and Carmen P. Escalante, MD

Most patients with cancer will ultimately receive some form of therapy, the goal of which is generally to cure the patient. Treatment modalities also may be used in the diagnosis, stabilization, or palliation of disease. Many patients additionally receive adjuvant therapy, which can be thought of as "insurance." For example, after surgical resection of a melanoma, a patient at high risk for recurrence of disease may receive adjuvant therapy with interferon to decrease that risk.

Of the four major therapeutic modalities for cancer—chemotherapy, surgery, radiation therapy, and biotherapy—surgery is the most commonly used, although many patients receive a combination of several types of therapy. For example, a woman with breast cancer may first have surgery to remove the breast mass, followed by radiation therapy and chemotherapy. A newer although at times controversial cancer treatment is bone marrow transplantation (BMT). These treatments, although necessary to manage the patient's disease, often are associated with side effects and complications that may be physical, emotional, or social in nature. A multidisciplinary team is vital to effectively manage both the treatment-associated complications and the emotional responses that accompany the diagnosis and treatment of cancer.

This chapter outlines the principles of management of the cancer patient and provides an overview of each of the major cancer treatment modalities, examples of their use in clinical practice, common therapy-related complications, and important points for educating patients and families about their therapy. Brief discussions of the psychosocial changes related to a diagnosis of cancer and the late complications of cancer therapy are provided to assist midlevel providers in preparing patients and their families to cope with the complications of cancer treatment.

PRINCIPLES OF MANAGEMENT OF THE CANCER PATIENT

Several key areas are important to the comprehensive management of patients receiving cancer therapy: physical assessment, treatment of therapy-related complications, and patient education. A complete patient assessment, before, during, and after therapy, forms the cornerstone of management. A thorough pretherapy assessment using a body systems approach provides a baseline for evaluating complications that may arise from therapy. Important areas to include in such an assessment are a history of the patient's prior treatment or chronic illnesses, current symptoms, functional and psychosocial status, and factors such as age or alterations in organ function (renal or hepatic) that may affect his or her tolerance to therapy. As therapy progresses, an evaluation of the patient's adherence to plan and tolerance of the therapy is vital. One of the most important roles of the midlevel provider is prompt recognition of therapy-related side effects (e.g., lowered blood cell counts, signs and symptoms of infection) so that these complications can be treated in a timely manner and further complications (e.g., sepsis) can be avoided. Many scales available in the oncology literature, such as those from the Eastern Cooperative Oncology Group and the World Health Organization, can assist in quantifying the severity of symptoms.[1-3] Patient education also should be a priority in management, because patients and families are assuming an increasing responsibility for managing therapy in the home setting. Important education topics to consider are the rationale for therapy, understanding of the treatment plan, expected side effects and management strategies, signs and symptoms that should be reported to the health care team, self-care skills such as self-administration of medication or central venous catheter care, coping skills, and identification of resources. Midlevel providers in primary care settings can do much to reinforce information provided by the oncology specialty team.

CHEMOTHERAPY

Chemotherapy treats malignancies systemically. The principal goal of chemotherapy is to destroy malignant cells without harming normal cells or the host. However, most chemotherapeutic agents are nonspecific and therefore affect both malignant and normal cells.

Both pharmacologic and biochemical factors determine a cancer cell's sensitivity and resistance to chemotherapy. A cell's ability to repair chemical injury and to metabolize chemotherapeutic agents allows recovery from drug-induced tissue damage. Successful therapy requires that cellular repair mechanisms in malignant cells be inadequate and that those of normal cells be sufficient to allow cell survival.

The cell cycle is composed of four phases during which the cell prepares for and enters mitosis (cell division). This concept is important because actively dividing cells are the most sensitive to chemotherapy. The efficacy of chemotherapy depends on the number of cells undergoing active cell division. Nondividing cells remain relatively resistant to chemotherapy unless treatment continues until those cells enter the cell cycle.

Tumor growth is related to the proportion of cells actively dividing, the length of the cell cycle, and the rate of cell loss. Because of variations in these three factors, variable rates of tumor growth are observed among tumors from different histologic tissue types and among metastatic and primary tumors having the same histology. Small tumors (i.e., those with a small tumor volume) have the most rapid growth. As tumors get larger, growth slows based on a complex process that depends on cell loss and on the supply of blood and oxygen to the tumor.

In the "log kill" hypothesis of chemotherapy, some constant fraction of malignant cells die with each such treatment. Therefore, chemotherapy models have been developed to employ alternating non-cross-resistant therapies (e.g., combinations of chemotherapy agents), induction-intensification approaches, and adjuvant chemotherapy regimens.

Chemotherapy may be used to cure cancer, to palliate or stabilize disease as preliminary therapy before BMT, or as adjuvant therapy. Responses to chemotherapy include complete response, partial response, stable disease or minimal response, and disease progression. Complete response is defined as the disappearance of all evidence of disease and no new appearance of disease for a specified interval (usually 4 weeks). Partial response is defined as reduction by at least 50% in the sum of the products of the two longest diameters of all lesions, maintained for at least one course of therapy with no new appearance of disease. Minimal response is any response less than a partial response; it usually is not reported in clinical trials. Progression is defined as growth of disease during chemotherapy. Tumors for which chemotherapy may be curative include testicular cancer and certain hematologic malignancies such as Hodgkin's disease. In many solid tumors (e.g., breast cancer, prostate cancer, non-small cell lung cancer), chemotherapy has been proven to induce a complete remission with increased patient survival.[4-6]

MECHANISM OF ACTION

Deoxyribonucleic acid (DNA) synthesis is the principal target for most anti-neoplastic agents. Ribonucleic acid (RNA) transcription and microtubular binding are additional targets. Chemotherapy agents are often divided into classes, each having a unique mechanism of action. Cell cycle-nonspecific agents, such as alkylating agents, damage DNA and need not be administered during the DNA synthesis (S) phase of the cell cycle. The affected cells die when attempting to replicate with defective DNA. Cell cycle-nonspecific agents have a linear dose-response curve; the greater the dose of drug, the greater the fraction of cell kill. Other examples of such agents include the antitumor antibiotics, nitrosoureas, and hormone and steroid drugs. Cell cycle-specific drugs have a plateau in cell killing; beyond this plateau, cell kill does not increase with further increases in drug dosage. Classes of cell cycle-specific agents include antimetabolites, which interfere with DNA synthesis, and the vinca plant alkaloids, which interfere with the cell's ability to divide.[7]

TOXIC EFFECTS OF CHEMOTHERAPY AND THEIR MANAGEMENT

Chemotherapeutic agents cause injury to both normal and malignant tissues. Those normal cells most often affected are rapidly dividing cells such as hematopoietic cells, hair, and cells lining the gastrointestinal tract. Often the injury results in expected side effects such as mucositis, diarrhea, nausea and vomiting, alopecia, and anticipated intervals of bone marrow suppression. Possible complications of bone marrow suppression include infection related to a lowered white blood cell count, anemia due to a low red blood cell count, and bleeding caused by a lowered platelet count. See Table 21–1 for a review of the most common therapy-related side effects.

Certain chemotherapeutic agents can cause serious toxic effects to specific organ systems. This often occurs with prolonged therapy. Serious chemotherapy toxicity is one of the most significant barriers to delivery of curative doses of treatment. The following discussion and Table 21–2 summarize by organ system the most important of these effects and the drugs involved.

Table 21–1. Common Side Effects with Cancer Therapies

CHEMOTHERAPY	SURGERY	RADIATION THERAPY	BIOTHERAPY
Fatigue	Fatigue	Fatigue	Flu-like symptoms
Changes in hematologic values	Pain	Changes in hematologic values	Fatigue
Low white blood cells	Changes in mobility	Low white blood cells	Loss of appetite
Low red blood cells	Changes in nutrition	Low red blood cells	Altered taste sensation
Low platelets	Potential for postoperative infections	Low platelets	Slowed thinking
Nausea and vomiting		Skin changes	Memory problems
Mucositis: oral, rectal, and vaginal		Dry desquamation	Reversible changes in liver enzymes and hematologic values
Skin changes		Moist desquamation	Inflammatory reactions at injection sites
Alopecia		Site specific side effects	
Darkened nail beds			
Changes in sexuality			

Table 21–2. Organ Toxicity of Chemotherapeutic Agents

CARDIAC	PULMONARY	RENAL	HEPATIC
Amsacrine	Bleomycin	Carboplatin	Asparaginase
Busulfan	Busulfan	Carmustine	Azathioprine
Cisplatin	Carmustine	Cisplatin	Busulfan
Cyclophosphamide	Chlorambucil	Cyclophosphamide	Carboplatin
(high dose)	Cyclophosphamide	Ifosfamide	Carmustine
Daunorubicin	(high dose)	Methotrexate	Cyclophosphamide
Doxorubicin	Cytarabine	Mitomycin	Cytarabine
Fluorouracil	Melphalan (high	Streptozocin	Dacarbazine
Mitomycin	dose)		Dactinomycin
Mitoxantrone	Methotrexate		Hydroxyurea
Paclitaxel	Mitomycin		Mercaptopurine
Vinblastine			Methotrexate
Vincristine			Mitomycin
			Nitrosoureas
			Plicamycin
			Streptozocin
			Thioguanine

CARDIAC TOXICITY

Anthracyclines (doxorubicin, daunorubicin, mitoxantrone) are the chemotherapeutic agents most commonly associated with cardiac toxicity. These agents can result in acute cardiac dysfunction and supraventricular tachycardia. However, chronic anthracycline-associated toxicity, occurring weeks or months after drug administration, is of greatest significance. This chronic toxicity, usually manifested as cardiomyopathy, is dose and schedule dependent. Cumulative bolus doses greater than 550 mg/m^2 increase the risk of congestive heart failure with cardiac toxicity that is only minimally reversible.[8]

PULMONARY TOXICITY

Pulmonary toxicity from chemotherapy is relatively uncommon but potentially fatal. Bleomycin, an antibiotic antitumor agent, may produce severe pulmonary fibrosis. Risk factors associated with bleomycin pulmonary toxicity include a total administered dose of more than 400 U, older age of the patient, baseline pulmonary function abnormalities, prior or concomitant radiotherapy, exposure to high-dose oxygen, and concomitant administration of other chemotherapeutic agents. Monitoring for toxicity includes pulmonary function testing with discontinuation of the drug if change in pulmonary function is greater than 10% to 15%.[9]

RENAL TOXICITY

Most agents causing renal toxicity produce injury to the renal tubules. Some chemotherapeutic agents can cause acute and irreversible renal failure. Cisplatin-induced nephrotoxicity is dose-limiting and ranges from mild reversible azotemia to tubular necrosis and irreversible renal failure. It causes injury to both the proximal and distal tubules.

Cisplatin nephrotoxicity is reduced by aggressive hydration of the patient with saline (2 to 3 L over 8 to 12 hours) on the day of therapy. Mannitol may also be added. Cisplatin-induced acute toxicity may be managed by reducing the dose or discontinuing the drug and aggressively hydrating the patient. Dialysis is poorly effective in reversing cisplatin-induced renal failure; chronic renal failure may persist. Electrolyte imbalances, particularly hypomagnesemia and hyponatremia, are also associated with cisplatin administration. Treatment of these includes replenishment with oral or intravenous magnesium, depending on the patient's serum level and clinical presentation, and careful replacement of sodium or free water.

Hemorrhagic cystitis is associated with the alkylating agents cyclophosphamide and ifosfamide. It occurs in approximately 10% of patients who receive standard therapy. However, the incidence of hemorrhagic cystitis may be as high as 40% in patients who receive high-dose chemotherapy for BMT. Microscopic hematuria is present in 93% of those with hemorrhagic cystitis, and gross hematuria in 78%. Mesna, a uroprotective agent, is often given with ifosfamide and cyclophosphamide to prevent the accumulation of acrolein, a metabolite that is toxic to bladder mucosa and causes hemorrhagic cystitis. Recommended doses of mesna range from 60% to 160% of the cyclophosphamide dose, but controversy exists. Administration of mesna should begin before or during administration of the alkylating agent. Once hemorrhagic cystitis has developed, treatment includes clot evacuation, continuous bladder irrigation with saline or hydrocortisone or systemic aminocaproic acid.[10]

HEPATOTOXICITY

The majority of chemotherapeutic agents are metabolized in the liver, and many are directly hepatotoxic. Hepatotoxicity, which can be either acute or chronic, is noted when liver transaminase levels increase. Veno-occlusive disease of the liver may occur with high-dose chemotherapy in patients undergoing BMT or with radiation therapy to the liver. Methotrexate in daily oral doses can cause hepatic fibrosis and cirrhosis. This is less common with parenterally administered doses; however, acute hepatocellular injury can occur with high-dose methotrexate. Hepatotoxicity can be detected early by careful monitoring of liver function test results during administration of potentially hepatotoxic agents. Dose modification of various agents is necessary if increases in liver enzymes are noted on liver function tests.

SURGERY

Surgery is the oldest treatment for cancer and at one time was the only effective treatment. Over the last several years, surgical treatment of cancer has changed dramatically. It is still the preferred therapy for many cancers, with more than 60% of cancer patients treated surgically. However, today surgery is often combined with other treatment modalities. Moreover, it is also used in the diagnosis and staging of more than 90% of all cancers[11, 12] (Fig. 21–1). Advances in surgical techniques and a better understanding of patterns of spread in different cancers have allowed surgeons to perform successful tumor resections in an increased number of patients. Also, improvement and development of successful alternative treatment strategies able to control microscopic disease

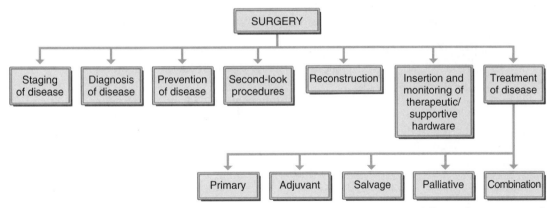

Figure 21-1. Applications of surgery in cancer care. (From Pfeifer KA: Surgery. In Otto SE (ed): Oncology Nursing, 2nd ed. St. Louis, Mosby–Year Book, 1994.)

have allowed surgeons to reassess the degree of surgical intervention necessary and to perform less radical surgeries than were done in the past.

Surgical treatment of cancer has both advantages and disadvantages for the patient. Among the advantages is that tumor heterogeneity, often encountered in other cancer treatment modalities, is not a factor in surgical interventions. Tumors offer no biologic resistance to surgery, and there are no potential carcinogenic effects of this treatment. Surgery provides the most accurate evidence of the extent of disease by pathologic staging and allows a description of the histology of the malignancy. It also offers potential cure to a large portion of patients with undisseminated tumors.

There are also disadvantages to surgery. During surgical resection both normal and neoplastic tissues are damaged, which can cause significant morbidity, deformity, and/or loss of function. Patients may experience a significant change in body image. Surgery also can result in mortality for some patients. Moreover, nonlocalized cancers usually are not amenable to surgical therapy. Also, because malignancy often involves unresectable vital organs, curative resections may be limited.

SURGERY FOR CANCER PREVENTION

There are situations in which surgery can prevent or reduce the risk for development of cancer, and it is important that primary care providers recognize these situations. They include the following:

Cryptorchidism is associated with an increased risk of testicular carcinoma. The risk is reduced if orchiopexy is performed at an early age.
Ulcerative colitis often is associated with colon cancer in patients with a 10-year or longer history of the disease. A colectomy is indicated in certain situations.
The majority of patients with familial adenomatous polyposis develop colon cancer by 40 years of age. By age 70, virtually all patients with familial polyposis will develop colon cancer. Colectomy is often beneficial in this group, and it is advisable for all patients with the mutant gene (APC gene) for familial polyposis to undergo prophylactic colectomy before the age of 20.
Patients with multiple endocrine neoplasia (MEN) (type 2 or type 2A or 2B) are at risk for development of medullary thyroid carcinoma. These patients should

be screened for the presence of C-cell hyperplasia using pentagastrin-stimulation tests. If thyrocalcitonin levels are increased, thyroidectomy should be performed to prevent possible development of medullary thyroid carcinoma. In MEN-2A, DNA analysis for the detection of the RET gene is highly reliable for identifying individuals with MEN-2A.

Leukoplakia is a risk factor for the development of squamous cell carcinoma of the oropharynx. Close monitoring is necessary, as is termination of other potentially harmful risks such as tobacco use. If tissue dysplasia is severe, surgical intervention may be required to prevent the development of squamous cell cancer.

SURGERY FOR CANCER TREATMENT

The role of surgery in cancer treatment can be divided into six separate areas. Approximately 70% of patients with solid tumors who present for the first time to the physician already have micrometastases beyond the primary site. Therefore, again a combination of antineoplastic treatment modalities is often essential for a successful outcome.

CURATIVE SURGERY

The basic principle of curative oncologic surgery is the ability of the surgeon to remove all malignant tissue. This concept is based on the belief that malignant tissue is capable of unlimited proliferation and growth from a few or even a single malignant cell. The surgeon should have a reasonable expectation that the involved neoplastic tissue can be completely resected with a normal tissue margin and with acceptable morbidity. Curative surgery should offer results that are equivalent or superior to those of comparable treatment options in terms of quality of life and life expectancy. Curative surgery is based on the stage and type of tumor, the tumor biology, and the clinical setting. It may be combined with other adjuvant treatments.

CYTOREDUCTIVE SURGERY

The ability to control residual disease may be improved by resecting bulk disease in certain advanced malignancies. Cytoreductive surgery is an option only when other effective treatment modalities are unable to control the unresected residual disease. This treatment option is commonly used in Burkitt's lymphoma and ovarian carcinoma.

SURGERY FOR METASTATIC DISEASE

Patients with a single focus of metastatic disease often can undergo resection with acceptable morbidity. Factors for consideration before surgical intervention in metastatic disease include histology of the tumor, disease-free interval, tumor doubling time, and location, size, and number of sites of metastatic disease. Examples wherein surgical intervention for metastatic disease may be appropriate are soft tissue and bony sarcomas with pulmonary metastases.

SURGERY FOR ONCOLOGIC EMERGENCIES

Oncologic emergency situations in which surgical intervention may be appropriate involve hemorrhage, perforation, or infection. However, consideration should be given to prognosis and avoidance of the patient's suffering.

PALLIATIVE SURGERY

The principle of palliative surgery is to provide benefit even though cure is not an option. These benefits may include removal of tumors that threaten a vital function, relief of intolerable symptoms, production of transient regression of disease, or prophylaxis to prevent the onset of symptoms. Examples of palliative surgical interventions are resection or bypass of tumor to prevent obstruction of the intestinal tract, resection of tumor mass to control hemorrhage, and resection to treat perforation of a hollow viscus.

RECONSTRUCTIVE AND REHABILITATIVE SURGERY

Because quality of life is extremely important to cancer patients, surgery for reconstruction and rehabilitation is an essential aspect in treatment planning. Some of the newer surgical techniques that are improving cancer patients' quality of life include the use of transabdominal myocutaneous flaps after modified radical mastectomy, free transfer of tissue after head and neck surgery, and continent ileostomies and sigmoidoscopies.

SURGICAL COMPLICATIONS IN THE CANCER PATIENT

Surgeons are often called to provide surgical therapy for complications related to a malignancy or to assist in the diagnosis of infectious complications. Because of lower surgical risks owing to improved postoperative care, use of surgical intervention in these instances has increased. Table 21–3 outlines some complications in the cancer patient that require surgical evaluation.

RADIATION THERAPY

Radiation therapy is the use of high-energy ionizing rays or particles to treat cancer. Ionizing radiation is energy that causes the ejection of an orbital electron

Table 21–3. Complications in the Cancer Patient Requiring Surgical Evaluation

ORGAN DYSFUNCTION	ETIOLOGY
Acute abdomen	Abscesses (hepatic and splenic)
	Fungal infections (aspergillosis and mucormycosis)
	Hemoperitoneum
	Neuropathy (*Vinca* alkaloids)
	Pancreatitis
	Peritonitis
	Pneumonia
	Splenic infarcts
	Tumor lysis
	Typhlitis and enterocolitis
	Usual causes of acute abdomen (e.g., appendicitis, cholecystitis, bowel obstruction)
Perianal	Abscesses (unusual in neutropenic patient)
	Fissure or fistula
	Inflammed hemorrhoids
Pulmonary	Fungal pneumonia (aspergillosis, phycomycosis)
	Interstitial pneumonitis
Skin	Cellulitis
	Embolic lesions (endocarditis)
	Extravasation of vesicant drugs
	Infections of decubitus ulcers or tumor masses
	Postoperative wound infection
	Systemic infections causing skin lesions
Central nervous system	Brain abscess
	Intracranial hemorrhage
	Intracerebral metastases
	Leptomeningeal carcinoma
	Meningitis
	Paraneoplastic syndromes

during absorption. This process is associated with a large amount of energy. The most common form of radiation used in practice today is the high-energy photon. γ-Rays and roentgen rays are both photons; they differ only in their origin. γ-Rays are produced intranuclearly, whereas roentgen rays are produced extranuclearly. γ-Rays used in radiation therapy are produced by the decay of radioactive isotopes; almost all roentgen rays used in radiation therapy are produced electronically by machines and are known as x-rays.

Both γ-rays and x-rays are part of the electromagnetic spectrum and move at the speed of light. Penetration of tissues in the body is determined by the transfer of the energy from these γ-rays and x-rays. Higher-energy x-rays retain greater amounts of their original dose at a specific depth than do lower-energy x-rays. The biologic effects of ionizing radiation are dose dependent, a measure of the energy absorbed, and independent of the energy of the incident beam.[13] Different types of cells have different degrees of radiosensitivity.

The intensity of an x-ray beam is governed by the inverse square law, which states that the radiation intensity from a point source is inversely proportional to the square of the distance away from the source. For example, if a source of radiation is 10 cm from a surface, the intensity at a point 10 cm below the surface would be one fourth of the intensity on the surface.

Radiation is a localized therapy that may be used to cure by eradicating disease, to control the growth and spread of disease, to control microscopic disease, or to palliate and reduce symptoms. Examples of tumors that are curable by irradiation include skin tumors, early-stage Hodgkin's disease, laryngeal cancer confined to the vocal cords, and early-stage breast cancer after lumpectomy.[14-16]

TOXIC EFFECTS OF RADIATION THERAPY AND THEIR MANAGEMENT

There are three separate phases of radiotherapy effects. Early effects usually are observed during treatment or within the first few weeks after its completion. Acute radiation effects occur largely in renewing tissues such as skin, oropharyngeal mucosa, small intestine, rectum, bladder mucosa, and vaginal mucosa. These tissues proliferate rapidly. Often the radiotherapist makes a small decrease in radiation fraction size or allows a short treatment break to permit rapid resolution of an excessive reaction. Intermediate effects usually occur several weeks to months after completion of therapy, and late effects usually are encountered many months to years after treatment. Late effects are actually the dose-limiting factor in radiation therapy. These effects include necrosis, fibrosis, fistula formation, nonhealing ulceration, and specific organ damage. Oncogenesis is also a late effect of radiotherapy. Clinically, late effects appear to depend on the total dose of radiation and the amount of the radiation fraction.

The incidence and severity of normal tissue toxicity from irradiation depend on numerous treatment factors, including total radiation dose, fraction size, interval between fractions, quality and type of radiotherapy, dose rate, intrinsic radiosensitivity, and the specific tissues irradiated. The most common toxic effects, divided by organ system, are outlined in Table 21–4 along with the recommended treatments.

BIOTHERAPY

Biotherapy, or biologic therapy, is the use of agents derived from biologic sources or agents affecting biologic responses.[17] Historically, this type of therapy has focused on altering or enhancing the response of the immune system in battling cancer. The primary mode of action for many of these agents centers on immune responses, but other mechanisms of action include antiproliferative activity, changes in the differentiation or maturation of cells, and alterations in the process of tumor metastasis.

Several categories of agents are used in cancer therapy today: interferons, interleukins, hematopoietic growth factors, and monoclonal antibodies. See Table 21–1 for the most common side effects of biotherapy and Table 21–5 for a list of biologic agents and their most common uses in cancer therapy. Although most biologic agents are used in the treatment of cancer, some are used as supportive therapy to diminish the toxicity associated with other treatment modalities (e.g., the hematopoietic growth factors) or to diagnose and detect cancer (e.g., monoclonal antibodies).

The interferons are a family of proteins having antiviral, antiproliferative, and immunomodulatory effects. There are three major types (α, β, and γ), with interferon-α being the most commonly used in cancer therapy. Interferon usually is given as a subcutaneous injection. The side effects associated with this therapy include flu-like symptoms, fatigue, decreased appetite, changes in mental status, and alterations in white blood cell counts and liver enzyme profiles.[18]

The interleukins are natural body proteins that have been named in sequence as they are identified. To date, there are 18 interleukins. One of their primary roles is in signaling and communication between cells of the immune system. Many also affect the maturation and differentiation of hematopoietic cells. As of May 1998, only interleukin 2 (aldesleukin) had received regulatory approval.

Table 21-4. Toxic Effects of Radiotherapy: Treatment and Prevention

ORGAN	EFFECTS	TREATMENT/PREVENTION
Head and neck Oropharyngeal mucosa	Acute effects Mucositis	Saline/bicarbonate solution swish q.i.d. Sucralfate solution swish q.i.d. Topical viscous lidocaine/ diphenhydramine/simethicone solution swish or gargle 10–15 mL/q.i.d. for analgesia Systemic analgesics p.r.n. Antifungals p.r.n.
	Late effects Thin oral mucosa Chronic ulceration and necrosis	Systemic or topical anesthetics Excellent hygiene Antibiotics p.r.n. Occasionally pentoxifylline 400 mg b.i.d. Surgical intervention p.r.n.
Esophagus	Acute effects Esophagitis	Lidocaine/diphenhydramine/ simethicone solution 10–15 mL q.i.d. for analgesia Sucralfate solution swish and swallow q.i.d. Systemic analgesics p.r.n. Antifungals p.r.n. Nasogastric or gastrostomy feeding tube for severe esophagitis
	Late effects Strictures Chronic dysphagia	Esophageal dilatation Metoclopramide 10 mg t.i.d. or q.i.d. for reflux symptoms
Salivary glands	Acute effects Parotitis	Aspirin/NSAIDs
	Late effects Xerostomia	Sialagogues Pilocarpine 5 mg PO t.i.d. Fluoride gel for prevention of dental caries
Taste buds	Acute effects Loss of taste (usually sour and bitter are suppressed greater than sweet and salty)	Education of patient before therapy Encouragement in continuing adequate oral intake despite loss of appetite in conjunction with taste loss
	Late effects Loss of taste can be permanent	
Ear	Acute effects Otitis externa Serous otitis media	Hydrocortisone/neomycin/ polymyxin B ear drops t.i.d. Decongestants, antibiotics p.r.n., myringotomy p.r.n.
Skin	Acute effects Erythema and dry desquamation	Nonionic moisturizers t.i.d. Hydrocortisone cream (1%) applied topically t.i.d. p.r.n. Gentle washing Avoid skin irritants
	Moist desquamation	As above and normal saline compresses before creams Polymyxin B/neomycin cream t.i.d.
	Ulceration, necrosis	Treat infections as appropriate Normal saline compresses Polymyxin B/neomycin cream t.i.d.
	Late effects Chronic skin changes	Moisturizers Sun block

Table 21–4. Toxic Effects of Radiotherapy: Treatment and Prevention *Continued*

ORGAN	EFFECTS	TREATMENT/PREVENTION

Gastrointestinal Stomach	Acute effects
	  Nausea and vomiting
	
	  Gastritis
	
	Late effects
	  Dyspepsia
	  Gastritis
	  Ulceration
	  Perforation
		Antiemetics p.r.n., nausea and
		  vomiting
		Fluid replacement
		Electrolyte repletion
		Sucralfate elixir 1 g q.i.d.
		H₂ blocker for gastritis
		Sucralfate 1 g q.i.d.
		H₂ blocker
		Surgery

Intestines	Acute effects
	  Nausea and vomiting
	  Early satiety
	  Anorexia and fatigue
	  Proctocolitis
	  Hematochezia
	  Radiation enteritis
	
	Late effects
	  Obstruction
	  Perforation
	  Bleeding
	  Malabsorption
	  Fistulas, strictures
	  Tenesmus, cramps, obstipation,
	    diarrhea, rectal urgency
		Diarrhea treated with low-residue
		  diet
		Antiemetics p.r.n.
		Fluid replacement
		Electrolyte repletion
		Loperamide or diphenoxylate, 1–2
		  tabs PO q.i.d. p.r.n. (infection
		  should be excluded)
		Proctitis treated with
		  hydrocortisone cream or
		  suppositories
		Blood transfusion p.r.n.
		Low-residue diet and stool
		  softeners
		Loperamide or diphenoxylate with
		  atropine
		Fiber laxatives
		Endoscopic laser surgery for
		  bleeding from ulceration and
		  telangiectasias
		Surgery p.r.n.

Genitourinary Bladder	Acute effects
	  Cystitis
	
	Late effects
	  Decreased bladder capacity
	  Hematuria from telangiectasias
	  Chronic irritative or obstructive
	    urinary symptoms
	  Fistulas
		Phenazopyridine hydrochloride
		  100–200 mg PO t.i.d. p.r.n.
		  dysuria
		Oxybutynin chloride (Ditropan) 5
		  mg PO t.i.d. p.r.n. frequency/
		  urgency
		Flavoxate hydrochloride (Urispas)
		  200 mg PO t.i.d. p.r.n.
		  frequency/urgency
		Drugs to increase bladder storage:
		  propantheline bromide,
		  oxybutynin chloride, imipramine
		  hydrochloride
		Drugs to increase outlet resistance:
		  ephedrine hydrochloride,
		  pseudoephedrine hydrochloride,
		  phenylpropanolamine
		Surgery
		Bleeding treated with cystoscopy
		  and selective cauterization,
		  followed by irrigation with
		  various agents (alum, silver
		  nitrate, or dilute formalin)
		Vesicovaginal fistulas treated with
		  surgery (may require
		  construction of continent urinary
		  reservoirs with intestine)
		Table continued on following page

Table continued on following page

Table 21–4. Toxic Effects of Radiotherapy: Treatment and Prevention *Continued*

ORGAN	EFFECTS	TREATMENT/PREVENTION

Vulva	Acute effects
	  Erythema, moist desquamation, usually greatest in intertriginous areas
	  Skin edema of vulva and mons pubis
	  Streptococcal lymphangitis
		Aggressive personal hygiene; twice-daily sitz baths and gentle skin cleansing followed by complete drying of vulvar region
		Topical steroid and antibiotic creams are applied for symptomatic relief and prevention of infection
		Whirlpool baths may be beneficial
		Ulceration or necrosis requires debridement
		Myocutaneous flaps may be necessary
		Atrophic vulvar skin after healing may benefit from topical estrogen or testosterone creams
		Dilatation of the introitus to prevent fibrotic stenosis may be necessary
		Streptococcal lymphangitis is treated with high-dose penicillin followed by prophylactic low-dose penicillin for a minimum of 6–12 mo

	Late effects
	  Vulvar skin thinning, atrophy, dryness
	  Pain, pruritus, telangiectasias
	  Skin hyperpigmentation
	  Fibrosis of underlying subcutaneous tissues may result in dyspareunia if involving the clitoris or vaginal introitus
	  Late ulceration with chronic serous drainage may occur 1–2 yr after treatment	

Vagina	Acute effects
	  Erythema, moist desquamation
	  Confluent mucositis
	  Severe congestion
	  Submucosal hemorrhage
	  Progressive vascular damage and ischemia
	  Epithelial sloughing, ulceration, and necrosis
		Vaginal douching with hydrogen peroxide and water
		Daily vaginal dilatation after acute reaction resolved
		Intravaginal estrogen cream twice weekly to promote healing, prevent vaginal atrophy, and improve lubrication
		Fistula formation treated with periodic debridement and antibiotics
		Urinary and fecal diversion sometimes required

	Late effects
	  Thinning and atrophy, telangiectasias
	  Dyspareunia
	  Adhesions or synechiae
	  Fusion of vaginal walls
	  Vaginal ulceration or necrosis	

Cervix and uterus	Acute effects
	  Superficial ulceration of cervix
	  Rarely hematometra
	  Necrosis
		Douching with hydrogen peroxide and water 2–3 times daily
		Debridement p.r.n.

	Late effects
	  Cervical os stenosis
	  Uncommonly high-grade endometrial carcinoma or uterine sarcoma
		Dilatation of stenotic cervical os
		Surgery, chemotherapy, and/or radiation therapy

Table 21–4. Toxic Effects of Radiotherapy:
Treatment and Prevention *Continued*

ORGAN	EFFECTS	TREATMENT/PREVENTION
Ovary	Acute effects Premature menopause Uncommonly ovarian carcinoma after treatment for cervical cancer Sexual dysfunction	Protection of ovaries by transplantation to sites distant from irradiation site Sexual dysfunction history using available psychological instruments Improving personal hygiene Hormones Vaginal lubrication Routine use of a vaginal dilator Hormonal replacement with oral conjugated estrogens and progesterone p.r.n.
Male reproductive system	Acute effects Testicular dysfunction with azoospermia, oligospermia, hormonal changes Late effects Recovery of sperm count Sterility	Appropriate radiotherapy field shielding Sperm banking

Aldesleukin is administered as an intravenous infusion or subcutaneous injection. Complications of interleukin therapy include flu-like symptoms, fatigue, changes in mental status, nausea, vomiting and loss of appetite, a capillary leak syndrome that leads to fluid retention and weight gain, hypotension and oliguria resulting from decreased renal perfusion, skin rashes, and changes in hematologic laboratory values.[18]

The hematopoietic growth factors are a family of proteins involved in the proliferation, maturation, and differentiation of blood cells. Two white blood cell growth factors (sargramostim and filgrastim), one red cell growth factor (epoetin alfa), and a platelet growth factor (opreleukin) are approved for use as supportive therapy after chemotherapy. Clinical trials continue to evaluate their use in the treatment of primary and secondary loss of bone marrow function. These growth factors usually are administered by subcutaneous injection. Of all the biologic agents, they are generally the best tolerated and have few associated side effects.

Monoclonal antibodies are antibodies produced from a single clone of cells that are highly specific in targeting cancer cells. Their use for the treatment of cancer remains investigational, although one antibody has received regulatory approval for the treatment of non-Hodgkin's lymphoma. Used alone, they interact with immune cells to kill cancer cells, or they can be used as carriers to deliver drugs or toxins to tumor cells. They can be used with low-dose radioisotopes to detect cancer. Historically, the majority of monoclonal antibodies were produced from murine (mouse) cells, thus the major anticipated side effect was allergic reactions ranging from hives and itching to anaphylaxis.° Monoclonal antibodies are most often infused intravenously.

BONE MARROW TRANSPLANTATION

One of the most common complications of cancer therapies is their negative impact on the functioning of the bone marrow. In BMT, first, higher doses of

---

°Recombinant DNA technology is now used to produce human/mouse chimeric antibodies with the intent of decreasing potential allergic reactions.

Table 21–5. Indications for the Use of Biotherapy in the Treatment of Cancer

AGENT	APPROVED INDICATIONS	TRADE NAME
Interferon-alfa 2a	Hairy cell leukemia, Kaposi sarcoma, chronic myelogenous leukemia	Roferon A (Roche Laboratories)
Interferon-alfa 2b	Hairy cell leukemia, Kaposi sarcoma, adjuvant therapy for melanoma, in conjunction with anthracycline chemotherapy for initial treatment of patients with non-Hodgkin's lymphoma	Intron A (Schering Corporation)
Interleukin 2 (aldesleukin)	Metastatic renal cell cancer, metastatic melanoma	Proleukin (Chiron Therapeutics)
Granulocyte colony-stimulating factor (filgrastim)	To decrease the incidence of infection in patients with nonmyeloid malignancies after myelosuppressive chemotherapy and bone marrow transplantation To promote the movement of peripheral blood stem cells (PBSC) into the circulation for autologous PBSC transplantation, to support treatment of patient with acute myeloid leukemia	Neupogen (Amgen)
Granulocyte-macrophage colony-stimulating factor (sargramostim)	To decrease the incidence of infection in patients with nonmyeloid malignancies after autologous bone marrow transplantation and to treat graft failure or engraftment delay To promote the movement of PBSC into the circulation for autologous PBSC transplantation After induction chemotherapy in older adults with acute myelogenous leukemia	Prokine (Immunex)
Epoetin alfa	Treatment of anemia in cancer patients on chemotherapy	Procrit (Ortho Biotech)
Interleukin 11 (Oprelvekin)	Prevention of severe thrombocytopenia and the reduction of the need for platelet transfusions following myelosuppressive chemotherapy in patients with nonmyeloid malignancies	Neumega (Genetics Institute)
Monoclonal antibody satumomab pendetide	Detection of colorectal and ovarian cancer	OncoScint CR/OV (Cytogen)
Capromab pendetide	Detection of prostate cancer	ProstaScint (Cytogen)
Rituximab	Treatment of CD 20-positive B cell non-Hodgkin's lymphoma	Rituxan (IDEC Pharmaceuticals and Genentech, Inc.)

chemotherapy, and on occasion radiotherapy, are given to kill tumor cells. Then, transfusions of bone marrow cells, either the patient's own or cells from a related or unrelated donor, are given to "rescue" or repopulate the damaged marrow with functioning cells. Several types of transplantation are used in cancer care today. Transplants are characterized by the relationship of the recipient to the donor. *Autologous* transplants use the patient's own bone marrow cells to repopulate the marrow after the conditioning regimen. This approach is frequently used in patients with breast cancer. A variation of this approach is the infusion of peripheral blood stem cells that are obtained by pheresis and usually are readministered in the ambulatory setting.

In *allogeneic* transplants, the patient receives someone else's bone marrow. There are several types of allogeneic transplants, but the major distinction is whether the donor of the marrow is related or matched but unrelated to the patient. Transplantation is often used in an attempt to achieve a cure in patients with hematologic malignancies such as acute myelogenous leukemia or chronic myelogenous leukemia.

The pretransplantation conditioning regimen uses high doses of chemotherapy with or without total body irradiation to destroy malignant cells, destroy the patient's pre-existing immunologic state, and create space in the marrow cavity for the transplanted cells. Complications to be expected are those commonly associated with these therapies, although they are more severe because of the high doses used. The most common complications unique to BMT are infectious sequelae related to immunosuppression and graft-versus-host disease (GVHD). In GVHD, the donor's immune cells (graft) recognize the patient's (host) cells as foreign and attack them. This complication has both acute and chronic components, distinguished by target organs, pathology, and the timing of their occurrence after transplantation. Symptoms seen with acute GVHD are severe skin changes and gastrointestinal problems (diarrhea, nausea, and vomiting). Chronic GVHD is characterized by scleroderma-like features that affect multiple organ systems and by persistent immunodeficiency. Treatment centers on early prevention and detection, supportive management, and immunosuppression.

Teaching priorities are numerous because of the intensity of this therapeutic modality. Areas to cover include the transplantation process, bleeding and infection precautions, management of symptoms and associated side effects, strategies for coping with alterations in body image and sexuality, medication schedules, and reportable signs and symptoms, especially those related to GVHD.[19, 20]

MULTIMODALITY THERAPY

The ultimate goal of cancer therapy is survival of the patient. To improve therapeutic indices, cancer therapies are often combined. Therapeutic approaches, each having a unique mechanism of action, collectively battle the cancer more effectively. In solid tumors such as breast, colon, or lung cancer, surgery is often used as first-line therapy to remove the tumor mass. Chemotherapy may then be given as adjuvant therapy to eliminate microscopic disease. Radiotherapy may be given after chemotherapy, as a more localized approach, to decrease the chance of disease recurrence. An example of this approach is the use of radiation therapy after lumpectomy in breast cancer. Another strategy used for larger tumor masses is to administer neoadjuvant chemotherapy first, to decrease the size of the mass, and then follow with a surgical procedure. Finally, multimodality therapies may be given concurrently. In the treatment of melanoma, for example, combination chemotherapy is given in concert with biotherapy (interferon and interleukin 2). The health care professional must be alert to the side effects and complications commonly expected with each therapeutic modality and must anticipate unusual or unexpected side effects that may result from the combination. In recent years, as supportive therapies have become available to manage side effects associated with cancer treatments, combination therapies and more aggressive approaches have become a clinical reality. Examples of these supportive therapies include hematopoietic growth factors to combat myelosuppression, new antiemetics such as granisetron and ondansetron to control nausea and vomiting, and chemoprotective agents such as amifostine and dexrazoxane to decrease nephrotoxicity and cardiotoxicity, respectively.[21]

PSYCHOSOCIAL IMPLICATIONS OF CANCER THERAPY

A diagnosis of cancer causes profound changes in the lives of patients and their families. Reactions and life changes experienced include fear of death, disfigurement or disability, anxiety related to living with uncertainty, strain on roles and relationships, spiritual distress, and social problems such as insurance cancellation, job discrimination, and reintegration into school or the workplace after treatment. Crucial points in the disease trajectory, when the patient's need for support is often the greatest, include diagnosis and initiation of treatment, recurrence of cancer, and the terminal phase of the disease.[22] The multidisciplinary health care team combines the skills and talents of each discipline to effectively support patients and families living with cancer. Effective care includes recognizing and responding to the changes mentioned.

Useful interventions include reinforcing existing or teaching new coping skills, acknowledging the patient's feelings, encouraging positive supportive relations, facilitating communication between the patient and the family and between the patient and the health care team, providing information, and recognizing the need for referral for more intensive counseling services.[23] Education is of utmost importance in empowering patients and families to cope with and manage cancer and treatment-related complications. See Table 21–6 for a review of patient education priorities for each major therapeutic modality. Awareness of support services that are available to patients, such as support groups and classes offered by the American Cancer Society or information hotlines (e.g., National Cancer Institute hotline, 1-800-4CANCER), is helpful in supporting the patient through diagnosis and treatment of cancer.

LONG-TERM COMPLICATIONS

Late complications of cancer treatment can affect a large variety of body systems and organs. These deleterious effects are observed 12 months or longer after cancer treatment. Perhaps the most important late side effect of cancer treatment is the induction of second cancers. Several epidemiologic studies have demonstrated increased risks of leukemia and solid tumors in patients given radiation therapy. Significant increases in leukemia risk have also been observed after chemotherapy with alkylating agents.

With increasing numbers of patients surviving decades after receiving initial cancer treatment, patients can now be monitored for longer time spans to detect complications arising from previous treatments. Table 21–7 outlines categories of late complications of cancer treatment.[24, 25]

SUMMARY

Over the last 50 years, significant progress has been made in the treatment of cancer. Today, the overall 5-year survival rate for all cancers is 50%.[26] Even though each major therapeutic modality for cancer carries with it complications that at times are significant, progress continues in developing strategies that lead to improved survival for patients. In the future, it is hoped that therapy will be

Table 21–6. Patient Education for Cancer Therapies

CHEMOTHERAPY	SURGERY	RADIATION THERAPY	BIOTHERAPY
Inform patient and family regarding chemotherapy treatment program, schedule of treatments, and diagnostic and laboratory tests Review prescribed drugs, expected side effects, and management strategies Assess demonstration of self-care skills (e.g., central venous catheter care, injections) Teach reportable signs and symptoms Signs and symptoms of infection (fever, chills, cough, diarrhea, inflammation); uncontrolled nausea and vomiting, bleeding or bruising, shortness of breath.	Inform patient and family regarding purpose, site, type, and extent of planned surgery Review anticipated side effects (e.g., pain, bodily changes, fatigue) Practice coughing and deep breathing exercises, incisional splinting, range of motion exercises Plan for progressive return to prior activities Teach self-care activities (e.g., wound and incisional care, drain care, ostomy care) Teach reportable signs and symptoms: uncontrolled pain, uncontrolled nausea and vomiting or inability to maintain food or fluid intake, signs and symptoms of infection (e.g., fever, inflammation at incision), bleeding	Inform patient and family regarding purpose, type, and procedures for receiving radiation therapy Review anticipated side effects and management strategies (e.g., skin care, alterations in food and fluid intake) Review delayed side effects (e.g., skin changes, fatigue) Teach reportable signs and symptoms (related to radiation port): signs and symptoms of infections, bleeding, uncontrolled nausea and vomiting or diarrhea, severe skin changes (moist desquamation)	Inform patient and family regarding goals of therapy and agent to be received, treatment setting, and duration of therapy Assure demonstration of self-care skills (e.g., injection technique) Review expected side effects and management strategies Teach reportable signs and symptoms: excessive fatigue, severe mental status changes (confusion or depression), cardiac symptoms, weight losses or gains of more than 10 pounds, allergic reactions, shortness of breath, decreased urine output, severe inflammatory reaction at the injection site, fevers uncontrolled with antipyretics or unrelated to normal pattern

Table 21–7. Categories of Late Complications of Cancer Treatment

CATEGORY	TYPE OF LATE COMPLICATION	CANCER TREATMENT
Second cancers	Leukemia Solid tumor	Radiation therapy (thyroid and breast are more radiosensitive) Chemotherapy (most important second cancer after chemotherapy is acute nonlymphocytic leukemia)
Hormonal and reproductive effects	Hypothalamic and pituitary dysfunction Change in gonadal histology and dysfunction in males Gonadal and reproductive dysfunction in females Infertility in males and females	Radiation therapy Chemotherapy
Immunologic effects	Immunosuppression Increased risk of infection after splenectomy	Radiation therapy Chemotherapy Surgery
Heart disease	Cardiomyopathy after doxorubicin Pericarditis Coronary artery disease Cardiac dysfunction	Chemotherapy Radiation therapy
Kidney and urinary bladder effects	Nephropathy Renal failure Cystitis Urinary bladder fibrosis Telangiectasia	Radiation therapy Chemotherapy
Gastrointestinal organs effect	Hepatic changes resulting in portal hypertension Damage to small intestine, colon, rectum	Chemotherapy Radiation therapy
Neurologic and psychological effects	Ataxia Changes in neuropsychologic function Decreases in IQ score and cognitive function	Chemotherapy Radiotherapy
Pulmonary effects	BCNU pulmonary toxicity Pulmonary fibrosis	Chemotherapy Radiotherapy
Bone effects	Osteonecrosis	Chemotherapy Radiotherapy

able more specifically to target cancer cells and spare normal cells. New discoveries in supportive therapies also will remain an active area of focus.

The importance of the midlevel provider's role in complementing and reinforcing information and care provided by the oncology specialty team cannot be stressed enough. Through awareness of potential complications associated with cancer therapy and early recognition of their occurrence, more serious complications can be avoided. The provision of education and supportive services to patients and families at one of the most difficult times anyone can face is invaluable. Together, the multidisciplinary team can meet the challenge of caring for patients during the treatment of cancer.

REFERENCES

1. Oken M, Creech R, Tormey D, et al: Toxicity and response criteria of the Eastern Cooperative Oncology Group. Am J Clin Oncol 1982;5:649.
2. Miller A, Hoogstraten B, Statquet M, et al: Reporting results of cancer treatment. Cancer 1981;47:207.

3. Kisner DL: Reporting treatment toxicities. In Buyse ME, Staguet M, Sylvester RJ (eds): Cancer Chemotherapy Trials: Methods and Practice. New York, Oxford University Press, 1984:178–190.
4. Krakoff I: Cancer chemotherapeutic and biologic agents. CA Cancer J Clin 1996;46:134–141.
5. L. Tenenbaum (ed): Cancer Chemotherapy and Biotherapy: A Reference Guide, 2nd ed. Philadelphia: WB Saunders, 1994.
6. Barton-Burke M, Wilkes GM, Ingwersen K (eds): Cancer Chemotherapy: A Nursing Approach, 2nd ed. Boston, Jones & Bartlett.
7. Epstein R: Drug-induced DNA damage and tumor chemosensitivity. J Clin Oncol 1990;8:2062–2084.
8. Schwartz RG, McKenzie WB, Alexander J, et al: Congestive heart failure and left ventricular dysfunction complicating doxorubicin therapy. Am J Med 1987;82:1109–1118.
9. Lehne G, Lote K: Pulmonary toxicity of cytotoxic and immunosuppressive agents. Acta Oncol 1990;29:113–124.
10. Fillastre JP, Viotte G, Morin JP, et al: Nephrotoxicity of antitumoral agents. Adv Nephrol Necker Hosp 1988;17:175–218.
11. American Cancer Society. Cancer facts and figures 1988. CA Cancer J Clin 1988;38:5–22.
12. Eberlein TJ, Wilson RE: Principles of surgical oncology. In Holleb AI, Fink DJ, Murphy GP (eds): American Cancer Society Textbook of Clinical Oncology. Atlanta, American Cancer Society, 1991:25–34.
13. Fowler JF: The linear quadratic formula and progress in fractionated radiotherapy. Br J Radiol 1989;62:679–94.
14. Prosnitz LR, Kapp DS, Weissberg JB: Radiotherapy. N Engl J Med 1983;309:771–77, 834–40.
15. Dow KH, Bucholtz JD, Iwamoto RR, et al (eds): Nursing Care in Radiation Oncology, 2nd ed. Philadelphia, WB Saunders, 1992.
16. Perez CA, Brady LW: Principles and Practice of Radiation Oncology, 2nd ed. Philadelphia, JB Lippincott, 1992.
17. Oldham RJ: Biotherapy: General principles. In Oldham RJ (ed): Principles of Cancer Biotherapy, 2nd ed. New York, Marcel Dekker, 1991:1–22.
18. Rieger PT: Patient Management. In Rieger PT (ed): Biotherapy: A Comprehensive Overview. Boston, Jones & Bartlett, 1995:195–219.
19. Whedon MB (ed): Bone Marrow Transplantation: Principles, Practice and Nursing Insights. Boston, Jones & Bartlett, 1991.
20. Keller C: Bone marrow transplantation. In Otto SE (ed): Oncology Nursing, 3rd ed. St. Louis, Mosby–Year Book, 1997:614–640.
21. Ethiofosin. In Dorr RT, Von Hoff D (eds): Cancer Chemotherapy. Stanford, CT, Appleton & Lange, 1994:453–459.
22. McCray ND: Psychosocial and quality-of-life issues. In Otto SE (ed): Oncology Nursing, 3rd ed. St. Louis, Mosby–Year Book, 1997:817–834.
23. Carroll Johnson R, Gorman L, Bush NJ (eds): Psychosocial Nursing Care along the Cancer Continuum. Pittsburgh, Oncology Nursing Press, Inc., 1998.
24. Boivin JF: Second cancers and other late side effects of cancer treatment. Cancer 1990;65:77–75.
25. Tucker MA, Coleman CN, Cox RS, et al: Risk of second cancers after treatment for Hodgkin's disease. N Engl J Med 1988;318:76–81.
26. American Cancer Society: Cancer Facts and Figures, 1998. Atlanta, American Cancer Society, 1998.

Chapter 22

Pain and Symptom Management

Deborah M. Thorpe, PhD, RN, CS, and
Richard Payne, MD

INTRODUCTION

One of the greatest tragedies of modern medicine is the needless suffering of countless patients from pain and other untreated symptoms.[1, 2] Because we live in an age when the issue of physician-assisted suicide is daily front-page news and because pain is a common factor in requests for assisted suicide, it is critical that health care providers develop greater skill in treating pain and other symptoms that interfere with quality of life. Pain is one of the most common symptoms of not only disease but also many treatments. An estimated 75% of all cancer patients experience significant pain. When disease is advanced, this figure rises to 95% or more.[3] However, despite considerable research, new knowledge, and the availability of many treatment options, pain continues to be undertreated. Basic pain management is reviewed in this chapter, with the greatest emphasis on pharmacologic management of pain and related symptoms, particularly basic principles and management of side effects related to opioid therapy. The reader is urged to consult the references for a variety of expert and timely resources for further study.

BARRIERS TO EFFECTIVE PAIN TREATMENT

CULTURAL AND ATTITUDINAL BARRIERS

Clinical decision making for pain management is greatly shaped by attitudes and concepts about pain. These in turn are influenced by factors that vary widely among health care professionals, patients, and family members.[4]

Attitudes, rather than scientific knowledge, are among the most influential forces in assessment of and decision making for pain management. One problem is that pain is a *subjective* experience that cannot be objectively or directly measured. Most health care providers are taught to focus on objective findings and to rely on diagnostic tests to confirm and validate assessments. They are given very little training in assessing and acting on subjective complaints. When a definite physical cause for a pain complaint cannot be identified and documented, health care professionals tend to assume that the pain is not real. This often contributes to the development of adversarial relationships between patients and their caregivers.[5]

A significant number of patients suffer unrelieved pain because they quietly accept the attitude that their pain is not real or because they lack the ability to express their pain convincingly. Others believe that pain is an inevitable consequence of cancer and fear that treatment, especially with opioids, will cause addiction or intolerable side effects. Patients, families, and caregivers alike tend to view opioid use as "bad" under any circumstance, leading to a tendency to avoid or underuse opioids. A key reason for undertreatment is the failure to distinguish legitimate from illegitimate opioid use.[4, 6]

KNOWLEDGE DEFICITS

Few health care professionals have had sufficient education in pain management to overcome the influence of the prevailing attitudes about pain and cultural barriers to the effective treatment of pain. Much of what is taught about pain is outdated and inaccurate. Early opioid studies often were conducted with subjects who were not experiencing pain. Some of the research consisted of single-dose studies in correctional institutions with subjects who were addicts. Subsequent research has shown that the pain stimulus is a critical factor in the pharmacokinetics and pharmacodynamics of opioids.[7] Despite the many advances in understanding pain mechanisms and the pharmacology of opioids, newer information has been incorporated into professional curricula slowly. Consequently, most graduates of health care programs are influenced by myths and misconceptions about opioids and know little about pain mechanisms and appropriate alternative treatments that may be required for some types of pain.

The following are major myths that interfere with effective treatment: (1) narcotics (opioids) carry a high risk for respiratory depression, even in opioid-tolerant patients; (2) opioids given orally are less effective; (3) opioid use to treat pain carries a significant risk of addiction; (4) "addiction" and "dependence" are the same; and (5) opioids should be reserved for terminally ill patients.

GOVERNMENTAL AND REGULATORY BARRIERS

Another significant barrier involves the influence on practice of the laws and regulations governing opioid use. The existence of drug abuse in society makes it necessary to strictly control and regulate the use of opioids. Unfortunately, many of the regulations are vague and ambiguous, and the regulators who enforce them are concerned primarily with numbers rather than clinical outcome when prescribing practices are challenged. Many states have laws requiring the use of triplicate prescriptions, with copies being kept by the prescriber, the dispensing pharmacy, and the state agency responsible for regulation of controlled substances. This requires the practitioner to obtain specially issued prescriptions and heightens the awareness that opioids receive a higher level of scrutiny. As a result, practitioners are often more reluctant to use this class of drug and instead prescribe them very sparingly or in amounts perceived to be acceptable—even though in most states there are no specific prescribing limits written into the regulations.[8, 9] In some states these prescriptions are monitored by police agents who have no training in the appropriate use of opioids. For example, in the state of Texas, the monitoring agency is the Department of Public Safety—the state police. This level of scrutiny has a chilling effect on willingness to prescribe opioids. In states with triplicate programs, many physicians or other practitioners eligible to prescribe do not obtain the appropriate forms and are thus spared the "risk" of being accused of or sanctioned for use that is deemed inappropriate. In addition to law enforcement officials' influence, medical and other professional licensing boards make decisions based on the same outdated information that influences clinical decisions. In a survey of medical licensing boards, Joranson and colleagues[10] found that even those with the authority to grant or remove a professional's license to practice did not have adequate knowledge of the laws or current research with respect to opioid prescribing.

To overcome these powerful influences on practice, it is imperative that all health care professionals become aware of the barriers, seek knowledge to support recommended practices, and participate in efforts to improve the treatment of pain for the patients for whom they care. The Wisconsin Cancer Pain

Initiative[11] was the first effort to organize cancer care specialists from all disciplines to take the lead in promoting awareness and removing barriers. Most states now have organized cancer pain initiatives. In 1989, the Texas legislature passed the Intractable Pain Treatment Act,[12] and California and several other states have enacted or are considering similar legislation. These laws emphasize the legitimate use of opioids and clarify ambiguous language in regulations that are often interpreted too narrowly. Another important event was the publication of cancer pain treatment guidelines by the Agency for Health Care Policy and Research.[13] Like the guideline *Acute Pain Management: Operative or Medical Procedures and Trauma*[14] published earlier, these guidelines are intended to reflect the state of knowledge about effective and appropriate care and to offer recommendations to improve clinical practice. These two documents are excellent resources for all health care providers, particularly those caring for cancer patients. Ordering information is provided in Figure 22–1.

PAIN ASSESSMENT AND MEASUREMENT

Although pain is a subjective experience that cannot be directly or objectively measured, there are techniques that provide meaningful and objective clinical information. Assessment of pain, like any other diagnostic process, should involve a comprehensive history, a thorough physical assessment, and a monitoring and documentation plan.

QUALITATIVE ASSESSMENT

Qualitative assessment includes basic information about the history and nature of the pain. Key points to assess include the location or locations of the pain, its onset and duration, its characteristics (e.g., sharp, dull, aching, burning), and factors affecting the pain (e.g., what makes the pain better or worse). The words

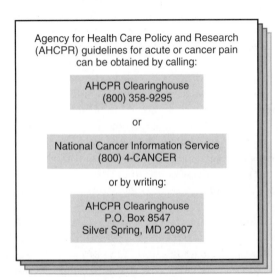

Figure 22–1. Ordering information for the Agency for Health Care Policy and Research (AHCPR) Guidelines.

a patient chooses to describe his or her pain are very helpful indicators. For example, the description of pain as "burning" frequently points to the diagnosis of neuropathic pain. Other words such as "horrible," "unbearable," or "exhausting" or other affective descriptions can reveal the impact that pain has on the individual. The mnemonic PQRST is a helpful guide to a comprehensive pain assessment (Fig. 22–2).

QUANTITATIVE ASSESSMENT

There are numerous quantitative assessment tools that help the patient estimate and communicate the intensity of his or her pain. These in turn can be used to monitor pain over time. The key to choosing a scale for clinical use is to select one that the patient can use effectively. For most patients, the scale of 0 to 10 (where 0 = no pain and 10 = the worst possible pain) is easy to understand and use. Other scales, such as the faces scale (Fig. 22–3), are helpful in communicating with young children (≥3 years) or patients with communication barriers. Patients with tumors of the head and neck who have undergone surgery or radiation treatments that affect the ability to speak and patients who speak a foreign language may be able to use a visual scale more readily. Some have difficulty translating their pain to raw numbers, particularly if they have memory or other cognitive deficits. In such situations, a simpler scale using descriptive words such as "none," "mild," "moderate," and "severe" may be most appropriate.

Cleeland and associates[15] showed in large-scale studies that pain intensity ratings of 1 to 4 (on a 0 to 10 scale) generally equate with mild pain, 5 to 6 with moderate pain, and 7 to 10 with severe pain. These groupings are also associated with significant declines in functional abilities as the intensity increases. However, these are subjective measures, and there are no "normal" values. For example, a pain rating of "5" for one patient cannot be assumed to be less than a rating of "8" by another patient. Nor can it be said that a particular pain problem

Figure 22-2. "PQRST" mnemonic for comprehensive pain assessments.

P: PATTERN/PLACE
  • Location
  • Timing (e.g., day vs night, constant, etc.)
  • Onset and duration

Q: QUALITIES
  • Characteristics (e.g., burning, sharp, dull)

R: RESPONSE/REACTION
  • Impact of pain (emotional, social)
  • Limitation of activity
  • Factors that make it better
  • Factors that make it worse

S: SEVERITY
  • Intensity ratings (e.g., 0–10, faces)

T: TREATMENT
  • Current treatments
  • Past treatments
  • What works/what doesn't

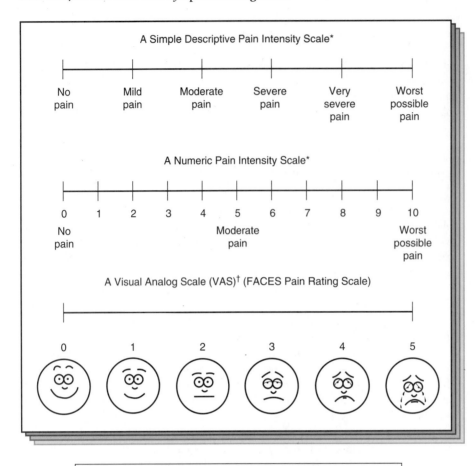

A Simple Descriptive Pain Intensity Scale*

| No pain | Mild pain | Moderate pain | Severe pain | Very severe pain | Worst possible pain |

A Numeric Pain Intensity Scale*

0   1   2   3   4   5   6   7   8   9   10

No pain — Moderate pain — Worst possible pain

A Visual Analog Scale (VAS)† (FACES Pain Rating Scale)

0   1   2   3   4   5

*If used as a graphic rating scale, a 10-cm baseline is recommended.
†A 10-cm baseline is recommended for visual analog scales.

Figure 22–3. Faces pain rating scale. (From Wong D, Whaley LF: Clinical Manual of Pediatric Nursing. St. Louis, CV Mosby, 1992.)

should have a certain level of pain. Individual patients interpret these scales from their own perspective, and between-patient comparisons in a clinical setting are not valid. Intensity scales are most helpful when monitoring for change over time as the patient's situation or response to treatment evolves.

When a patient is unable to communicate about his or her pain because of cognitive impairments or even coma, significant pain can still be a problem. In these situations, the health care professional has little to rely on but behavioral observation. Restlessness, agitation, moaning, and grimacing (particularly with movement) may indicate the patient's distress and can be used to monitor response to treatment. Conversely, alert and oriented patients do not have to demonstrate such behavior to confirm that their pain is real. Patients can cope with pain in various ways, and it is possible to suffer severe pain without any outwardly visible signs.

PAIN AS A VITAL SIGN

Systematic assessment of pain is vital to effective pain management, and pain should be considered a vital sign—as important to the patient's well-being as blood pressure and pulse. Many institutions have added pain intensity assessment to vital sign routines. In this manner, pain can be documented where the assessment is most likely to be noticed, such as on the graphic record with other vital signs. Frequency of assessment, as for any other parameter, depends on the severity and stability of the problem. In a pain crisis or after a painful event such as surgery, pain ratings should be made more frequently. When pain is stable and under control, it can be monitored on a more routine basis.

PAIN SYNDROMES COMMON IN CANCER

Pain may be acute and self-limited, or it may be chronic. Acute pain is associated with particular events such as trauma or surgery and under usual circumstances resolves within an expected time frame. A person in acute pain is more likely to present typical signs and symptoms of pain (e.g., guarding, grimacing, diaphoresis, altered pulse or blood pressure). With chronic pain, however, the physical signs are usually less obvious because the internal mechanisms that regulate vital functions adapt. Behavior adapts as well, and people learn to cope with pain in a variety of ways. The caregiver should remember that a patient need not look as if he or she is in pain to be experiencing significant pain. The guiding principle in responding to a patient's complaint of pain should be that "Pain is whatever the patient says it is."[16] Indeed, studies have shown a discrepancy in ratings of pain as assessed by patients' reports and their caregivers' estimates of their pain.[17] It is rare for patients to be deliberately deceptive about pain; therefore, the health care professional should accept the patient's assessment and use it as the basis for treatment.

NOCICEPTIVE PAIN

Nociceptive pain is a function of a normal nervous system. Nociceptors are the sensory receptors of the peripheral nerves that receive noxious stimuli and relay that message from the periphery to the spinal cord. There the message may undergo modulation and be transmitted to the brain, where the stimulus is ultimately interpreted in the cerebral cortex and appropriate motor responses are generated (e.g., withdrawing a hand from a hot stove). Nociceptive pain is *somatic,* arising from soft tissue and musculoskeletal structures, or *visceral,* arising from the autonomic fibers of the smooth muscle of the internal organs. Nociceptive pain serves a significant function as a warning mechanism in many cases. It is such pain, when acute, that alerts a person to seek care (e.g., chest pain in a patient with an impending myocardial infarction). Pain also is a common presenting symptom at the time a diagnosis of cancer is made.[18]

NEUROPATHIC PAIN

Neuropathic pain occurs as a result of injury to the nervous system (the peripheral nerves, spinal cord, or brain). Nerves can be injured or damaged by being cut, crushed, stretched, compressed, or exposed to toxic substances (e.g., chemotherapy agents, viruses). After injury to a nerve, a cascade of events results in anatomic as well as neurochemical changes in the neuron. A severed peripheral nerve may regrow, but it may branch out to cover a wider receptive field than before the injury. Neurotransmitters such as serotonin and norepinephrine may become depleted at the synapse, resulting in abnormal or aberrant impulse firing.[19] Characteristic examples of neuropathic pain include postherpetic neuralgia, phantom-limb pain, and peripheral neuropathy. Neuropathic pain usually is easy to identify by its characteristics. Patients typically refer to this type of pain as burning, tingling, shocking, or electric (e.g., "like my finger was stuck in a light socket"). The onset of pain may be delayed after the precipitating event. Patients may also experience allodynia (sensitivity to stimuli that are normally not noxious, such as touch). Neuropathic pain may also be accompanied by sympathetic dysfunction. As the injured nerve regrows, ephaptic connections are made with sympathetic nerves that subsequently provide constant stimuli into the peripheral nerve.[20] Reflex sympathetic dystrophy has been associated with crushing injuries and with tumor invasion or use of neurotoxic antineoplastic agents such as cisplatin in some cancer patients.

Neuropathic pain frequently is more difficult to treat than nociceptive pain and may require multiple modalities of treatment for effective control. In the past, neuropathic pain was considered to be not responsive to opioids, but responses have been seen. The difficulty lies in the fact that the doses required to relieve neuropathic pain are often substantially higher than for nociceptive pain and may be associated with increased risk of dose-limiting side effects. Other types of drugs, such as tricyclic antidepressants and anticonvulsants, and other modalities, such as transcutaneous electrical nerve stimulation, usually are needed.

BONE PAIN

Cancer that spreads to bone causes one of the most severe forms of pain experienced by cancer patients. If untreated, it can lead to disability and impair quality of life. Several factors are prominent in bone pain. One is the inflammation accompanying tumor growth. When there is metastatic spread to the spinal structures, even a slight degree of inflammation can cause intense pain due to swelling and compression of nerve roots against bone. When tumor extends into the epidural space, neurologic function ultimately is compromised if growth is unchecked. Pain may be exacerbated by movement, particularly with metastasis to weight-bearing regions. Liberal use of opioids usually is necessary to control bone pain, but adjuvant treatment with corticosteroids or nonsteroidal anti-inflammatory drugs (NSAIDs) is frequently required.

Bisphosphonates (etidronate, pamidronate) and calcitonin inhibit bone resorption and are useful in managing the hypercalcemia that often accompanies it. Some early evidence suggests that these agents may also relieve bone pain; however, more research is required to validate routine use.[20, 21]

Palliative radiotherapy is one of the most effective therapies in treating painful bone metastases.[22, 23] Treatment courses for palliation are significantly shorter than those used for other primary tumors. The most common treatment involves giving 30 Gy of radiation in 10 fractions. Radiotherapy controls and shrinks the tumor mass, allowing sufficient healing to take place to strengthen the bone. In weight-bearing bone, the issue of stability must always be addressed. If the tumor has eroded the cortical bone to the point that the risk of fracture increases, then surgical stabilization should be considered. If the patient is not a surgical candidate, specific immobilization and weight-bearing guidelines should be made, and the patient should be evaluated for appropriate assistive devices (e.g., crutches, walker) to promote safety in ambulation.

Strontium 89 (Metastron) is a radionuclide that can be used with radiation therapy or as an alternative, particularly when pain recurs in previously irradiated sites or with multiple sites of bone destruction. Localization of strontium to the cortical bone spares the marrow to a greater degree than radiation or chemotherapy; however, bone marrow toxicity is the principal effect of concern.[24] Strontium 89 should not be administered if the platelet count is below 60,000/L or if the white blood cell count is below 2400 cells/L. The nadir for both counts occurs at 4 to 8 weeks after treatment, and hematologic monitoring should be done at least monthly.[25]

Although most of the controlled trials of strontium 89 have focused on prostate cancer,[26] where tumor activity in bone is primarily osteoblastic, it has been effective in breast cancer, which typically produces more osteolytic activity. Other tumor types, including lung cancer, colon cancer, and adenocarcinomas, have been treated with success as well.

Because of the high incidence of spinal metastases, especially in breast, lung, and prostate cancer, spinal cord compression should be suspected until ruled out when a patient with one of the high-risk tumors complains of back or neck pain. In the event of cord compression, neurosurgical and radiotherapeutic consultation should be immediate and symptoms should be managed aggressively. Opioids should be freely titrated to pain relief, and dexamethasone should be given to control cord swelling and minimize neurologic dysfunction. Approximately 30% of patients who are diagnosed with cord compression present with pain but without neurologic signs. Early intervention is the key to preserving neurologic function.[27, 28]

TREATMENT-RELATED SYNDROMES

It should also be recognized that some of the pain problems seen in cancer patients result from the treatments rather than from the cancer itself. Virtually any of the current antineoplastic therapies may be associated with identified pain syndromes.[29] Surgery not only is responsible for acute postoperative pain but also may be associated with long-term sequelae. For example, patients undergoing mastectomy or thoracotomy may develop a complex of symptoms involving neuropathic and musculoskeletal pain; these are often referred to as postmastectomy or postthoracotomy syndromes. Many of the problems, particularly the musculoskeletal symptoms, can be controlled by a preventive approach. The exercises commonly taught to women after mastectomy can prevent the remaining underlying muscles from becoming painful by maintaining good muscle tone and flexibility. These same exercises would benefit patients undergoing thoracotomy, but they are not as routinely taught. A painful, frozen shoulder that can result from guarding and disuse is much more difficult to treat once it is well established.

The neuropathic component of these pain syndromes is more difficult to predict. Fortunately, not all patients who undergo surgical procedures develop neuropathic pain. In some, it is very mild and resolves over time; in others, it increases in intensity and persists for a long time. Although we have much to learn about the cascade of events leading to neuropathic pain syndromes, treatment is more successful when intervention occurs earlier rather than later, when the pain is well established.

Other treatment-related syndromes include peripheral neuropathies and plexopathy resulting from neural toxicities of many of the chemotherapy and biologic agents as well as late effects of radiation therapy.

PRINCIPLES OF PAIN MANAGEMENT

The method of pain management should be chosen only after a thorough assessment of the patient and the pain complaint. Patients with advanced disease often present with multiple pain complaints; each focus of pain should be examined, assessed, and taken into consideration in developing an appropriate plan of care. The guiding principle for treatment is to use the simplest, least invasive, and most cost-effective means of pain control (Fig. 22–4). Oral pharmacologic therapy forms the foundation and is likely to be effective in most patients.[13, 14, 29, 30] Only as the pain progresses in intensity and under selected circumstances is it necessary to progress to more invasive interventions that carry not only higher risks but also increased costs. Figure 22–4 also emphasizes the role of complementary and adjuvant treatments. Antineoplastic therapies

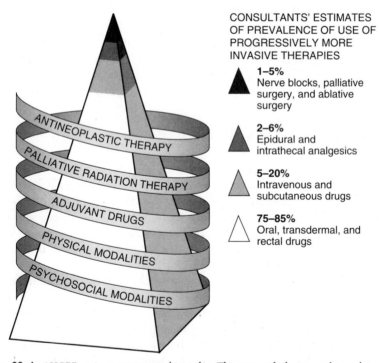

Figure 22–4. AHCPR pain management hierarchy. The pyramid depicts a hierarchy of pain management strategies from least invasive (at the base) to most invasive (at the apex). Therapies depicted on the ribbon may benefit many patients who are receiving concurrent treatments at any level of invasiveness. Estimates presented in the sidebar are based on published data and consultants' estimates for various clinical populations in industrialized nations but may not reflect all settings and do not necessarily reflect what is optimal. (From Jacox A, Carr DB, Payne R: Management of Cancer Pain: Clinical Practice Guideline No. 9. AHCPR Publication No. 94-0592. Rockville, MD, Agency for Health Care Policy and Research, U.S. Department of Health and Human Services, Public Health Service, 1994.)

such as radiation therapy, surgery, or chemotherapy are an important component of pain treatment. The underlying cause of the pain (e.g., tumor growth) should be treated whenever possible. However, because many of these therapies take time to yield an effect, it is important to treat the pain symptomatically, closely observe the patient, and make changes in the treatment as needed. When therapies available to treat the tumor have been exhausted, then the focus of management becomes palliation of the pain and other symptoms.[13]

TERMINOLOGY

Before one can understand the pharmacologic actions of opioids, it is essential to clarify some of the terms that are often misapplied and misunderstood in practice. The most problematic labels are addiction, dependence, and tolerance. In addition, pseudoaddiction is a recently recognized phenomenon that all health care providers should be alert to.

Addiction is primarily a psychological and behavioral problem in which obtaining and taking drugs, usually for reasons other than pain, becomes the paramount purpose in life. To that end, the addict may sacrifice everything, including work, resources, pleasure, values, and even life itself. The key distinguishing factor in addiction is the loss of ability to control the drug use despite known risks and potential harm. Few cancer patients fit this description, unless there is a pre-existing history of substance abuse. Such patients require additional care and a more stringent system of controls in treating pain; however, a history of addiction does not preclude the judicious use of opioids. Unfortunately, persons with a known history of addiction are among the least likely to receive effective pain control.

There is a common fear that exposure to opioids produces a euphoria that leads to the subsequent, compulsive use of the drug. In reality, the person experiencing pain rarely, if ever, experiences euphoria. Dysphoria, in fact, is a common and distressing side effect of opioids that may lead patients to stop using the drug or to use it in an ineffective manner because they do not like the way they feel. Another significant factor in distinguishing legitimate from illegitimate use of opioids is that patients who use these drugs and achieve satisfactory pain control are better able to function and enjoy a better quality of life. In stark contrast is the addict whose quality of life and ability to function are severely impaired with drug use.[31] In a large-scale study, Porter and Jick showed that the actual incidence of addiction as a result of treatment for pain is rare.[29]

Dependence is a physiologic process of adaptation to the presence of a drug. The terms addiction and dependence are *not* interchangeable. Both the addict and the patient requiring continued use of opioids for the treatment of pain may become dependent, but dependence does not preclude the legitimate use of opioids in the treatment of pain. The only clinical significance of dependence is the potential for a withdrawal reaction if the drug is stopped suddenly.[31] This is a familiar concept to most clinicians, who would not hesitate to use effective drugs that require careful tapering rather than abrupt discontinuation once the therapeutic effect is no longer required (e.g., corticosteroid therapy). An all too common scenario is the unnecessary experience of withdrawal in an opioid-dependent patient who decides to stop taking the medication because the pain has resolved.

Tolerance is another poorly understood term. Often patients resist taking opioids, even when their pain is severe, because they fear that they will become "immune" to the drugs' effects and that the drugs will not work when they are "really" needed. These patients may associate being tolerant with being addicted. Health care providers may also believe this and therefore hold back on offering opioids or escalating the dose. Although tolerance may occur to a degree, it is not a limiting problem; the pure agonist opioids (with the exception of meperidine) can be safely escalated to overcome tolerance, if necessary, because there is no ceiling or maximum dose limit.[32] However, experience with cancer patients has shown that tolerance, especially at stable chronic doses, does not occur to the degree that was once believed.[33] Many patients are able to remain on the same dose for long periods. If escalation of dose is required because of tolerance, it is usually in small increments. If a patient's dose requirement is increasing at a more rapid rate, one should evaluate the patient carefully for evidence of progressive disease with increased pain intensity.

Pseudoaddiction is seen in patients who may have become labeled as "difficult" or "drug-seeking" because of persistent and sometimes aggressive behavior in seeking treatment for their pain. On the surface, their behavior can be problematic, with frequent demands for refills of medications or increased dosage. However, after thorough assessment, many of these so-called drug seekers are found only to be seeking pain relief, and their behavior is actually a consequence of undertreatment.[34] Pseudoaddiction most commonly occurs when medications are given at intervals greater than their expected duration of action. Another common problem is giving a drug that is of insufficient potency for the intensity of the pain (e.g., acetaminophen and codeine for severe pain). The patient who has endured persistent, unrelieved pain may become more aggressive in seeking pain relief and may independently increase the dose in a desperate attempt to attain relief. This may lead to the need for frequent refills. Although some of these actions are "red flags" that should alert the practitioner to inappropriate drug use, a closer assessment is essential before labeling the patient an addict or drug seeker. For example, if a patient is given a prescription for 30 tablets of morphine with the instruction to take one every 4 hours as needed and the return appointment is in 1 month, unless only one dose is needed per day the patient will run out early. Care must be taken, especially when pain is persistent, to give an adequate supply of drug to last during the interval between visits.

TREATMENT OF PAIN IN PATIENTS WITH A HISTORY OF SUBSTANCE ABUSE

A history of substance abuse, whether active or inactive, is not an absolute contraindication to treatment with opioids. Many lifestyle behaviors associated with drug abuse put a person at greater risk for development of cancer or other life-threatening, painful conditions such as acquired immune deficiency syndrome (AIDS). Health care professionals should not judge or punish these patients but should attempt adequate treatment of pain. Pain and addiction are best addressed as separate entities, with appropriate interventions for each problem. As for any other patient, pain relief should be the primary goal.[35, 36] The same principles of opioid management apply, with additional limits and ground rules clearly outlined. A thorough assessment of the abuse history is important, as is talking with the patient in an open, straightforward manner. The patient should be provided with a clear outline of expected behaviors and guidelines. Close contact and continued assessment of the pain and drug use are essential. A written list of ground rules emphasizing the importance of safe-guarding medications and taking them exactly as directed should be given. A general policy of not replacing lost or stolen medications is one approach, although any patient is apt to lose or damage a supply of medication at one time or another. Repeated loss of prescriptions should not be tolerated, and patients who report that their drugs were stolen should be asked to file a police report.

It should also be recognized that patients who have abused drugs in the past are likely to have a degree of pre-existing tolerance, and the practitioner should anticipate that a higher dose of medication may be required, particularly for surgical or other painful procedures. Unfortunately, the tendency is to give these patients *lower* doses at *longer* intervals, which only heightens the problem behavior and adds to the development of adversarial relationships between patients and caregivers.

Once pain control has been achieved in the patient with a history of substance abuse and a stable dose has been identified, a verbal or written contract with the patient can be established. In most situations, liberal titrating instructions are given to patients to provide the flexibility needed to maintain adequate control; however, if the potential for abuse is expected, closer scrutiny of dose titration may be warranted, and the patient should be instructed to contact the provider for any dose adjustments. A contract might also stipulate that the patient receive pain prescriptions from only one source; if so, this stipulation must be communicated clearly to any other physicians and health care providers. Other stipulations might be that the patient refrain from any illicit substance (e.g., cocaine, heroin) or alcohol use and submit to random drug screening to determine whether the prescribed drug is actually being taken or whether illicit drugs are present. If behavior problems are not well controlled by these mea-sures, it is appropriate to refer the patient for psychiatric and/or concurrent substance abuse therapy.[37] It is important to seek a professional who is willing to take the pain treatment into account. Many substance abuse programs require strict abstinence from drugs, regardless of their therapeutic intent.

OPIOID PHARMACOLOGY

Opioids relieve pain by binding to the opiate receptor sites located in the brain and in the spinal cord. Although there are opiate receptors outside the central nervous system (CNS) and there is some evidence that there may be a peripheral mechanism of action, the primary mechanism is considered to be central.[38] Opioids are classified into several categories: (1) pure agonists, (2) mixed agonist/antagonists, (3) partial agonists, and (4) pure antagonists.[39]

Pure agonists bind to the opiate receptor sites to relieve pain, and there is no maximum or ceiling dose. With the exception of meperidine (Demerol), these drugs can be titrated freely to relieve pain. Meperidine has limited usefulness and is not recommended for chronic use. Unlike other pure agonists that have no end-organ toxicities, meperidine is associated with significant neurotoxicity, particularly from its metabolite, normeperidine. Normeperidine has a longer half-life than meperidine and is associated with nervous system excitability that can result in delirium, tremors, or seizures. This toxicity is an even greater risk in elderly patients and in those with renal insufficiency or hepatic impairment.[40]

Mixed agonist/antagonists such as pentazocine (Talwin) or nalbuphine (Nu-bain) bind with some opioid receptors and block others. Therefore, this category of drug can produce as well as antagonize analgesia. When a mixed agonist/

antagonist is given as a single agent, the analgesic effect predominates. However, when it is given in combination with or after a pure agonist drug, the antagonism predominates. These drugs provide poor pain control and can precipitate a withdrawal reaction in the opioid-dependent patient. This category of drug is not recommended for chronic use for cancer pain because of the mixed effect and because of a higher incidence of neurotoxicity and psychomimetic side effects.[39, 41]

Partial agonists such as buprenorphine (Buprenex) bind only to a single receptor type. This category of drug is not well understood and may have some antagonist activity. Therefore, its use in cancer patients is limited.

Opioid antagonists are essentially a safety net for opioid use. For example, the antagonist naloxone (Narcan) competes with pure agonists to bind opiate receptors and can reverse the effect of the pure or mixed agonist/antagonist opioids. Few other dangerous drugs have a drug that can reverse its action. However, naloxone is frequently misused and overused.[42, 43] Reversal of opioids should be done with great care. Rapid administration of naloxone reverses not only undesired effects such as respiratory depression but also the pain relief. Furthermore, it can precipitate a major pain crisis and significantly impair the patient's quality of life. In patients who have developed dependence, a profound withdrawal reaction can result. Withdrawal is not only unnecessary for reversing the unwanted side effect but can be devastating, particularly to the debilitated patient. Rapid injection of naloxone is not a benign experience. It has been associated with severe nausea, vomiting, cardiovascular stimulation including tachycardia, hypertension, pulmonary edema, and dysrhythmias resulting from a sudden increase in sympathetic nervous system activity.

Naloxone should be reserved for truly emergency situations such as significant respiratory depression with evidence of inadequate oxygenation. The decision to administer naloxone should not be based on respiratory rate alone, because this is an inadequate indicator of overall respiratory function. Although naloxone is often administered for a myriad of reasons including confusion, sedation, or somnolence, these are not sufficient indications. If sedation or somnolence is a problem, it is better treated by altering the dosage of the drug or managing related symptoms (see Management of Symptoms and Side Effects). Other causes of altered mental status should be pursued (e.g., hypercalcemia, other metabolic encephalopathies).[43] Naloxone is more likely to be indicated in the opioid-naive patient or in situations where analgesics have been combined with other drugs that enhance the respiratory-depressing effect (e.g., benzodiazepines). Naloxone should always be administered slowly in a dilute solution (e.g., 0.4 mg in 10 mL of normal saline solution).[42] The dose should be carefully titrated to reverse only the respiratory depression and to maintain pain relief. Once the critical situation is stabilized, patients should be carefully monitored, taking into consideration the half-life of the drug whose effect was reversed. In particular, when using drugs such as levorphanol (Levo-Dromoran) and methadone (Dolophine) that have long half-lives or sustained-release preparations (e.g., MS Contin, Oramorph, Oxycontin) with a prolonged duration of action, subsequent doses or a carefully titrated infusion of naloxone may be required.

EQUIANALGESIC DOSING GUIDELINES

The key to effective pain control is titration of the dose to a level that relieves pain. Opioids such as morphine and hydromorphone (Dilaudid) are considered "strong," and others such as codeine and hydrocodone are considered "weak"; however, all opioids are essentially capable of producing equally effective analgesia if given in equianalgesic doses.[13, 29, 42] The primary problem with the weak opioids is that they are usually combined with aspirin or acetaminophen, which means that the dose cannot safely be increased beyond a certain point because of dose-limiting renal and hepatic toxicity associated with the nonopioid drug.

The milligram strength or potency varies from one drug to another based on the molecular weight of the drug, but doses that are equally effective can be given. For example, only 1.5 mg of hydromorphone is required to produce the same degree of analgesia as 10 mg of morphine. Likewise, an orally administered drug can be equally as effective as a parenterally administered dose if it is adjusted to account for biotransformation. When an opioid is administered via the gastrointestinal tract, it is subject to greater biotransformation because of the *first-pass effect*. The circulation surrounding the upper gastrointestinal tract and, to some degree, the lower tract routes a significant portion of its blood directly into the hepatic circulation without reaching the systemic circulation. A portion of the drug taken by mouth (or administered through a feeding tube or rectally) is subject to metabolism into nonanalgesic substances. If a patient is getting good analgesia from 10 mg of parenteral morphine sulfate, it would take approximately 30 mg of oral morphine to produce the same effect, because as much as 20 mg is metabolized before it reaches the systemic circulation. The parenteral-to-oral ratio varies from drug to drug. The conversion chart shown in Table 22–1 can be used to facilitate changes in route of administration that may be needed as a result of side effects or change in patient status (e.g., changing from the oral to parenteral route because of a bowel obstruction). Morphine is the standard for comparison because it is one of the oldest and most widely used opioids and more is known about its pharmacology. It is also one of the most versatile drugs because preparations are available for most routes of administration.

ROUTES OF ADMINISTRATION

The oral route of administration is the preferred route because of its simplicity and cost-effectiveness.[13, 29, 42] However, opioids are extremely versatile drugs and can be given just as effectively by numerous other routes. The choice of route of administration should be based on factors such as (1) the nature and stability of the pain, (2) whether factors exist that preclude oral administration (e.g., bowel obstruction, impaired swallowing), (3) the functional status of the patient (whether the patient can mentally or physically comply with the regimen), (4) history of side effects, (5) availability of drug dosage forms, and (6) cost. Selection of the appropriate option also requires an understanding of the process of biotransformation and equianalgesic dosing guidelines (see previous discussion).

ORAL ROUTE

Oral administration is the route of choice because of its simplicity, convenience, and good tolerance by most patients. Furthermore, if the drug is given in equianalgesic doses, the oral route is as effective as any other. Long-acting forms of opioids such as morphine (MS Contin, Oramorph) and oxycodone

Table 22–1. Oral and Parenteral Analgesic Equivalencies and Relative Potency of Drugs Compared with Morphine

DRUG CLASSIFICATION	PARENTERAL (IV) (mg)	ORAL (PO) (mg)	CONVERSION FACTOR (IV to PO)	DURATION (PARENTERAL– ORAL) (hr)
Pure agonists				
Morphine	10	30	3–6°	3–4
Methadone (Dolophine)†	10	20	2	4–8
Hydromorphone (Dilaudid)	1.5	7.5	5	2–3
Fentanyl	0.1	–	–	1
Meperidine (Demerol)	75	300	4	2–3
Levorphanol (Levo-Dromoran)†	2	4	2	3–6
Oxymorphone (Numorphan)	1	6‡	6‡	3–6
Codeine	130	200	–	3–4
Oxycodone (e.g., Roxicodone, Percodan, Tylox)§	–	15	–	3–5
Hydrocodone (Vicodin, Lortab)‖	–	30–200¶	–	3–5
Propoxyphene (Darvon, Darvocet)	–	200	–	3–6
Partial agonist				
Buprenorphine (Buprenex)	0.4	–	–	6–8

°Conversion (oral-to-parenteral) ratio of 3:1 is required for chronic, around-the-clock dosing; single or intermittent dose conversion may require conversion ratio of 6:1.

†Long half-life; observe for accumulation of drug and side effects after 48–72 hours.

‡Available only in rectal form.

§Except for Roxicodone, oxycodone is combined with either aspirin (Percodan) or acetaminophen (Percocet, Tylox) in doses of 325–750 mg. **These drugs should not be taken in doses exceeding safe limits of aspirin or acetaminophen.**

‖All forms (Lortab, Vicodin) come combined with varying doses of acetaminophen. **Dosage should be controlled so as not to exceed the safe limit of acetaminophen.**

¶Equivalence data not substantiated; thought to approximate that of codeine, but may approach that of oxycodone.

Data from Jacox A, Carr B, Payne R: Management of Cancer Pain: Clinical Practice Guideline No. 9. AHCPR Publication No. 94-0592. Rockville, MD, Agency for Health Care Policy and Research, U.S. Department of Health and Human Services, Public Health Service, 1994; and Porter J, Jick H: Addiction is rare in patients treated with narcotics. N Engl J Med 1980;302:123.

(Oxycontin) allow greater dosing intervals and more sustained pain control. Additional opioids are being developed in long-acting forms that will enhance the ability to tailor drug delivery to patient needs. Oral administration is usually the most cost-effective route. For these reasons, the oral route should be used unless specific patient factors dictate the use of another route.

RECTAL ROUTE

The rectal route, although infrequently used, is a simple, cost-effective route for patients who cannot take oral medication. It is useful if the dose requirement is not very high because the dosages now commercially available are limited. Generally, the rectal dose is thought to be equivalent to the oral dose. The degree to which the colorectal circulation is subject to the first-pass effect may vary from patient to patient, so it is important to evaluate patients closely for their response and to adjust the dose as needed. Patients who are immunosuppressed are not suitable candidates for rectal administration because of an increased risk of trauma, bleeding, and subsequent infections. Medications also may be administered via stomas (e.g., colostomy), provided the suppository can be retained long enough to be fully absorbed.[44]

INTRAVENOUS ROUTE

The intravenous route provides the quickest response, with onset of activity within 10 to 15 minutes. The duration of effect, however, is shorter than for other routes. Intravenous administration is most appropriately used in acute situations when rapid titration is desirable or oral administration is not possible (e.g., bowel obstruction, severe nausea and vomiting).

SUBCUTANEOUS ROUTE

Although the subcutaneous route is often overlooked, it is an efficient and effective method of parenteral administration. Subcutaneous injections are less painful and more predictably absorbed than intramuscular injections. The subcutaneous route is also effective for small-volume, continuous infusion and is often used in the hospice setting when intravenous access is difficult or no longer required for administration of other drugs.[45]

INTRAMUSCULAR ROUTE

Because of injection-related pain and less predictable absorption, the intramuscular route is the least desirable route of administration. Intramuscular injections are also contraindicated in patients who are thrombocytopenic or neutropenic because of increased risk of bleeding and infection.

TRANSDERMAL ROUTE

The transdermal route is the newest route of administration. Currently, only fentanyl (Duragesic) is available for transdermal delivery through a patch. It takes about 8 to 14 hours after a patch is applied for the blood level of the drug to reach a steady state; therefore, the transdermal route is more appropriate for use after pain has been stabilized via another route. When transdermal fentanyl is discontinued, a subcutaneous reservoir of the drug remains and may take 16 hours or longer to be eliminated after the last patch is removed. Therefore, if a patient has experienced an untoward effect while a patch is on, close monitoring for an extended period is required after removal.[46]

EPIDURAL ROUTE

The epidural route was originally for short-term use (e.g., labor and postoperative pain), but it is increasingly employed in the management of chronic pain. Drugs administered epidurally are absorbed primarily through the dura and distributed in the cerebrospinal fluid to opiate receptor sites found in the brain and spinal cord. Although a small portion of the drug may be absorbed through the epidural capillary circulation, most of the drug is delivered directly to the CNS. As a result, very little of the drug is subject to biotransformation, and very small doses can provide analgesia equal to that achieved via other routes. This route is indicated for patients who require high doses and/or who have experienced intolerable opioid side effects that have not responded to treatment. Local anesthetic agents can be combined with opioids in epidural infusions to enhance analgesia.[47–49]

Patients must be carefully selected when long-term epidural administration is under consideration. The patient or caregiver must be capable of managing the techniques and equipment necessary (e.g., infusion pumps, catheter care). To decrease the risk of infection, catheters may be tunneled under the skin to place the exit port away from the insertion site. Infusion pumps requiring infrequent refilling can be fully implanted subcutaneously and filled with a concentrated drug; however, these devices cost more initially because they are more expensive than external pumps and require surgical placement. The implanted pumps usually are not cost-effective unless the patient is expected to live longer than 3 months. After 3 to 4 months, the higher initial costs tend to be offset by lower maintenance costs and lessened risk of morbidity (e.g., infection of an external catheter). External systems usually involve rental of a pump as well as continued maintenance costs for disposable tubing, dressings, and treatment of infections should they occur.

INTRATHECAL AND INTRAVENTRICULAR ROUTES

Drugs can be administered directly to the opiate receptor sites, without being subjected to biotransformation, by intrathecal or intraventricular routes. Intrathecal administration is done with a spinal catheter. Intraventricular administration is done with an implanted device such as an Ommaya reservoir (placed subcutaneously, usually in the frontal region, and connected to a catheter inserted through a bur hole in the skull to give access to the ventricles). These access devices can also be used in conjunction with implanted pumps. Consequently, intrathecal and intraventricular administration provides the most analgesia with the smallest dose and longest duration.[47]

Patients must be carefully screened to determine the appropriateness of any of the "high-tech" procedures (parenteral, epidural, and intrathecal infusions and implanted pumps). Other routes that are more cost-effective and carry fewer risks should be explored exhaustively by professionals skilled in pain management before these invasive, higher-risk measures are considered. Furthermore, cost issues related to pain management are emerging as the debate over health care reform continues and will remain an important focus for research and health policy development.[50]

SCHEDULE OF ADMINISTRATION

Schedule of administration is another important factor in tailoring drug dosing to individual patient needs. Providing medication on a *regular* rather than *as-needed* (p.r.n.) basis is recommended, even for short-term, acute pain such as postoperative pain. It takes less medication to control pain when it is given regularly around-the-clock than when given p.r.n. Dosing p.r.n. leads to greater peaks and valleys in analgesic blood levels between doses, especially when patients wait until the pain is severe before requesting medication.[13, 42] Administration p.r.n. is most appropriate for supplemental dosing for acute exacerbations or "breakthroughs" of pain—that is, it is used in addition to the scheduled medication. An important factor in tailoring drug therapy to individual patient needs is the schedule of administration.

Knowledge of the expected duration of action of each opioid is essential to successful pain management. If a short-acting drug such as hydromorphone (usually lasting only 2 to 3 hours, especially when given intravenously) is prescribed to be given every 6 hours, the patient will have to tolerate increasing pain for as long as 3 to 4 hours until another dose is given. A common mistake made when attempting to taper or wean a patient from an opioid is to increase the interval between doses. That approach usually makes the pain problem worse. The preferred method is to decrease the dose while maintaining the appropriate interval based on the expected duration of action of the drug.

The most reasonable approach to pain control is to give whatever dose is needed to relieve the pain and to select a management strategy that sustains control for the required length of time. When rapid titration is necessary, as for postoperative pain or severe pain that is out of control, a patient-controlled analgesia (PCA) pump is most appropriate.[51] Most pumps can provide a continuous (basal) infusion that may be combined with a p.r.n. dose the patient self-administers. This provides more highly individualized dosing and continuous analgesia. Some studies have even shown not only improved pain control but also reduced morbidity with PCA. Patients with less pain can move more readily and therefore reduce their risk of postoperative complications such as impaired gastric motility and respiratory compromise.[52]

As the acute pain-causing problem resolves (e.g., healing takes place) and pain lessens, patients require fewer doses, allowing the dose to be tapered as rapidly as the patient tolerates it. When tapering the dose administered by a PCA pump, it is best to begin by decreasing the basal rate gradually (e.g., 50% every 12 to 24 hours). If the number of p.r.n. doses required does not increase significantly, the patient will probably be able to tolerate further dose reduction. If the number of p.r.n. doses increases, then the basal rate should not be reduced further until the patient is able to tolerate it and requires fewer p.r.n. doses. Dose titration always requires frequent assessment of the patient's pain intensity to guide the process.

ADJUVANT ANALGESICS

NONSTEROIDAL ANTI-INFLAMMATORY DRUGS

The inflammation that accompanies many painful conditions triggers the release of prostaglandins, which are thought to facilitate transmission of nociceptive stimuli by activating and sensitizing peripheral nociceptors. The NSAIDs are believed to reduce inflammation, pain, and fever by inhibiting production of prostaglandins. NSAIDs alone may be effective in relieving mild to moderate pain when inflammation is a significant factor underlying the pain. For moderate to severe pain, they may be used in combination with opioids. The peripheral mechanism of prostaglandin inhibition appears to enhance the opioid action, providing greater analgesia.

Though this category of analgesics is very useful in relieving pain, cautious use and careful monitoring for side effects are critical.[53] Most NSAIDs have a significant potential for gastrointestinal, renal, and/or hepatic toxicity that limits their use in some patients, particularly the elderly and those with impaired renal or hepatic function. In addition, with the exception of choline magnesium trisalicylate (Trilisate) and diflunisal (Dolobid), most NSAIDs interfere with platelet aggregation, increasing the risk of bleeding in patients who are receiving chemotherapy and in those who have blood or bone marrow disease. Response to NSAIDs varies, and it is not easy to predict which drug will be useful in any given patient. An NSAID should be given regularly for a 7- to 10-day trial period before judging it to be ineffective.

CORTICOSTEROIDS

The corticosteroids, like the NSAIDs, are useful in treating pain in which inflammation is a primary or contributing factor; these drugs also interfere with prostaglandin production. The more potent steroids, such as dexamethasone, are important in acute situations such as epidural spinal cord compression by bone metastases. Potent steroids relieve pressure on the cord and traction on nerve roots caused by peritumoral edema or trauma to the spine. Other benefits of steroids include their euphoric effects and stimulation of appetite, both of which enhance the patient's sense of well-being. Improvement in sense of well-being is an added benefit for the debilitated, cachectic cancer patient with metastatic disease. However, corticosteroid use often is limited by potentially serious side effects such as immunosuppression, gastrointestinal bleeding, myopathy, hyperglycemia, and psychological disturbances.

TRICYCLIC ANTIDEPRESSANTS

The tricyclic antidepressants play several roles in pain control. Although patients with chronic pain may become clinically depressed and could benefit from the tricyclics for their antidepressant effect, the primary indication for a tricyclic in pain management is its intrinsic analgesic effect. In neuropathic pain syndromes such as postherpetic neuralgia or brachial plexopathy, the tricyclic antidepressants are often the front-line therapy. The mechanism of analgesia is thought to be neurochemical (i.e., inhibition of serotonin reuptake at the synapse). The newer, serotonin-specific antidepressants such as fluoxetine (Prozac) have not been found to be as effective as the first-generation tricyclic antidepressants such as amitriptyline (Elavil), nortriptyline (Pamelor), or desipramine (Norpramin), suggesting that additional mechanisms are at work in the modulation of pain. Tricyclics also can potentiate analgesia by increasing plasma levels of opioids, thereby increasing the bioavailability of the opioids.[54, 55]

Thorough patient education about the use of tricyclic antidepressants is essential. Often, patients who have experienced a caregiver's attitude that their pain is not real may have their fears that the pain is psychological reinforced when an antidepressant is prescribed. It should be stressed to the patient that the medication is being given for its analgesic effect. The patient also should be informed that, because tricyclics work by a different mechanism than opioids, the response pattern will be different. Usually the response to tricyclics is much more subtle. Patients do not feel a quick or dramatic analgesic effect, and, when questioned about relief, the patient may not be able to detect a noticeable change until the dose has been slowly titrated to effect. It is helpful for patients to know this so that they do not stop taking the medication because it does not seem to be helping the pain as expected. Side effects that may be dose-limiting or problematic to the patient include dry mouth, cardiac arrhythmias, and postural hypotension. The tricyclics should be used with caution in elderly patients and in those with a history of cardiac problems, especially arrhythmias.

ANTICONVULSANTS

Anticonvulsants such as carbamazepine (Tegretol), phenytoin (Dilantin), and valproic acid (Depakene) are indicated in the treatment of neuropathic pain, particularly when the pain is shooting or lancinating. The anticonvulsants are thought to work by suppressing the aberrant neuronal firing that occurs after nerve injury. Like the tricyclics and NSAIDs, the anticonvulsants produce significant side effects that necessitate close monitoring. Among the potentially most serious side effects are bone marrow suppression and hepatic impairment. Other less serious ones are ataxia and diplopia. Regular monitoring of blood counts and liver function, combined with careful dose titration and monitoring of the drug levels in the blood, is necessary.

ORAL AND PARENTERAL LOCAL ANESTHETICS

The infusion of local anesthetics such as lidocaine (Xylocaine) and bupivacaine (Marcaine) has been effective in the management of diabetic neuropathy.[56] Mexilitine (Mexitil), an oral form of lidocaine, is one of the newer sodium-channel-blocking agents and has been found to be effective in the treatment of neuropathic pain syndromes such as diabetic neuropathy and trigeminal neuralgia.

PSYCHOTROPICS

Psychotropic drugs, when appropriately used, are significant adjuncts in the management of pain. However, these agents are not substitutes for analgesic medication. Many health care providers believe that benzodiazepines such as lorazepam (Ativan) and diazepam (Valium) relieve pain. They do not. Anxiety and emotional distress often exacerbate pain and lower the patient's ability to tolerate pain; therefore, concurrent rather than alternative treatment of anxiety enhances pain control and improves the patient's quality of life. Psychological symptoms such as anxiety, panic, depression, and other mood disorders should be recognized, targeted, and treated appropriately with pharmacologic and/or psychosocial interventions. The underlying pain problem must also be addressed and treated appropriately. If the needed analgesics are not provided, neither problem is likely to be resolved, because the continued pain will exacerbate the psychological symptoms and vice versa.

The benzodiazepines, particularly diazepam, are also useful for muscle spasm, a type of pain that is less likely to respond, if at all, to analgesics alone. Diazepam and clonazepam (Klonopin) in relatively low doses are also helpful in managing myoclonus, a less common side effect but one seen more frequently at high-dose opioid levels. Phenothiazines have often been thought of as potentiators of analgesia, but there is little objective evidence to support this.[57] Methotrimeprazine (Levoprome), however, is an exception. Not only is it a potent antiemetic, but it has also been shown to produce analgesia comparable to that produced by opioids.[58] Phenothiazines and other antiemetic drugs play an important role when used for their specific actions. For example, nausea with or without vomiting may be a concurrent problem associated with chemotherapy or constipation, necessitating appropriate antiemetic therapy.

CENTRAL NERVOUS SYSTEM STIMULANTS

Sedation is one of the most common side effects of opioid use. It is frequently responsible for patients' undermedicating themselves. Sedation is frequently a response to extended sleep deprivation, which resolves as pain is relieved and normal sleep is restored. In some patients, however, somnolence is persistent and may be relieved by giving a CNS stimulant to avoid risking loss of good pain control.

The first step in treating persistent sedation is to encourage the patient to increase caffeine intake, which alone may be enough to counteract the sedating effects of the opioids. Relatively few patients will require the addition of a stimulant such as dextroamphetamine or methylphenidate (Ritalin). If they do, such drugs should be given in the lowest dose that effectively reverses the sedation. Stimulants should be taken when the patient awakens in the morning and again at noon or in the early afternoon, depending on the patient's usual sleep and activity pattern. They should not be taken later than 2 or 3 PM because they may interfere with normal sleep. CNS stimulants may also enhance opioid analgesia and may even permit reduction of the opioid dose. Giving a stimulant may also contribute to the well-being of the patient, especially the terminally ill patient, by improving not only pain control but also activity and appetite.[59]

MANAGEMENT OF SYMPTOMS AND SIDE EFFECTS

The key side effects to be expected with opioid medications include constipation, nausea with or without vomiting, sedation, myoclonus, urinary retention, and, rarely, respiratory depression. Most of these side effects can be readily prevented and/or controlled with careful assessment and management.

CONSTIPATION

Constipation is an anticipated side effect of all opioids, and an aggressive approach to its prevention and management is essential.[60] An effective, commonly used regimen consists of taking two to four Senokot-S tablets twice a day. The patient should be instructed to adjust the dose to that which produces a regular, comfortable bowel movement at least every other day. The actual dose varies widely among patients and is not related to the opioid dose. If patients are unable to have normal bowel movements on this regimen, 1 to 2 ounces of lactulose (Cephulac) at bedtime can be added to the regimen on a regular or p.r.n. basis depending on individual patient needs.

If the patient has not had a bowel movement in more than 3 days or is known to be impacted, an aggressive attempt to clean out the bowel from above and below is essential. This can be accomplished by administering lactulose (1 to 2 ounces) every 4 hours and giving milk-and-molasses enemas (Table 22–2) every 6 hours until no more formed stool is passed. If the patient is experiencing nausea and/or vomiting, one or two milk-and-molasses enemas should be given before starting the lactulose.[61]

Occasionally, particularly in patients with intra-abdominal disease and pressure on the bowel from a tumor mass, the regimen just described is not enough. If the patient is not obstructed, addition of an agent that stimulates bowel motility, such as metoclopramide (Reglan) or cisapride (Propulsid), may be helpful.

NAUSEA WITH OR WITHOUT VOMITING

Nausea with or without vomiting is most often a transient side effect associated with initiation of therapy or increases in dose. It is best managed by first ensuring that the patient's bowels are properly functioning, because constipation is often a principal cause or major contributing factor. Patients should be started on a bowel program such as the one specified in the previous section. For some patients, a good bowel cleanout and prophylaxis is all that is needed. Others require antiemetics. If vomiting is persistent, and particularly if medications cannot be retained reliably, the regular use of a suppository is recommended. If nausea is the primary problem and the patient can tolerate oral medications,

---

Table 22–2. Instructions for Milk-and-Molasses Enemas

Ingredients and supplies
  8 oz warm water
  3 oz powdered milk
  4.5 oz molasses
  Enema bag with a long, soft tube (e.g., red rubber catheter) attached
Directions
  Put water and powdered milk into a jar
  Close the jar and shake until the water and milk appear to be fully mixed
  Add molasses and shake the jar again until the mixture is evenly colored
  Pour the mixture into the enema bag
  Gently introduce the tube into the rectum about 12 inches, but do not push beyond resistance
  Administer the enema with the bag held high
  Repeat every 6 hr until good results are achieved
  May be altered with lactulose or sorbitol taken orally

Bisanz A: Managing Bowel Function When Taking Pain Medicine: A Patient Guide. Houston, The University of Texas M. D. Anderson Cancer Center, 1996.

then the antiemetic should be administered on a schedule (e.g., Compazine 10 mg every 6 hours or 15 mg sustained-release Compazine every 12 hours).

Tolerance to this side effect may develop after pain control is achieved and a stable opioid dose is reached. Once the nausea has been controlled by bowel cleanout and appropriate antiemetic medication, the dose can be changed to p.r.n. Many patients are able to manage without antiemetics as long as the opioid dose remains stable. If titration to higher opioid doses is required, further antiemetic therapy may be required.

SEDATION

Sedation is likewise most often a transient side effect. It is also often a function of pre-existing sleep disturbance and may abate once more normal sleep patterns are restored. Patients should be instructed to anticipate sedation during the dose titration period and to allow themselves to get as much rest as possible. If sedation persists it can be treated with caffeine or CNS stimulants, as described previously. If sedation is not relieved but the patient has achieved good pain control, the dose may be reduced gradually until sedation is relieved without sacrificing pain control. If satisfactory alertness has not been achieved despite the addition of a CNS stimulant, changing to another opioid may help.

MYOCLONUS

Myoclonus is a fairly common opioid side effect, especially with higher doses. The patient may experience mild to moderate muscle jerks, most commonly during sleep but occasionally throughout the day. If the jerking is mild and not bothersome to the patient, nothing needs to be done other than reassuring the patient that this is a minor side effect. If it is bothersome, e.g., disrupts sleep or increases pain, the drug can be changed or a low dose of benzodiazepine can be prescribed, as described previously.

URINARY RETENTION

Urinary retention is a less frequently seen but often transient side effect. It may manifest as difficulty in urinating or frank inability to do so. The patient should be instructed to turn on the water faucet to assist in stimulating micturition. Other techniques include pouring warm water over or gently massaging the bladder area. If these simple measures do not work and the patient is uncomfortable and completely unable to empty the bladder, straight catheterization and change to another opioid may be required. In rare situations where urinary retention persists despite trying different opioids and other pain-relief measures, the patient may be taught intermittent self-catheterization.

RESPIRATORY DEPRESSION

Respiratory depression is a rare side effect in the presence of severe, unrelieved pain, even in the opioid-naive patient. Most patients become tolerant of the respiratory-depressant effects within a few days of initiating opioids. However, since this is the most potentially serious untoward effect, opioid-naive patients should be carefully monitored when opioid therapy is begun, particularly if other drugs such as anesthetic agents and/or sedative agents (especially benzodiazepines) are also administered (see Opioid Pharmacology).

REFERENCES

1. Melzack R: The tragedy of needless pain. Sci Am 1990;262:27.
2. Marks RM, Sachar EJ: Undertreatment of medical inpatients with narcotic analgesics. Ann Intern Med 1973;78:173.
3. Bonica JJ: Cancer pain. In Bonica JJ (ed): The Management of Pain, 2nd ed. Philadelphia, Lea & Febiger, 1900:400.
4. Hill CS, Fields WS, Thorpe DM: A call to action to improve relief of cancer pain. In Hill CS, Fields WS (eds): Drug Treatment of Cancer Pain in a Drug-oriented Society: Advances in Pain Research and Therapy, vol 11. New York, Raven Press, 1989:353.
5. McCaffery M, Thorpe DM: Differences in perception of pain and the development of adversarial relationships among health care providers. In Hill CS, Fields WS (eds): Drug Treatment of Cancer Pain in a Drug-oriented Society: Advances in Pain Research and Therapy, vol 11. New York, Raven Press, 1989:113.
6. Foley KM: The "decriminalization" of cancer pain. In Hill CS, Fields WS (eds): Drug Treatment of Cancer Pain in a Drug-oriented Society: Advances in Pain Research and Therapy, vol 11. New York, Raven Press, 1989:5.
7. Hill CS: Oral opioid analgesics. In Patt RB (ed): Cancer Pain. Philadelphia, JB Lippincott, 1993:129.
8. Hill CS: A review and commentary on the negative influence of licensing and disciplinary boards and drug enforcement agencies on pain treatment with opioid analgesics. Journal of Pharmacy Care in Pain and Symptom Control 1993;1:33.
9. Angarola RT, Wray SD: Legal impediments to cancer pain treatment. In Hill CS, Fields WS (eds): Drug Treatment of Cancer Pain in a Drug-oriented Society: Advances in Pain Research and Therapy, vol 11. New York, Raven Press, 1990:213.
10. Joranson DE, Cleeland CS, Weissman DE, Glison AM: Opioids for chronic cancer and noncancer pain: A survey of state medical board members. Federation Bulletin: The Journal of Medical Licensure and Discipline 1992;79:15.
11. Dahl JL, Joranson DE, Engber D, Dosch J: The cancer pain problem: Wisconsin's response. A report on the Wisconsin Cancer Pain Initiative. J Pain Symptom Manage 1988;3:S1.
12. Texas Acts 1989, 71st Legislature, First Called Session, Ch. 5, Sec. 1, effective November 1, 1989. Codified at Article 4495c, Vernon's Civil Statutes.
13. Jacox A, Carr DB, Payne R: Management of Cancer Pain: Clinical Practice Guideline No. 9. AHCPR Publication No. 94–0592. Rockville, MD, Agency for Health Care Policy and Research, U.S. Department of Health and Human Services, Public Health Service, 1994.
14. Acute Pain Management Guideline Panel: Acute Pain Management: Operative or Medical Procedures and Trauma (Clinical Practice Guideline). AHCPR Pub. No. 92–0032. Rockville, MD, Agency for Health Care Policy and Research, U.S. Department of Health and Human Services, Public Health Service, 1992.
15. Cleeland CS, Gonin R, Hatfield AK, et al: Pain and its treatment in outpatients with metastatic cancer: The Eastern Cooperative Oncology Group's Outpatient Pain Study. N Engl J Med 1994;330:592.
16. McCaffery M, Beebe A: Pain: A Clinical Manual for Nursing Practice. St. Louis, CV Mosby, 1989.
17. Grossman SA, Sheidler VR, Swedeen K, Mucenski J, Piantadosi S: Correlation of patient and caregiver ratings of cancer pain. J Pain Symptom Manage 1991;6:53.
18. Bonica JJ: Anatomic and physiologic basis of nociception and pain. In Bonica JJ (ed): The Management of Pain, 2nd ed. Philadelphia, Lea & Febiger, 1990.
19. Fields HL: Pain. New York, McGraw-Hill, 1987.
20. Elomaa I, Blomqvist C, Grohn P, et al: Long-term controlled trial with diphosphonate in patients with osteolytic bone metastases. Lancet 1983;1:146.
21. Roth A, Kolaric K: Analgesic activity of calcitonin in patients with painful osteolytic metastases of breast cancer. Oncology 1986;43:283.
22. Bates T: A review of local radiotherapy in the treatment of bone metastases and cord compression. Int J Radiat Oncol Biol Phys 1992;23:217.
23. Arcangeli G, Micheli A, Arcangeli G, et al: The responsiveness of bone metastases to radiotherapy: The effect of site, histology and radiation dose on pain relief. Radiother Oncol 1989;14:95.
24. Blake GM, Zivanovic MA, McEwan AJ, Ackery DM: Sr-89 therapy: Strontium kinetics in disseminated carcinoma of the prostate. Eur J Nucl Med 1986;12:447.

25. Metastron Prescribing Information. Arlington Heights, IL, Amersham Healthcare/Medi-Physics, 1993.

26. Porter AT, McEwan AJB, Powe JE, et al: Results of a randomized phase-III trial to evaluate the efficacy of strontium-89 adjuvant to local field external beam irradiation in the management of endocrine resistant metastatic prostate cancer. Int J Radiat Oncol Biol Phys 1993;25:805.

27. Clouston PD, DeAngelis LM, Posner JB: The spectrum of neurological disease in patients with systemic cancer. Ann Neurol 1992;31:268.

28. Byrne TN: Spinal cord compression from epidural metastases. N Engl J Med 1992;327:612.

29. Porter J, Jick H: Addiction is rare in patients treated with narcotics. N Engl J Med 1980;302:123.

30. Jaffe JH: Drug addiction and drug abuse. In Gilman AG, Rall TW, Nies S, Taylor P (eds): Goodman and Gilman's Pharmacological Basis of Therapeutics, 8th ed. New York, Pergamon Press, 1990:522.

31. Foley KM: The treatment of cancer pain. N Engl J Med 1985;313:84.

32. Foley KM: Changing concepts of tolerance to opioids: What the cancer patient has taught us. In Chapman CR, Foley KM (eds): Current and Emerging Issues in Cancer Pain: Research and Practice. New York, Raven Press, 1993:331.

33. Cherny JI, Portenoy RK: The management of cancer pain. CA Cancer J Clin 1994;44:262.

34. Weissman DE, Haddox JD: Opioid pseudoaddiction: An iatrogenic syndrome. Pain 1989;35:363.

35. Portenoy RK, Payne R: Acute and chronic pain. In Lowinson JH, Ruiz P, Millman RB (eds): Substance Abuse: A Comprehensive Textbook, 2nd ed. Baltimore, Williams and Wilkins, 1992:691.

36. Wesson DR, Ling W, Smith DE: Prescription of opioids for treatment of pain in patients with addictive disease. J Pain Symptom Manage 1993;8:289.

37. Savage SR: Pain medicine and addiction medicine: Controversies and collaboration [preface]. J Pain Symptom Manage 1993;8:254.

38. Hargraves KM, Jorris JL: The peripheral analgesic effects of opioids. American Pain Society Journal 1993;2:51.

39. Jaffe JH, Martin WR: Opioid analgesics and antagonists. In Gilman AG, Rall TW, Nies S, Taylor P (eds): Goodman and Gilman's Pharmacological Basis of Therapeutics, 8th ed. New York, Pergamon Press, 1990:485.

40. Kaiko RF, Foley KM, Grabinski PY, et al: Central nervous system excitatory effects of meperidine in cancer patients. Ann Neurol 1983;13:180.

41. Benedetti C, Butler SH: Systemic analgesics. In Bonica JJ (ed): The Management of Pain, 2nd ed. Philadelphia, Lea & Febiger, 1990:1640.

42. American Pain Society: Principles of Analgesic Use in the Treatment of Acute Pain and Chronic Cancer Pain: A Concise Guide to Medical Practice. Skokie, IL, American Pain Society, 1992.

43. Manfredi PL, Ribeiro S, Chandler SW, Payne R: Inappropriate use of naloxone in cancer patients with pain. J Pain Symptom Manage 1996;11(2):131–134.

44. McCaffery M, Martin L, Ferrell BR: Analgesic administration via rectum or stoma. ET Nursing 1992;19:114.

45. Bruera E, Ripamonti C: Alternate routes of administration of opioids for the management of cancer pain. In Patt RB (ed), Cancer Pain. Philadelphia, JB Lippincott, 1993:161.

46. Payne R: Transdermal fentanyl: Suggested recommendations for clinical use. J Pain Symptom Manage 1992;7(s3):40.

47. Cousins MJ, Mather LE: Intrathecal and epidural administration of opioids. Anesthesiology 1984;61:276.

48. DuPen S, Williams AR: Management of patients receiving combined epidural morphine and bupivacaine for the treatment of cancer pain. J Pain Symptom Manage 1992;7:125.

49. Hogan Q, Haddox JD, Abram S, Weissman D, Taylor ML, Janjan N: Epidural opiates and local anesthetics for the management of cancer pain. Pain 1991;46:271.

50. Ferrell BR, Griffith H: Cost issues related to pain management: Report from the Cancer Pain Panel of the Agency for Health Care Policy and Research. J Pain Symptom Manage 1994;9:221.

51. Ferrante FM, Ostheimer GW, Covino BG (eds): Patient-controlled analgesia. Boston, Blackwell Scientific Publications, 1990.

52. Wasylak TJ, Abbott FV, English MJ, Jeans ME: Reduction of post-operative morbidity following patient-controlled morphine. Can J Anaesth 1990;37:726.

53. Roth SH: Merits and liabilities of NSAID therapy. Rheum Dis Clin North Am 1989;15:479.

54. Max MB: Effects of desipramine, amitriptyline, and fluoxetine on pain in diabetic neuropathy. N Engl J Med 1992;326:1250.

55. Botney M, Fields HL: Amitriptyline potentiates morphine analgesia by a direct action on the central nervous system. Ann Neurol 1983;13:160.

56. Bach FW, Jensen TS, Kastrup J, Stigsby B, Dejgard A: The effect of intravenous lidocaine on nociceptive processing in diabetic neuropathy. Pain 1990;40:29.

57. McGee JL, Alexander MR: Phenothiazine analgesia: Fact or fantasy. American Journal of Hospital Pharmacy 1979;36:633.

58. Lasagna RG, DeKornfeldt TJ: Methotrimeprazine: A new phenothiazine derivative with analgesic properties. JAMA 1961;178:887.

59. Bruera E, Miller MJ, Macmillan K, Kuehen N: Neuropsychological effects of methylphenidate in patients receiving a continuous infusion of narcotics for cancer pain. Pain 1992;48:163.

60. Levy MH: Constipation and diarrhea in cancer patients. Cancer Bulletin 1991;43:412.

61. Bisanz A: Managing Bowel Function When Taking Pain Medicine: A Patient Guide. Houston, The University of Texas M. D. Anderson Cancer Center, 1996.

Chapter 23

Medical Decision Making at the End of Life: Hospice Care and Care of the Terminally Ill

Mary K. Hughes, BS, MS, and Sharon Weinstein, MD

Table 23–1. Estimated Frequencies of Death from Cancer at Most Frequent Sites by Sex, 1998

Male		Female	
Lung	32%	Lung	25%
Prostate	13%	Breast	16%
Colon and rectum	9%	Colon and rectum	11%
Pancreas	5%	Pancreas	5%
Leukemia	4%	Ovary	6%

Data from Landis SH, Murray T, Bolden S, Wingo PA: Cancer statistics 1998. CA Cancer J Clin 1998;46:14.

Despite ever-advancing strides in its treatment, cancer remains a life-threatening disease. There are times when technology does not prolong an acceptable quality of life but simply prolongs the process of dying. In such cases, decisions that are never easy become even harder to make. When does the physician decide that treatments are no longer effective and that aggressive medicine should be abandoned in favor of palliative care?

Often there is a turning point in the patient's condition when it becomes clear that death is near. This does not mean that the patient's situation is hopeless but that the nature and focus of hope has changed. There is no longer an expected cure or remission but the hope for symptom control. This can be a very meaningful time in the patient's life despite the poor prognosis. Yet, in Western society, death has become a topic that cannot be discussed or referred to openly. This makes decision making about a change from active to palliative treatment even harder.[1]

EPIDEMIOLOGY

Parker and colleagues[2] predicted that in the United States, almost 1,360,000 new cancer cases would be diagnosed in 1996 and that, despite all the therapeutic modalities available, more than half a million people would die of cancer. Table 23–1 lists, for 1998, the estimated frequencies of death due to cancer at the five most common sites for each sex.[2] Walsh[4] estimated that 250,000 patients annually will choose hospice care but that many others will not know that it is an option. Table 23–2 lists the 5-year relative survival rates in the United States according to anatomic site.[3] If the predicted survival rate is high, it may prevent the physician from referring the patient to a hospice despite his or her physical condition.

Table 23–2. Five-Year Survival Rates for Frequently Diagnosed Cancers

SITE	PERCENT
Bladder	81
Colon and rectum	61
Corpus uteri	83
Female breast	83
Lung	13
Lymphoma	50
Ovary	44

Data from American Cancer Society: Cancer Facts and Figures 1996. American Cancer Society, 1996:16.

END-OF-LIFE ISSUES: WHEN TO REFER

APPROACHES TO THERAPY

There are four basic approaches to cancer therapy: surgery, chemotherapy, radiation therapy, and biologic therapy. Each approach can be used alone or in combination with the others. Treatment can be curative, salvaging, or palliative. In each cancer, the most effective treatments known are used initially, followed by the next line of therapy if the first proves ineffective.

As disease progresses, choices of treatment become more and more limited until there are no choices left. When metastatic disease progresses after initial chemotherapy, patients can receive additional salvage regimens sequentially and be treated with chemotherapy until death. The patient may seek treatment at other facilities if the primary facility exhausts its treatment options. This depends on the resources available to the patient and the desires of patient and family. Sometimes the search is futile, and the patient progresses to the terminal phase of cancer. By focusing on sequential treatment, both the health care team and the patient can avoid more difficult issues, such as declining health and approaching death. However, the time for hospice care may come sooner than the health care team or patient expects. Consequently, according to Kitzbrunner,[5] 50% of terminally ill cancer patients in the United States are not being given the option of hospice care or are referred too late to take full advantage of the support a hospice program can offer.

Breitbart and associates[6] describe patients as being terminally ill if they have a life expectancy of 3 to 6 months and have been switched to the palliative mode of care. However, Lesko and Holland[7] point out that when medical symptoms significantly intensify, patients often view themselves as terminally ill. At this point, a referral to hospice care is appropriate.

HOSPICE CARE

Hospice is a program of palliative and supportive services that provides physical, psychological, social, and spiritual care for the dying and their families.[8] The philosophy of such programs is to affirm life. The goal is to help the dying patient maintain quality of life, comfort them with dignity, allow them autonomy, and give loved ones the opportunity for emotional closure. A hospice program offers palliative care to any person who has opted to discontinue curative treatment. The hospice movement grew in part out of a reaction to the perception of modern medical care as aggressive, impersonal, and insensitive. Hospice care requires a blending of professional roles, thus transforming the multidisciplinary team into an interdisciplinary one.

Table 23–3 lists and describes the role of each interdisciplinary team member.[9, 10] However, many hospice programs do not have the luxury of employing the various therapists to augment the interdisciplinary team. According to the World Health Organization,[11] palliative care is the active total care of patients whose disease is unresponsive to treatment. Symptom control as well as psychological, social, and spiritual care is paramount. Hospice affirms life and regards dying as a normal process, neither hastens nor postpones death, and offers a support system to help the family with its grief during and after the patient's death. Through the effort to control symptoms, palliative care may reduce tumor burden and prolong life. It is active, compassionate care given at a time when

Table 23–3. The Hospice Interdisciplinary Team

MEMBER	ROLE
Attending physician	• Brings continuity of care • Addresses patient's physical and emotional needs
Hospice team physician	• Addresses palliative care needs of the individual • Educates rest of the team • Consultant to the attending physician
Nurse	• Provides and coordinates care, ensuring quality of life for both the patient and family • Most frequent contact with patient and family in home and institution • Helps patient cope with advancing disease • Educates both family and patient • May be specialized in certain aspects of patient care
Social worker	• Assesses needs of patient and family and identifies resources • Caregiver and educator • Intervenes via either instrumental services or emotional support • Link between the hospice team and other community services • Essential before death and during bereavement
Clergy	• Must be a good listener • Facilitates spiritual guidance between the patient and family as well as their religion • May perform funeral or memorial services
Physiotherapist	• Helps plan activities aimed at maximizing patient's resources • Relaxes patient through massage • Educates patient about transfers or positioning
Occupational therapist	• Assesses patient function and recommends adaptive equipment • Makes play and leisure activities available in inpatient setting
Music therapist	• Uses music in a deliberate way to reduce patient's anxiety and physical symptoms
Art therapist	• Provides patient with a variety of forms of self-expression
Dietitian	• Informs patients about basic nutrition and ways of meeting patient's nutritional needs • Has good quality of life as goal
Pharmacist	• A resource to physicians about drug interactions and side effects
Volunteer	• Assists the medical and paramedical staff in providing quality of life for patient and family • Bridges the gulf between the professionals and the community

Adapted from Ajemian I: The interdisciplinary team. In Doyle D, Hanks GWC, MacDonald N (eds): Oxford Textbook of Palliative Medicine. New York, Oxford University Press, 1995:17; and Eng MA: The hospice interdisciplinary team: A synergistic approach to the care of dying patients and their families. Holistic Nursing Practice 1993;7(4):49. © 1993 Aspen Publishers, Inc.

the goals of cure and prolonging life are not the most important ones or may not be possible.[12]

Many patients and family members are unaware of the option for hospice care. They instead view the hospital as the place to go to die when all other treatment has failed or when the family can no longer care for the patient at home. Often the physician may view a referral to hospice as "doing nothing" instead of as an integral component of comprehensive cancer care. When chemotherapy may not provide a meaningful therapeutic result, the oncologist should offer the option of hospice services as early in the terminal phase of cancer as possible.

CULTURAL ISSUES

Previous generations have taught individual members how to behave during illness and suffering. It is very uncommon for a person to go against his or her cultural, religious, or ethnic beliefs when dying.[13] Therefore, it is important for the practitioner to be familiar with the traditions of various cultures and religions when offering palliative care to patients. However, the patient's personal preference is very powerful in determining palliative care options. Prejudging patients leads to their depersonalization and is to be avoided when offering palliative care treatment choices.

ETHICAL ISSUES

According to Williams,[14] ethics is the study of morality, the good and the bad, the right and the wrong, in human decision making and behavior. Medicine has probably been subject to more ethical analysis throughout history than any other discipline. Historically, physicians' ethical behavior was the primary concern, but now the rights and duties of other health care workers and of patients are equally important. Now, owing to expanding technology and diminishing resources, the ethics of limiting life-sustaining treatment (bioethics) is being explored. This interdisciplinary field requires the participation of experts in both biomedicine and ethics and is characterized by a great diversity of opinion on almost every issue. Bioethics is a set of moral principles that govern the behavior of physicians and other health professionals.

Table 23–4 lists and describes ethical principles used in determining whether a palliative care referral is needed.[15] One of the most influential principles is that of informed consent. By accepting this principle, the physician shifts the power in the physician-patient relationship toward the patient; physicians sometimes find this uncomfortable.[15] The American Nurses Association mandates that nurses uphold the patient's right to autonomy by becoming the patient's advocates in the matter of informed consent.[16]

When offering information, physicians and nurses must recognize that a patient's choices should be respected not because they agree with those choices but because it is the patient's right to know or not to know.[17] The medicalization of dying deprives the dying person of autonomy and can result in wasteful medical care. Therefore, some hospitals have adopted futile-care policies to decrease physical and psychological suffering for the patient and the family when there is no possibility of a favorable outcome for the patient. These policies also have economic effects on society, institutions, families, and patients.

Table 23–4. Ethical Principles for Use in Determining Need for Hospice

PRINCIPLE	DEFINITION
Autonomy	Respect for the patient's capacity of self determination and exercise of personal informed choice
Nonmaleficence	Obligation not to intentionally inflict harm
Beneficence	Obligation to promote good and remove and prevent harm
Justice	Fair allocation of medical resources, impartiality, and fairness
Fidelity	Obligation to be truthful and keep promises
Paternalism	Making decisions for others without their input
Informed consent	Disclosure, comprehension, voluntariness, and competence
Veracity	Obligation to tell the truth
Confidentiality	Obligation to keep information shared, in a professional relationship, private
Sanctity of life	Belief that human life has intrinsic worth and value and the obligation to preserve and protect a person's meaningful life as defined by that person

Data from Luce JM: Physicians do not have a responsibility to provide futile or unreasonable care if a patient or family insists. Crit Care Med 1995;23:760.

Table 23–5. Patient Self-Determination Act

Hospitals, skilled nursing facilities, home health agencies, health maintenance organizations, and
  certain preferred provider organizations must
• provide patients written information about their rights under state law to make decisions about
  medical care—including the right to formulate advance directives—as well as the written policies
  of the provider that implement these rights
• document in patients' medical records whether patients have advance directives
• not condition the provision of care or otherwise discriminate against patients based on whether
  they have advance directives
• ensure compliance with state law, respecting advance directives by provider organizations
• provide education for staff and community on advance directives

Adapted from Omnibus Reconciliation Act of 1990. Congressional Record, U.S. House of Representatives.
Sections 4206, 4751. October 26, 1990.

MEDICAL-LEGAL ISSUES

Table 23–5 lists the mandates imposed by the National Patient Self-Determination Act of 1990.[18] The act mandates that all institutions inform patients of their right to set up formal advance directives such as living wills, durable powers of attorney for health care decisions, and do-not-resuscitate directives. Every state has legislated the right to such directives. Because the patient's autonomy is held and even extended by means of an advance directive, it can be ethically and legally dangerous to treat a patient without consent.[19]

Table 23–6 describes the two types of advance directives and gives examples of each. The patient must be competent when completing these forms. Tables 23–7 and 23–8 list the advantages and disadvantages of advance directives, respectively. Tables 23–9 and 23–10 do the same for proxy directives. Table 23–11 describes the five elements of competency. Determining competency is essential since a competent patient has the right to refuse treatment at any time.

It is important for the patient to have both types of directives to reduce the problems of each. For example, Emanuel and coworkers[20] found that 93% of medical outpatients and 89% of the general public want advance directives, regardless of age, health, or other demographics. Nevertheless, only a small minority of Americans have written advance directives, and often their physicians are not aware of them. When several physicians are involved in the patient's care, communication about advance directives may not be a priority. It is very important, then, for the physician to include the competent patient in any discussion about do-not-resuscitate decisions. This is not a decision the physician can make cavalierly without regard to the patient. Ultimately, the physician decides whom to treat and how to treat them, but when deciding to withhold treatment (e.g., resuscitation) it is important to get the patient's input or at the very least to inform the patient about the decision. This cannot be a paternalistic

Table 23–6. Advance Directives

TYPES	DEFINITION	EXAMPLES
Instructional Directive	Gives the patient's treatment preferences when the patient has a specific request, fear, or religious concern he or she wants to protect	Living will, advance directive, do-not-resuscitate order
Proxy Designation	Names a person to make health care decisions; especially useful when the patient doesn't want family to become automatic surrogate	Durable power of attorney for health care

Table 23–7. Advantages of Advance Directives

Protect moral and legal rights of self-determination
Diminish uncertainty about what patient wants done
Reduce conflict among decision makers
Relieve anxiety of families and practitioners about making life-and-death decisions
Relieve patient's fears about overtreatment
Facilitate altruism by
  • allowing patients to donate organs
  • relieving families of economic burden of unnecessary treatment

Data from Emanuel LL, Barry MJ, Stoeckle JD, et al: Advance directives for medical care. N Engl J Med 1991;324:889.

Table 23–8. Problems with Advance Directives

Incompetent patient is a different person with different preferences than when competent
Unanticipated therapeutic options may emerge
Patient's actual condition may be different than anticipated
Patient's interests may have changed dramatically
Advantageous treatment may be precluded if an advance directive overrules the physician and the family or if preferences are too detailed
Tend to focus on cessation of treatment rather than continued treatment
Not nuanced to fit patient's needs at the time of the actual decisions
Usually does not go into effect unless the patient is terminally ill
May demand care that is judged medically futile

Table 23–9. Advantages of Proxy Directives

Greater flexibility
More relevance to the patient's actual condition
Greater personal involvement of the decision-maker
Rests on principle of substituted judgment (another judgment substituted for the patient's)

Table 23–10. Problems with Proxy Directives

Patient's wishes may be misinterpreted by proxy who incorporates his or her own personal quality-of-life preferences or best-interest standards into the decision-making process
Serious financial or emotional conflict of interest may cause the proxy to misconstrue or misrepresent the patient's wishes

Table 23–11. Five Elements of Competency

Age	18 years old
Communicating choices	Able to maintain and communicate stable choices long enough for them to be implemented
Understanding relevant information	Able to understand relevant information (if not, then cannot make choices)
	Can remember words, phrases, ideas, and sequences of information
	Can comprehend the fundamental meaning of information about treatment
	Can understand causal relations and the likelihood of various outcomes
Appreciating the situation and its consequences	Can understand specific implications that the choices carry for one's future
Manipulating information rationally	Can use logical processes to compare benefits and risks of various treatment options, weighing information to reach a decision
	Can form a chain of reasoning

Data from Beauchamp TL, Childress JF: Principles of Biomedical Ethics, 4th ed. New York, Oxford University Press, 1994:144.

decision but must take into account the ethical principles of informed consent, sanctity of life, and veracity.

The patient's right to prepare advance directives hinges on how the right to die is viewed. Thanatologic totalitarianism is the belief that there is only one right way to die. But there are many ways to die with dignity. Being resigned to an imminent death is no more an expression of human dignity than fighting until the last breath. Advocating for the patient is extremely important to ensure patient autonomy and avoid paternalistic decision making. Thanatologic liberalism, on the other hand, is the belief that there is more than one way to die and that each person should have choices about certain aspects of dying.

A dilemma is posed by active euthanasia, the deliberate termination of a person's life to prevent further suffering. This is different from withholding of life-sustaining treatments or administration of medications that may hasten death, because the latter two acts have another primary purpose (e.g., to decrease respiratory distress). The dilemma, then, is between the ethical imperative to alleviate suffering, especially in terminally ill patients who make a conscious decision to end their lives, and the proscription against physicians' and nurses' helping to take a life. Sometimes patients feel that, instead of prolonging life, physicians and nurses prolong suffering and then abandon them in the state of extended suffering.

PSYCHOLOGICAL ISSUES

The physician and nurse who have provided cancer treatment to the patient may find it difficult to refer the patient to hospice because of their emotional involvement with the patient and patient's family. Contemporary Western society's virtual denial of death makes it difficult for the physician to talk to the patient about it. Such denial by the health care providers may affect the prognosis of the patient. For example, the physician and nurse may use denial to deal with the patient's progressing disease. At times the focus may be so much on the disease that the patient is not viewed holistically. The patient may trust the physician to do what is best and so not challenge or question the physician's actions.

Sometimes the physician and nurse may feel guilty because they cannot cure the patient, and this guilt may make them focus even more on the treatment of the disease instead of on the patient. This may make it even harder for the physician and nurse to talk with the patient. When the cancer progresses despite treatment, the physician and nurse may feel helpless to control the disease and the patient's symptoms.

The physician and nurse may fear being blamed for the patient's deteriorating condition, for not doing enough. The physician who feels like nothing more can be done to help the patient live may feel embarrassed and withdraw from the patient. The practitioner may also fear his or her own mortality, which makes it more difficult to deal with someone else's dying.

Palliative care decisions have to be made not only with outpatients but also with inpatients in various states of acuity. Some physicians regard withdrawal of life support as murder despite there being no difference ethically between withdrawing and withholding it. Withholding more treatment in favor of palliative care may add to the physician's guilt. Reasons for a reluctance to withdraw care include the caregiver's inappropriate fear of litigation, a reluctance to formally accept responsibility for terminal-care decisions, and a lack of comfort in acknowledging and implementing the decision to withdraw care.[21] There may be regret about what could not be done. According to a survey by Solomon and Moos,[22] 34% to 50% of the responding nurses and physicians believed that they had acted against their consciences in providing care to the terminally ill.

The anger that physicians and nurses may feel may be directed at the patient (for getting sicker), at the disease (for existing), or at themselves (for letting the patient down). Anger can distance the physician and nurse from the patient. By being emotionally distant, they are not as affected by the patient's death. This anger, however, may delay a hospice referral.

Both physicians and nurses grieve for the patient. Besides denial, guilt, fear, and anger, grief also involves sadness. This sadness can be exhibited by crying, withdrawal from others, or a desire to be alone, which can interfere with patient interaction. Often, crying in front of others, especially patients, is quite uncomfortable for the practitioner. Crying also contributes to the physician's or nurse's feeling out of control. This feeling is one of the most difficult to deal with and can be compounded by caring for patients with cancer. The disease, the side effects of treatments, the patient's wishes, the family's wishes, and the practitioner's feelings all add to this.

SPIRITUAL ISSUES

Only recently have people discerned the difference between religious and spiritual issues. Religion is more a formalized set of beliefs, rites, and ritual, whereas spirituality is the soul's search for meaning in any given experience.[23] The practice or nonpractice of religion (e.g., going or not going to church) is often associated with guilt. Spirituality is often confused with religion. Helping a patient deal with spiritual issues without the guilt associated with religion can be very rewarding for the health care giver. Helping the patient to resolve or let go of problem relationships can be very enriching to the patient. The practitioner's own spiritual issues may, however, interfere with referral of the patient to hospice care. The practitioner may feel an unrealistic need to "save" the patient from death and may be unable to let go of this expectation. The caregiver's religious beliefs may contribute to this inability to let go and refer the patient. Moreover, the practitioner's emotional suffering may be interpreted as part of his or her own spiritual journey and that to refer is to "get rid" of the patient instead of fulfilling the obligation to treat.

PARADIGM SHIFT FOR PHYSICIANS

In Western society, a death before 60 years of age is often considered premature, whereas a death after age 70 is considered timely and fitting.[24] Perhaps because death is less frightening and more salient for the older person, it is often easier to tell such a patient about a poor prognosis. In contrast, practitioners often attempt more heroic measures in the younger patient and may be less likely to refer such a patient to hospice.

The awareness of one's own death—a quality not shared with other members of the animal kingdom—produces an amazing range of responses in both the patient and the caregiver.[24] The patient's responses include anticipation of rest and peace, of drifting into nothingness, as well as fear and anxiety to the point of dread. Even though the old have had more experience with death and dying and think more about it than the young, they do not think death should come too soon.[24] Furthermore, as Kalish and Reynolds[24] found, young adults are more fearful of death and dying, dream more about death, are more desirous of dying quickly, and are more likely to fight death than to accept it peacefully.

The practitioner's feelings about death and dying influence how he or she delivers bad news to the patient and family. Physicians favor an open approach for themselves but a protective approach for their patients. Nurses believe it is important to inform the patient and family when aggressive treatment fails but also to keep some hope of cure alive.[25] Table 23–12 lists the sources of difficulty in communicating bad news.[26] These difficulties are complex and involve both patients and practitioners. The physician may initiate the discussion about hospice care, but often it is the nurse who helps the patient process this information. The physician may have a difficult time changing the focus of treatment from cure to comfort, and sometimes others on the health care team must help the physician recognize that treatment expectations have changed. Ultimately, the aggressive pursuit of survival must be balanced with the acceptance of death.

PALLIATIVE TREATMENT

SETTING

In 1994, some 300,000 Americans died at home under hospice care, and more than 1 million ended their lives in hospitals.[27] Different ethnocultural groups differed greatly in their choice of where to die. Practitioners are frequently confronted with decisions about sending terminal cancer patients home to die, transferring them to a hospice or palliative-care bed, or keeping them in an acute-care hospital. When patients believe that hospitalization is reserved for the dying, the suggestion to hospitalize is open to considerable misinterpretation. For instance, in the current health care reform environment, a dying patient may not be eligible for hospitalization. Conversely, when home hospice care is

Table 23–12. Sources of Difficulty in Communicating Bad News

The social denial of death	Lack of experience of death in the family
	High expectations of health and life
	Materialism
	Changing role of religion in caring for the dying
Patient's fears about dying	Suffering
	Never feeling better
	Uncontrolled pain
	Abandonment
	Isolation
	Spirituality issues
Factors originating in the practitioner	Sympathic pain
	Fear of being blamed
	Fear of the untaught
	Fear of eliciting a reaction
	Fear of saying "I don't know"
	Fear of expressing emotions
	Ambiguity of the phrase "I'm sorry"
	Own fears of illness/death
	Fear of the medical hierarchy

Data from Buckman R: Communication in palliative care: A practical guide. In Doyle D, Hanks GWC, MacDonald N (eds): Oxford Textbook of Palliative Medicine. New York, Oxford University Press, 1995:47.

offered, this may be misinterpreted by the patient and family because hospitalization was not offered.

Some patients and relatives, given adequate support and preparation, can continue to manage the patient's care at home, whereas others may require access to urgent admission or continuous home nursing support. It is important for the hospice team to work closely with the primary care team. In many cases, the primary care team signs off the case when the patient is treated by a hospice. This can contribute to feelings of abandonment by the patient, so it is important for the primary care physician to explain fully the reasons for this change in care and physicians. There may be times when the patient must be admitted on an emergency basis to an inpatient hospice unit or hospital in order to get problematic symptoms under control. During these times, good communication between the home care staff, the patient, the family, and the inpatient staff is extremely important. In the outpatient setting, nurses have more independence and autonomy, but with them comes more responsibility—for symptom management, for emotional support, and for family education. Hull[28] found that the hospital nurse focuses on direct patient care, while the home care nurse focuses primarily on consultation, with the family providing most of the care.

PHYSICAL SYMPTOM CONTROL

Culture influences the meaning of symptoms, the way a person reacts to symptoms, and the way symptoms are treated. Table 23–13 lists physical symptoms in terminally ill cancer patients.[6]

PAIN

Pain is the most common problem that cancer patients experience. It is more than just a symptom; it is an all-consuming experience. Many patients view pain as a direct result of cancer; for them, an increase in pain means the cancer has recurred or progressed.[29] Pain can make the patient, the family, and the practitioner feel out of control and frustrated.

To deal with such pain, programs like the World Health Organization three-step analgesic ladder (Table 23–14) have been set up.[30] A major thrust of the program is based on the belief that nothing has a greater impact on the quality of life of cancer patients than pain control. Therefore, cancer pain relief must be seen not in isolation but as part of a comprehensive palliative care program.

Table 23–13. Physical Symptoms in Terminally Ill Cancer Patients

VERY COMMON (40%–70%)	COMMON (10%–40%)	LESS COMMON (<10%)
Pain	Dyspnea	Dysphagia
Constipation	Nausea/vomiting	Pulmonary congestion
Weakness	Insomnia	Dry and/or sore mouth
Anorexia	Lethargy and/or sedation	Decubitus
Weight loss		

Data from Breitbart W, Levenson JA, Passik SD: Terminally ill cancer patients. In Breitbart W, Holland JC (eds): Psychiatric Aspects of Symptom Management in Cancer Patients. Washington, DC, American Psychiatric Press, 1993:173.

Table 23-14. World Health Organization's Three-Step Analgesic Ladder for Cancer Pain*

Mild pain	Nonopioids (e.g., aspirin, nonsteroidal antiinflammatory agents)
Moderate to severe pain	Weak opioids (e.g., codeine, oxycodone)
Severe pain	Strong opioids (e.g., morphine)

*Adjuvant analgesics may also be used at any of the three stages.
Adapted from World Health Organization: Cancer Pain Relief. Geneva, World Health Organization, 1986.

The treatment of pain is paramount regardless of how the cancer is being treated. Moreover, it is very important that the practitioner believe a patient's complaint of pain. The pain is what the patient says it is, regardless of objective criteria. Pain is a subjective experience. Aggressive pharmacologic pain management is mandatory, although the nurse also can help the patient with nonpharmacologic interventions such as visual imagery to provide a feeling of control. After pain control is achieved, educating the patient about the causes of pain and overcoming barriers to effective analgesic use also help to empower the patient. Establishing trust between the nurse and the patient helps the patient report pain, trusting that it will be treated. But it is also important for the patient to take an active part in pain control: to report it, to treat it quickly, and to report the effectiveness of the interventions. Finally, because pain has different meanings for each person, it is important that the nurse help the patient process the meaning found in the pain experience.

CONSTIPATION AND DIARRHEA

Bowel problems are common and distressing for patients with advanced cancer. The best treatment for constipation is prophylactic treatment. The practitioner can encourage the patient to increase fluid and fiber intake and to increase activity. Patients who are receiving opioids should be treated with stool softeners and laxatives. As for diarrhea, it should be treated as aggressively as possible as soon as it occurs. If the diarrhea is persistent, it is important to determine the cause so as to prevent dehydration in patients with advanced cancer.

ANOREXIA, WEIGHT LOSS, AND WEAKNESS

According to Breitbart and associates,[6] anorexia in advanced cancer patients can result from specific physical difficulties such as poorly controlled pain, mouth discomfort, difficulty in swallowing, nausea, and constipation. Anorexia and weight loss can also be caused by psychological factors including anxiety, depression, and conditioned food aversions.[7] Small, frequent feedings, nutritional supplements, and fluids can be prescribed to help patients gain weight. Sometimes steroids are administered to help increase appetite and produce a sense of well-being in patients with advanced cancer. Weakness can be the result of poor nutritional intake, advancing cancer, or decreased activity. Helping the patient to recognize times when he or she has more energy can help the patient to schedule the day for activities that are also pleasurable.

DYSPNEA

Breathlessness (dyspnea) is another common and distressing symptom for the patient with advanced cancer. It can be caused by primary disease, metastatic disease, or other medical conditions unrelated to cancer. Dyspnea inevitably causes anxiety that can overwhelm the patient, family, and caregiver. Breathing can be improved by radiation treatment if the cancer is causing the problem or by thoracentesis to remove fluid. Other measures include oxygen administration, relaxation exercises, and medications such as morphine, steroids, and anxiety-reducing drugs.

NAUSEA AND/OR VOMITING

With the altered taste, poor nutrition, chemotherapy, radiation therapy, metabolic imbalances, and side effects of certain medications associated with cancer treatment come nausea and vomiting. The treatment depends on the cause of the nausea. Steroids, antiemetics, surgery, lorazepam, and behavioral techniques may be helpful in controlling nausea and vomiting.

SLEEP DISORDERS

Sleep deprivation can result in a wide variety of psychological and physiologic changes in patients with advanced cancer. Table 23–15 lists several sleep disorders and their causes.[31] Insomnia can be defined as a subjective complaint of the patient who sleeps poorly; as such, it is a symptom, not a diagnosis. Treatment for insomnia includes sleep hygiene and other behavioral interventions (Table 23–16).[31] Treatment with hypnotic medications, benzodiazepines, neuroleptics, or antidepressants may be indicated when the cause is a physiologic or concomitant psychiatric disorder. Excessive daytime sleepiness can cause inactivity, poor motivation, decreased participation in treatment, poor social interactions, depression, and irritability.

Other less common physical symptoms the terminally ill patient experiences

Table 23–15. Sleep Disorders in Patients with Advanced Cancer

INSOMNIA	EXCESSIVE DAYTIME SLEEPINESS	DISORDERS OF THE SLEEP-WAKE CYCLE
Is a subjective complaint	Is common and frequently overlooked	Is due to frequent disruptions of nighttime sleep and relative inactivity during daytime
Is a symptom, not a diagnosis		
Has physiological, psychological, and environmental causes	Is often not seen as a problem by caretakers	Normal circadian rhythm may disappear
Can alter immune function	Compromises terminally ill patient	Increases caregiver burden

Data from Sateia MJ, Silberfarb PM: Sleep in palliative care. In Doyle D, Hanks GWC, MacDonald N (eds): Oxford Textbook of Palliative Medicine. New York, Oxford University Press, 1995:472.

Table 23-16. Sleep Hygiene for Patients with Advanced Cancer

RECOMMENDATION/COMMENTS

Maintain anchor points in the sleep-wake cycle
  Go to bed at the same time each night
  Get up at the same time each morning
Do not stay in bed for more than 30 minutes if unable to fall asleep at night
  If bedridden, read a book, work a puzzle, until drowsiness occurs
  Do not work at going to sleep
Eliminate late daytime napping
Take a warm bath 1 hour before bedtime if possible
  Since the body cools down during sleep, warming it before sleep time will allow it to begin
    cooling as patient is preparing for sleep
Drink warm milk or eat cheese and crackers, if not lactose intolerant
  Dairy products may be soporific
  Satiation helps with sleep
Use behavioral techniques to help with relaxation before bedtime
  Audiotapes may be helpful
Try to exercise a little each day
  Isometric exercises or passive exercises can be performed
  If possible, get out of bed each day
  Keep the mind stimulated as much as possible during the day
Avoid late-evening caffeine intake
Take medications for sleep as needed
  Avoid overusing sleep medications

Data from Sateia MJ, Silberfarb PM: Sleep in palliative care. In Doyle D, Hanks GWC, MacDonald N (eds): Oxford Textbook of Palliative Medicine. New York, Oxford University Press, 1995:472.

include dysphagia, sore mouth, dry mouth, pulmonary congestion, and decubiti (bed sores). If the dysphagia is caused by external compression, palliative radiation may be helpful. Use of a soft, pureed, or liquid diet and avoidance of oral medications may also be helpful to the patient. Taking a viscous lidocaine solution before meals may help the patient to tolerate meals.

Decubitus occurs as a result of a patient's inactivity, immunosuppressed condition, pain, dehydration, and anemia; it creates another source of pain and infection. It can be prevented by keeping the skin clean and dry, frequently turning the patient, ensuring good nutrition, and educating family members on their role in its prevention. Any treatment should be aimed at removing the source of irritation, necrotic tissue, and infection and protecting new healthy tissue.[32]

A frightening sound called the "death rattle" is frequently encountered at the terminal stage of dying. It is caused by the patient's difficulty in clearing the large airway secretions that accumulate. Because the terminally ill patient's senses and reflexes usually are dulled before this happens, the patient probably is not suffering. The patient's family should be told this. Treatment for the "death rattle" may include respiratory physiotherapy and a scopolamine patch to help dry up secretions and relax the smooth bronchial muscles.[6]

INFECTIONS

Several factors predispose cancer patients to infections, including the failure of anatomic barriers in the host, poor granulocyte functions, poor humoral immunity, weakened cellular immunity, bacterial colonization, and concomitant drug therapy. Table 23–17 lists the common infectious diseases encountered in patients with advanced cancer.[33] Central nervous system infections are often

Table 23–17. Common Infections in the Patient with Advanced Cancer

SITE	TYPE	TREATMENT
Respiratory tract	Pneumonia	Depends on results of sputum culture
	Fungal infection	Amphotericin-B
Gastrointestinal tract	Oral cavity infection–herpes, fungal	Acyclovir; nystatin suspension for candidiasis
	Esophagitis–fungal, herpes	Nystatin suspension for candidiasis; acyclovir
	Hepatitis	Interferon *not* indicated
	Diarrhea	Discontinuance of antibiotics, if possible
Urinary tract	Blockage	Removal of blockage, if possible
	Long-term catheterization	If symptomatic, antibiotics
Skin	Decubitus	Agents that treat cause of infection
	Lymphedema	Agents that treat cause of infection
	Herpes zoster infection	Acyclovir, analgesics
Central nervous system	Meningitis	Agents that treat cause of infection
	Viral encephalitis	Acyclovir, analgesics
Septicemia	Gram-negative bacterial infection	Appropriate antibiotics
	Staphylococcus infection	Appropriate antibiotics

Data from Morant R, Senn H: The management of infections in palliative care. In Doyle D, Hanks GWC, MacDonald N (eds): Oxford Textbook of Palliative Medicine. New York, Oxford University Press, 1995:378.

difficult to differentiate from other diseases. The first symptom may be dementia or delirium, and systemic infection must always be considered when these conditions appear. As for the bacterial infections, septicemia is often fatal: it can be caused by contamination at indwelling venous catheters, but any tubes are a potential entry port for infection. A blood culture identifies the cause of a bacterial infection so that it may be aggressively treated.

PSYCHIATRIC SYMPTOM CONTROL

Table 23–18 lists psychiatric symptoms frequently seen in patients with advanced cancer.[6] Terminal illness is not a psychiatric disorder. Because one is terminally ill, it should not be assumed that major depression should also be present. Therefore, when a psychiatric disorder is present in a terminally ill patient, it should be treated.

ORGANIC MENTAL DISORDERS: DELIRIUM AND DEMENTIA

In a study done by Massie and colleagues,[34] delirium was found in more than 75% of terminally ill patients. This supports the notion that medications given to the patient with multiorgan failure and a fragile state of physiologic functioning can be enough to cause delirium. Unfortunately, the treatment of delirium is difficult because the condition has many causes and because it may be irreversible. Also, workup may be limited by the setting and the patient's comfort level.

Table 23-18. Frequent Psychiatric Symptoms of the Patient with Advanced Cancer

SYMPTOM	ONSET	SIGNS & SYMPTOMS	TREATMENT
Delirium	Acute onset	Agitation Impaired cognitive function Altered attention span Fluctuating level of consciousness Change in sleep-wake cycle	Neuroleptics (i.e., haloperidol) Sedatives Supportive techniques Reversible effect, but not during last 24–48 hr of life Limited treatment choice
Dementia	Slow onset	Relatively alert status Less sleep-cycle impairment Short- and long-term memory deficits Impaired judgment Impaired abstract thinking Disturbed higher cortical functions	Depends on cause
Anxiety	Acute onset	Feeling agitated Poor concentration Increased worry Insomnia	Depends on cause (hypoxia, sepsis, pain, drug reactions) and presentation Opioid analgesics Benzodiazepines Neuroleptics Antihistamines Antidepressants

Depression	Slow onset	Hopelessness
		Worthlessness
		Excessive guilt
		Dysphoric mood
		Suicide ideation
		Anhedonia
		Neurovegetative symptoms
		  Fatigue
		  Poor appetite
		  Sleep disorder
		  Feeling helpless
		  Poor concentration
			Supportive psychotherapy
			Cognitive-behavioral techniques
			Antidepressants

Data from Breitbart W, Levenson JA, Passik SD: Terminally ill cancer patients. In Breitbart W, Holland JC (eds): Psychiatric Aspects of Symptom Management in Cancer Patients. Washington, DC, American Psychiatric Press, 1993:173.

ANXIETY

Anxiety can have many causes but is most likely to be caused by medical complications. Adverse drug reactions include delirium, akathisia, and withdrawal states.[6]

DEPRESSION

Patients with advanced cancer may experience depression and sadness. This can be an appropriate response to their condition. As Breitbart has shown,[35] even rather mild and passive thoughts of suicide are very likely to be associated with significant degrees of depression in terminally ill patients. This is important to remember because depression is a factor in 50% of all suicides.[36]

Helping the patient explore his or her depression and sadness and process these feelings can be part of the evaluation or treatment process. For instance, the patient may have no hope for a cure but can always hope for good symptom control. If drugs are to be used as treatment, then the prognosis and time frame for treatment are important factors in determining the type of drug to use. Effective medications to give include tricyclics (e.g., amitriptyline, desipramine, nortriptyline, imipramine), which also may help with pain control; second-generation antidepressants (e.g., trazodone, bupropion, fluoxetine), which are less cardiotoxic; and psychostimulants (e.g., dextroamphetamine, methylphenidate, pemoline), which are much faster working and energizing.[36]

SUICIDE

The suicide risk in terminally ill patients is greater than in the general population. The patients at highest risk are those with advanced disease who are also suffering from pain, depression, and delirium. According to a study by Faberow and coworkers,[37] 86% of patients who committed suicide did so in the preterminal or terminal stages of illness despite greatly reduced physical capacity. Hopelessness is the link between depression and suicide and is a significantly better predictor of completed suicide than depression alone.

Breitbart reports that fatigue, in the form of physical, emotional, spiritual, financial, familial, communal, and other exhaustion, increases the risk of suicide in cancer patients.[35] Since cancer is often a chronic illness, the longer a patient survives, the more hospitalizations, complications, and expense he or she may face. Also, if the dying process is long and drawn out, family and others may withdraw prematurely from the dying patient, contributing to the patient's feelings of abandonment and isolation.

Consequently, it is very important to assess the suicide risk and make the appropriate interventions. High-risk patients should be identified by early psychiatric intervention. A rapport should be established with the patient, especially by the nurse assessing the patient for suicidal thoughts or behaviors. The patient should be allowed to talk about suicidal thoughts, because this may decrease the suicide risk. Appropriate medications should be used to control symptoms. A close family member or friend should be involved by the medical staff in supporting the patient and reporting symptoms (this is an important part of treatment planning). Usually, psychiatric hospitalization is not desirable in terminally ill patients. Instead, the patient should be helped to gain and keep as much control as possible. The goal of the intervention should be to relieve suffering and thus prevent suicide, especially suicide that is driven by desperation.[36]

SYMPTOM CONTROL IN THE PATIENT WITH ADVANCED CANCER

CHEMOTHERAPY

In some circumstances, chemotherapy and hormonal therapy may offer relief of physical and psychiatric symptoms at little cost to the patient.[38] Low-dose reduced-toxicity regimens whose objective is to control symptoms and increase quality of life may be useful.

RADIATION THERAPY

The value of radiation therapy in palliative medicine lies in controlling local symptoms resulting from the effects of a tumor at a specific site.[39] Local irradiation of a patient with metastatic disease affects the irradiated site and does not influence the natural history of disease outside this area. The goal is to delay tumor growth, relieve pain, and stop bleeding. The treatment usually takes place within a short period (1 to 2 weeks).

SURGERY

The role of surgery in symptom relief is to gain control of the local disease, relieve obstruction (debulking), control discharge and bleeding, and control pain.[40] Palliative surgery can be used in reconstruction as part of a psychological rehabilitation to improve quality of life. Palliative surgery treats the patient first and the cancer second.

BEHAVIORAL INTERVENTIONS

Relaxation, distraction, and visual imagery are useful in managing a wide range of symptoms experienced by the terminally ill cancer patient. As part of a multimodal approach, behavioral therapy can be used to treat anxiety, pain, insomnia, anticipatory nausea and vomiting, and eating disorders.[41] Some techniques are primarily cognitive, focusing on perceptions and thought processes, while others are directed at controlling behavior patterns in an effort to improve the patient's coping abilities and relieve symptoms. Both elements (for example, muscular relaxation and cognitive distraction) are used in hypnosis, biofeedback, and systematic desensitization. These techniques can be learned by the nurse and taught to patients to give them more control in their lives as well as improve their quality of life.

TREATING THE FAMILY UNIT

Good palliative care includes attention to symptom control, counseling for the patient and family, and support for the medical staff.[12] It is important to help the family understand the illness and to support the family in coping with it. Because decision making in the care of the dying patient involves both the patient and the family, it is important to understand the roles and lines of authority within the family system. Who makes decisions for whom? Who can be involved in family meetings? Why are some apparently important participants not included in discussions?

The degrees of involvement and patterns of communication vary greatly. Gender may be one of the factors that defines roles in family systems.[12] Family problems can influence the patient's mood, cause role conflicts in the family, and also distress the patient.[42] Family members who provide practical and emotional support to the patient may find this support to be emotionally costly to themselves. For example, a study by Keitel and colleagues[43] showed that spouses may be more distressed than the patients even fairly early in the cancer process. By the time the patient enters the palliative phase of cancer, the family's emotional resources may be exhausted. This is especially true if there have been many hospitalizations and frequent expectations of death; the family members have a hard time believing that death will really happen now. On the other hand, if the disease or recurrence has a rapid trajectory, the family may still be in shock about the diagnosis of cancer while trying to make decisions about impending death. If the nurse notices this in family members, it is important to get feedback from the family about any new information that they are given (e.g., failure of the treatment). Written instructions to the family are often helpful, as is frequent reinforcement of new information.

SPIRITUAL ISSUES

Care during the final phase of cancer means helping the patient deal with spiritual and existential issues while providing the prerequisite physical comfort. During this transition, the meaningfulness of life is challenged by the patient's own suffering, which also confronts each person with his or her own vulnerability. Meaningless suffering can cause the patient to question his or her religious and spiritual beliefs. Consequently, the patient may become demanding, especially nonverbally, thereby making it difficult for the nurse and physician to stay with the patient.[44]

Table 23–19 presents several general truths about suffering.[45] These may apply also to nurses, since at times they suffer in response to suffering they encounter in the patient.[45, 46]

GRIEF

As Lindemann[47] points out, grief is an acute psychosocial process characterized by rapid onset, serious conditions, and treatable symptoms. Furthermore, grief is an observable syndrome with psychological and somatic symptoms that may appear immediately, be delayed, be exaggerated, or seem absent.[47] From the time of diagnosis, the patient may begin grieving for all the losses that have occurred or will occur as a result of having cancer.

Table 23–19. General Truths about Suffering

Suffering is a private lived experience of a whole person, unique to each individual.
Suffering results when the most important aspects of a person's identity are threatened or lost.
Because suffering is dependent on the meaning of an event or loss for the individual, it can not be assumed to be present or absent in any given clinical condition.
Possible sources of suffering are countless.
The expression of suffering is more accessible to nurses than the experience.
As a fundamental human experience, suffering has a basic structure.
The experience of suffering involves the person in a larger process that includes the person's own coping with suffering and the caring of others.
The caring environment in which the processes of suffering occur can influence a person's suffering either positively or negatively.

Adapted from Kahn DL, Steeves RH: The significance of suffering in cancer care. Semin Oncol Nurs 1995;11:9.

ANTICIPATORY GRIEF

Rando[48] describes anticipatory grief as the anticipation of a future loss that includes many of the signs and symptoms of grief. Anticipatory grief is considered to be an adaptive mechanism for the surviving individual and is the beginning of a grieving process that will end at the patient's death. This type of grief usually accelerates as death nears, whereas conventional grief decelerates over time. For example, the normal feelings of ambivalence towards the dying person may increase the griever's burden of guilt during the anticipatory period. Dying patients as well as family members experience this; they are struggling to accept the reality of separation before the death occurs. Health care practitioners can help the patient anticipate future losses (e.g., alopecia, amputation) before they occur so that the patient is more prepared for them.

FORMS OF DEATH

Sweeting and Gilhooly[49] described three forms of death: clinical, biologic, and social. Each can be viewed as a different form of loss. In Western society, social death precedes the other two, with the terminally ill person losing his or her social identity first. For example, the person is too ill to socialize as he or she did in the past. Grieving for these losses may take place during the terminal phase of the patient's illness.[50]

EMOTIONS OF GRIEF

Rando[48] lists some of the emotions experienced while grieving.[48] These emotions include depression, anger, apathy, fear, sadness, despair, guilt, anxiety, loneliness, and denial. These emotions do not necessarily happen in any order, and they wax and wane during the course of grieving. Anger and guilt may be more difficult to cope with than some of the other emotions. When the patient is angry, the anger may be directed toward the practitioner; knowing that this is part of grief can help the patient explore this feeling instead of feeling guilty. When the patient is feeling guilt, whether justified or not, the focus should be on how anger can be worked through instead of ignored and suppressed. At times, the fear of dying causes the patient to feel very lonely and isolated. Allowing the patient to talk about those feelings validates them.

COPING MECHANISMS

Rando[48] lists three main coping mechanisms of dying patients: retreat from, exclusion of, and mastery and control over the threat of death. In retreating, the patient's regression can be therapeutic if it helps the patient give up some independence and accept some restrictions in order to receive treatment. It also gives the person an altered sense of time; instead of looking forward in terms of months and years, the patient can take the future one day at a time.

Denial occurs more or less in all patients with a terminal illness. It helps to make life more bearable. Weisman differentiated three types of denial: type I, denial of the specific facts of the illness; type II, denial of the implications and extensions of the illness; and type III, denial of extinction.[51] Patients may also deny their concerns about the illness and their own emotional reactions to it. However, denial is usually more worrisome for the family and the practitioner than for the patient.

Patients who intellectualize their feelings are trying to reduce their anxiety by distancing themselves from the anxiety. This can help them feel more in control and allow them to see the disease as more predictable.

All patients employ coping mechanisms in coping with the stress of dying. If these responses are so strong that they interfere with the patient's ability to function, increase the pain, or prevent the patient from seeking medical treatment, then they are considered maladaptive.

BEHAVIORS

According to Rando[48] the behaviors associated with grief include crying, agitation, withdrawal, shouting, changes in sleeping or eating, poor concentration and memory, and fatigue. Knowing what behaviors to expect from the dying patient and from his or her family can help the practitioner plan for their care and recognize what is within normal parameters. Therefore, the relationship between the dying patient and the practitioner is very important. The main goals are to reduce the patient's physical and emotional suffering and to help the patient die with dignity.

Understanding the problems that confront the terminally ill patient is important for health care practitioners. Recognizing when to initiate appropriate interventions for patients and their family members is paramount, especially because treatment decisions at the end of life are never easy to make. We hope that the guidelines we have outlined in these chapters can help the practitioner collaborate in making these important decisions.

REFERENCES

1. Kastenbaum RJ: Death, Society and Human Experience. Columbus, Charles E. Merrill Pub Co, 1986.
2. Landis SH, Murray T, Bolden S, Wingo PA: Cancer statistics, 1998. CA Cancer J Clin 1998;46:14.
3. American Cancer Society: Cancer Facts and Figures 1996. American Cancer Society 1996:16.
4. Walsh D: Palliative care: Management of the patient with advanced cancer. Semin Oncol 1994;21:100.
5. Kitzbrunner BM: Ethical dilemmas in hospice and palliative care. Support Care Cancer 1995;3:28.
6. Breitbart W, Levenson JA, Passik SD: Terminally ill cancer patients. In Breitbart W, Holland JC (eds): Psychiatric Aspects of Symptom Management in Cancer Patients. Washington, DC, American Psychiatric Press, 1993:173.
7. Lesko L, Holland JC: Psychosocial complications of leukemia. In Henderson ES, Lister TA (eds): Leukemia, 5th ed. Philadelphia, WB Saunders Co, 1989:769.
8. National Hospice Organization: Standards of a Hospice Program of Care. Arlington, VA, National Hospice Organization, 1981.
9. Eng MA: The hospice interdisciplinary team: A synergistic approach to the care of dying patients and their families. Holistic Nursing Practice 1993;7:49.
10. Ajemian I: The interdisciplinary team. In Doyle D, Hanks GWC, MacDonald N (eds): Oxford Textbook of Palliative Medicine. New York, Oxford University Press, 1995:17.
11. Cancer Pain Relief and Palliative Care. Technical Report Series 804. Geneva, World Health Organization, 1990.
12. Latimer E, Lundy M: The care of the dying: Multicultural influences. In Masi R, Mensah L,

McLeod KA (eds): Health and Culture: Exploring the Relationships. Vol 2: Programs, Services and Care. New York, Mosaic Press, 1993:41.

13. Neuberger J: Cultural issues in palliative care. In Doyle D, Hanks GWC, MacDonald N (eds): Oxford Textbook of Palliative Medicine. New York, Oxford University Press, 1995:505.

14. Williams JR: Ethics in cross-cultural health. In Masi R, Mensah L, McLeod KA (eds): Health and Cultures: Exploring the Relationships. Vol 1: Policies, Professional Practice and Education. New York, Mosaic Press, 1993:255.

15. Miyaji NT: The power of compassion: Truth-telling among American doctors in the care of dying patients. Soc Sci Med 1993;36:249.

16. American Nurses Association: Code for Nurses with Interpretation Statements. Kansas City, MO, American Nurses Association, 1985:1.

17. Asai A: Should physicians tell patients the truth? West J Med 1995;163:36.

18. Omnibus Reconciliation Act of 1990. Congressional Record, U.S. House of Representatives. Sections 4206, 4751. October 26, 1990.

19. Beauchamp TL, Childress JF: Principles of Biomedical Ethics, 4th ed. New York, Oxford University Press, 1994:144.

20. Emanuel LL, Barry MJ, Stoeckle JD, et al: Advance directives for medical care. N Engl J Med 1991;324:889.

21. Koch KA, Rodeffer HD, Wears RL: Changing patterns of terminal care management in an intensive care unit. Crit Care Med 1994;22:233.

22. Solomon GF, Moos RF: A psychoneuroimmunologic perspective on AIDS research: Questions, preliminary findings and suggestions. In Temoshok L, Baum A (eds): Psychosocial Perspectives on AIDS. Hilldale, NJ, Lawrence Erlbaum, 1990:239.

23. Speck PW: Spiritual issues in palliative care. In Doyle D, Hanks GWC, MacDonald N (eds): Oxford Textbook of Palliative Medicine. New York, Oxford University Press, 1995:515.

24. Kalish RA, Reynolds DK: Death and Ethnicity: A Psychocultural Study. Farmingdale, NY, Baywood Publishing Company, 1981.

25. McClement SE, Degner LF: Expert nursing behaviors in care of the dying adult in the intensive care unit. Heart Lung 1995;24:408.

26. Buckman R: Communication in palliative care: A practical guide. In Doyle D, Hanks GWC, MacDonald N (eds): Oxford Textbook of Palliative Medicine. New York, Oxford University Press, 1995:47.

27. Jones TL: When less is more: Physicians turn to hospice care to help dying patients. Tex Med 92;1:42.

28. Hull M: Family needs and supportive nursing behaviors during terminal cancer: A review. Oncology Nursing Forum 1989;16:787.

29. Ferrell BR, Dean G: The meaning of cancer pain. Semin Oncol Nurs 1995;11:17.

30. World Health Organization: Cancer Pain Relief. Geneva, World Health Organization, 1986.

31. Sateia MJ, Silberfarb PM: Sleep in palliative care. In Doyle D, Hanks GWC, MacDonald N (eds): Oxford Textbook of Palliative Medicine. New York, Oxford University Press, 1995:472.

32. Miller CM, O'Neill A, Mortimer PS: Skin problems in palliative care: Nursing aspects. In Doyle D, Hanks GWC, MacDonald N (eds): Oxford Textbook of Palliative Medicine. New York, Oxford University Press, 1995:395.

33. Morant R, Senn H: The management of infections in palliative care. In Doyle D, Hanks GWC, MacDonald N (eds): Oxford Textbook of Palliative Medicine. New York, Oxford University Press, 1995:378.

34. Massie MJ, Holland JC, Glass E: Delirium in terminally ill cancer patients. Am J Psychiatry 1983;140:1048.

35. Breitbart W: Suicide in cancer patients. Oncology 1987;1:49.

36. Breitbart W, Passik SD: Psychiatric approaches to cancer pain management. In Breitbart W, Holland JC (eds): Psychiatric Aspects of Symptom Management in Cancer Patients. Washington, DC, American Psychiatric Press, 1993:49.

37. Faberow NL, Schneidman ES, Leonard CV: Suicide Among General Medical and Surgical Hospital Patients with Malignant Neoplasms. Medical Bulletin 9. Washington, DC, U.S. Veterans Administration, 1963.

38. MacDonald N: Principles governing the use of cancer chemotherapy in palliative medicine. In Doyle D, Hanks GWC, MacDonald N (eds): Oxford Textbook of Palliative Medicine. New York, Oxford University Press, 1995:105.

39. Hoskin PJ: Radiotherapy in symptom management. In Doyle D, Hanks GWC, MacDonald N (eds): Oxford Textbook of Palliative Medicine. New York, Oxford University Press, 1995:117.

40. Baum M, Breach NM, Shepherd JH, et al: Surgical palliation. In Doyle D, Hanks GWC, MacDonald N (eds): Oxford Textbook of Palliative Medicine. New York, Oxford University Press, 1995:129.

41. Horowitz SA, Breitbart W: Relaxation and imagery for symptom control in cancer patients. In Breitbart W, Holland JC (eds): Psychiatric Aspects of Symptom Management in Cancer Patients. Washington, DC, American Psychiatric Press, 1993:147.

42. Vachon MLS: Emotional problems in palliative care: Patient, family, and professional. In Doyle D, Hanks GWC, MacDonald N (eds): Oxford Textbook of Palliative Medicine. New York, Oxford University Press, 1995:575.

43. Keitel MS, Zevon MA, Rounds JB, et al: Spouse adjustment to cancer surgery: Distress and coping responses. J Surg Oncol 1990;43:148.

44. Diehl V: Controversies in terminal cancer care. Support Care Cancer 1994;2:82.
45. Kahn DL, Steeves RH: The significance of suffering in cancer care. Semin Oncol Nurs 1995;11:9.
46. Steeves RH, Kahn DL, Benoliel JQ: Nurses' interpretation of the suffering of their patients. Western Journal of Nursing Research 1990;12:715.
47. Lindemann E: The symptomatology and management of acute grief. Am J Psychiatry 1944; 101:141.
48. Rando TA: Grief, Dying and Death. Champaign, IL, Research Press, 1984:37.
49. Sweeting HN, Gilhooly MLM: Doctor, am I dead? A review of social death in modern societies. Omega 1992;24:251.
50. Rando TA: Grief, Dying and Death. Champaign, IL, Research Press, 1984:252.
51. Weisman AD: On Dying and Denying: A Psychiatric Study of Terminality. New York, Behavioral Publications, 1972.

Chapter 24

Health Promotion for Cancer Survivors

Jeanette Adams McNeill, DrPH, MSN

Of the estimated 1.4 million persons diagnosed with cancer in 1996, approximately one half will survive at least 5 years beyond their cancer diagnosis.[1] Some 10 million people alive today have a cancer history; 70% were diagnosed more than 5 years ago. The projections are that, among these survivors, women will outnumber men three to one because of the prevalence of female reproductive cancers that have relatively favorable prognoses.[2] Increasingly, however, men will survive colorectal, prostate, and bladder cancers. In addition, the ranks of elderly cancer survivors are anticipated to increase significantly. By the year 2025, the population older than 55 years of age is expected to increase by 75%, which will cause a corresponding increase in the number of persons living with cancer or with cancer in remission.[3]

In view of these trends, the importance of health promotion and screening for cancer survivors cannot be overemphasized. Persons with cancer are also at risk for development of acute and other chronic illnesses because the risk factors for some malignant diseases are also those of other conditions. Smokers who have lung cancer, for example, are also at risk of developing chronic pulmonary disease. Injury, substance abuse, and individual and family violence are additional sources of health problems. Despite their cancer history, survivors engage in risky behaviors with the same frequency as do their unaffected counterparts: unprotected sexual activity, failure to use seatbelts, and poor nutrition are some examples. As "cure" for cancer becomes more common, the overall health maintenance of the cancer survivor increases in importance.[4]

CLINICAL GUIDELINES FOR PROMOTION, PREVENTION, AND SCREENING

During the past few years, several initiatives have highlighted the health promotion needs of individuals and groups at risk and set goals for the efforts of health professionals. The first of these, *Healthy People 2000*,[5] is a product of an intensive national study that outlined the desired health outcomes and health services each population group needs. The cancer-related objectives of *Healthy People 2000* are as follows[5]:

- Reversing the rise in cancer deaths—particularly from lung, breast, cervical, and colorectal cancer
- Reducing the prevalence of cigarette smoking to less than 15% among those 20 years of age and older
- Reducing dietary fat intake to less than 30% of total calorie consumption, and increasing consumption of foods containing complex carbohydrates and fiber
- Increasing to 60% the proportion of persons of all ages who limit sun exposure, use sunscreens, wear protective clothing, and avoid artificial sources of ultraviolet light
- Increasing to 75% the proportion of primary care providers who routinely counsel patients about tobacco use, diet modification, and cancer screening recommendations
- Increasing to 80% the proportion of women aged 40 years and older, and to 60% the proportion of women aged 50 years and older who receive age-appropriate clinical breast examinations and mammograms
- Increasing to 95% the proportion of women with a uterine cervix who receive Pap tests

- Increasing to 50% the proportion of people older than 50 who have had a fecal occult blood test within the past 1 to 2 years, and to 40% the number older than age 50 who have had proctosigmoidoscopy
- Increasing to at least 40% of those older than 50 years of age visiting a primary care provider who have received oral, skin, and digital rectal examinations.

In addition, morbidity from other chronic illnesses can be reduced by preventive and screening activities related to decreasing cholesterol levels, reducing the incidence of obesity, increasing participation in regular exercise, and advocating safe sex behaviors.

The U. S. Preventive Services Task Force *Guide to Clinical Preventive Services* provides assistance for clinicians in planning preventive services such as screening tests and immunizations and in counseling patients concerning risk reduction.[6] The task force recommendations include the following: (1) assessment of a patient's personal health practices, (2) shared decision making by clinician and patient, (3) selective use of diagnostic and screening services, and (4) consistent provision of preventive services, particularly to individuals and families whose access to health care is limited. Health care providers are advised to support community-level interventions in lieu of individual preventive services, such as fluoridation of the water supply and immunization campaigns, when these are known to be effective in avoiding certain health problems.[6]

Finally, the American Nurses Association compiled a useful reference work, *Clinician's Handbook of Preventive Services: Put Prevention into Practice*, which, like the *Guide to Clinical Preventive Services*, categorizes preventive and screening activities according to their proven effectiveness, assists clinicians to determine the risk status of the client or community and to base screening recommendations on scientific knowledge, and recommends counseling to modify risk.[7]

RISK REDUCTION AND HEALTH PROMOTION ACTIVITIES

An important component of health promotion is education of the client regarding risk of cancer and other illness and the health-promoting activities that could modify such risks. A study of 40 adult survivors of childhood cancer revealed that 17.5% reported using tobacco and 72.5% reported using alcohol.[8] Sixty percent of these survivors believed that staying healthy was more important for them than for most other people; however, this belief was not necessarily expressed in health-promoting or risk-avoiding behaviors. High-risk behaviors tend to be interrelated—examples are alcohol use with unsafe sexual practices; drug use with poor nutrition; and lack of exercise with a high-fat, low-fiber diet. High-risk behavior is particularly common among young people.[8]

Communicating with patients about risk status and risk reduction is vital for health care providers and particularly so with patients who have survived cancer. Rowan[9] counsels that communication of risk and recommendations for risk reduction are "high stakes" activities. Sharing risk assessment and risk reduction recommendations with clients empowers clients to act. Giving a person specific rather than general information about risks is more likely to stimulate the client to change risky behavior and to adhere to recommendations. The National Cancer Institute conducted focus groups to evaluate various techniques of communicating with older people about cancer risk and prevention behaviors. Acknowledging the fear of cancer and of other diseases the older persons may have and then helping them to take charge of prevention and screening activities turned out to be a successful strategy.[10] Counseling of adults must be based on theories of how and why adults learn: they want to acquire information and skills to enhance their independence and ability to solve problems; what is learned is immediately applicable; and the new skills fit their life experience and role demands.[11]

CULTURALLY COMPETENT HEALTH PROMOTION

An important variable in providing health care to cancer survivors is the survivor's cultural group. Health care providers must take into account the influence of their client's cultural background and beliefs during risk assessment and in making specific health promotion recommendations. In assessing a patient, his or her ethnic group should be taken into account because it may affect cancer risk. African American men, for example, are at greater risk of developing prostate cancer and at lower risk of testicular cancer than are Anglo American men. Similarly, Hispanic women have a greater risk of cervical cancer than do Anglo American women.[12] Not enough research has been done to determine the origin of these risks; some are believed to arise from lifestyle (e.g., nutrition, sexual practices), and some are believed to be related to socioeconomic factors that may make it difficult for clients to obtain timely health care. The primary care provider's task is to include in a comprehensive assessment the cancer survivor's and the family's cultural beliefs and practices, their views of health and health care, and their use or nonuse of folk or culturally prescribed methods of treating symptoms of illness and promoting health. Frank-Stromberg and Olsen[13] published a useful guide for conducting preventive and screening activities with members of various ethnic groups.

Culturally sensitive strategies in working with individuals, families, and groups of various ethnic backgrounds may include the involvement of representatives of the client's cultural group in designing individual and public education programs and inviting traditional healers and community leaders to participate whenever possible. An example of this approach was the work of Castro and colleagues,[14] who examined the outcome of a 3-year project funded by the National Cancer Institute to reduce the risk of breast, cervical, and diet-related cancers in Latino women. Church-sponsored services delivered by a *promotora* (a peer health worker) were used to influence the participants to adopt cancer-preventing behaviors.

The provision of health promotion and education is inevitably influenced by language. Verbal and written instructions may need to be translated and clarified. Some health promotion materials can be written in the language of the target group, with input by group representatives to ensure relevance to the group's culture and beliefs. Avoiding stereotypes and generalizations about any ethnic group or person is essential to all assessment and intervention efforts.

HEALTH PROMOTION RECOMMENDATIONS

NUTRITION

The American Cancer Society, the American Heart Association, and the U.S. Preventive Services Task Force recommend that individuals consume a high-fiber, low-fat diet (Table 24–1). Fat intake is targeted at less than 30% of the total calories, although the average intake of persons in the United States is 36%.[6] Being overweight is a problem for about 25% of American adults, and the incidence is slightly higher in women.[6] Obesity poses risks of hypertension, cardiovascular disease, diabetes, colon and reproductive cancers, and gall bladder disease. Women who are 40% or more and men who are 33% or more over their ideal body weight have a mortality rate from cancer up to 55% higher than that of persons of normal weight, and lower levels of obesity are associated with a higher prevalence of certain cancers, such endometrial and prostatic cancer.[12] Lower socioeconomic status and some ethnic dietary customs are linked to high fat intake.[6]

LESS DIETARY FAT

Recommendations to limit fat intake come from clinical trials in which reduction of total or saturated fat intake was examined. As part of a multifactorial intervention, the study showed that lowered fat intake can reduce mortality rates

Table 24–1. Preventive Recommendations for Cancer Survivors

TOPIC	RECOMMENDATIONS/INTERVENTIONS
Nutrition	Daily: 25 g of fiber; <30% of total calories from fat. Weekly: 5–6 servings of vegetables and fruits; 6–11 servings of whole grains, breads, and pasta; limited consumption (2–3 servings) of red meat, poultry, eggs, and dairy products.
Exercise	Three to four times per week for 30 minutes: consistent exercise such as brisk walking or swimming, with attention to safety measures and general health maintenance.
Tobacco avoidance	Consistently assess clients regarding tobacco use and interest in tobacco use cessation; if applicable, provide regular tobacco cessation counseling and advice on pharmacologic and behavioral interventions for smoking cessation. Childhood cancer survivors should receive antitobacco messages based on the clients' characteristics and individual risk.
Immunizations	Provide individual intervention regarding access to and maintenance of immunizations, particularly with live-virus vaccines such as measles-mumps-rubella and polio. Boosters against tetanus and diphtheria should be maintained. Primary series should be completed by those who have not done so. Hepatitis and influenza immunizations should be obtained. Persons older than 65 years of age and those older than 50 living in institutional settings should obtain pneumococcal vaccination.
Substance abuse	Assess clients for signs and symptoms of substance use. Advise them about adverse health consequences of alcohol and drug use; monitor for problems with alcohol and drugs.
Stress and mental health issues	Assess clients for signs of depression or other mental health problems, including suicidal ideation; counsel them regarding stress management, strategies of stress reduction, and resources for assistance with psychosocial problems.
Workplace exposures and injury	Assess clients for risk factors of injury and exposure to dangerous substances or troubling conditions in the workplace.
Dental care	Advise clients to undergo regular annual dental examinations and perform daily flossing and brushing with fluoridated toothpaste.
Sexuality and family planning	Provide counseling about risk of HIV and other sexually transmitted diseases (STD) and measures to reduce risk; specifically, counsel individuals identified as intravenous drug users regarding HIV and STD risk and refer them to appropriate treatment facilities; offer testing to persons at risk of specific STD; provide periodic counseling about effective contraceptive methods.

from cardiovascular disease by 5% to 20% overall, with the most benefit seen in high-risk persons. But it was mainly the accompanying increased exercise that lowered the subjects' risk and raised their high-density lipoprotein cholesterol levels.[6]

MORE FIBER

The American Cancer Society recommends a fiber intake of 25 g/day. Fiber intake and colon cancer are significantly associated: high fiber consumption is correlated with lower colon cancer incidence. High fiber intake also is associated with a lowering effect on low-density lipoprotein cholesterol, successful weight reduction, treatment of glucose intolerance, and control of hyperlipidemia.[12]

MORE CALCIUM

Supplementation of dietary calcium for certain population groups (adolescents, young adult women, and postmenopausal women) has been recommended, although the direct benefit in slowing bone loss is inconsistently demonstrated by clinical studies. Calcium supplementation has been shown to be effective in reducing the incidence of fracture among postmenopausal women, although it is not as effective as estrogen replacement.[6]

IRON AND VITAMINS

Adequate dietary iron is important for menstruating women and for children, but iron therapy (the prescription of large amounts of iron) for these groups has not been supported in prospective studies (except for young children).[6] Counseling regarding normal sources of iron in the diet is recommended, however. Recommendations for vitamin supplements (e.g., β-carotene and other antioxidants) await more definitive study. Cancer survivors need an adequate dietary intake of vitamins and minerals as part of good nutritional practice. Current recommendations from the U.S. Department of Health and Human Services and the Department of Agriculture are based on a nutritional pyramid for diet planning. As Figure 24–1 shows, the base of the pyramid is fruits, vegetables, whole grains, and pasta, while the top shows limited consumption of fats, meats, and sugars.

PHYSICAL FITNESS AND EXERCISE

A national survey revealed that 58% of Americans engage either in little or irregular physical activity. A sedentary lifestyle and concomitant obesity have been linked to cardiovascular disease, cancer, diabetes, and other chronic illnesses.

Following a regular exercise program tends to reduce not only the risks of cardiovascular disease and cancer but also those of noninsulin-dependent diabe-

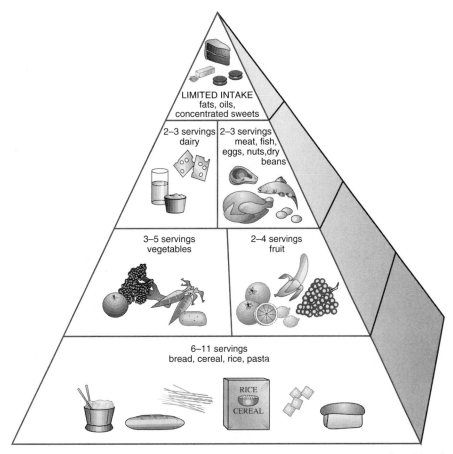

Figure 24–1. Food pyramid: a guide to daily food choices. (From U.S. Department of Health and Human Services.)

tes mellitus, diabetes, osteoporosis, and mental health disorders.[15] The estimate is that sedentary persons could reduce their risk of cardiovascular disease by 35% by starting an exercise program.[6] Despite demonstrated benefits, however, the risks of exercise must also be weighed. Persons who are obese and have had cardiovascular disease or hypertension or both should be evaluated thoroughly before beginning an exercise program. Furthermore, exercisers need advice and coaching to do warm-up and stretching exercises before vigorous workouts, avoid overexercising to the point of exhaustion or pain, and take basic precautions to avoid injury. Exercise is beneficial for cancer patients even during their treatment periods because it counteracts muscle wasting, loss of appetite, and depression.[16]

AVOIDING TOBACCO

Smoking or chewing tobacco is the single greatest cause of chronic illness, death, and disability in this country.[17] Despite a significant decline in tobacco use to the current level of about 30% of the population, some population groups, particularly young people, still use tobacco, and others have shown increased rates of smoking. The prevalence of tobacco use is inversely related to education and socioeconomic status; certain forms of tobacco, such as pipes, cigars, and smokeless tobacco, are primarily used by men.

Smoking among cancer patients has not been extensively researched, but one study at a large cancer center revealed usage rates that varied by ethnic group. Rates were approximately 30% among white men and white women, 22% among Hispanic women versus 44% among Hispanic men, and 28% among African American women versus 35% of African American men.[18] The number of cigarettes smoked per day increased with age, a finding that is of particular concern because older, heavier smokers have a more difficult time if they decide to stop smoking.

During cancer treatment, the adverse effects of tobacco use include increased risk and duration of oral mucositis, suppression of immunity with resulting negative effects on antitumor therapy and survival rates, and increased risk of a second malignancy.[19]

The mortality and morbidity of smokers are significantly higher than for nonsmokers or those who have managed to quit. Cancer (particularly of the respiratory tract), cardiovascular disease, gastric ulcer, postmenopausal osteoporosis, and low birth weight in babies of pregnant smokers are the major health risks firmly associated with smoking.[6] Passive smoking also has been documented to have adverse health consequences, such as chronic lung disease, coronary artery disease in spouses of smokers, and asthma and respiratory infections in children of smokers. Young people, primarily teens and preteens, are often influenced by their peers to start smoking. Other factors that predispose to chronic tobacco use include family history, gender (although the male predominance is rapidly decreasing), and use of other harmful substances.[17] Benefits of smoking cessation include immediate reduction in cardiovascular workload, improved respiratory function with decreased risk of infection, and long-term stabilization of pulmonary function with reduced respiratory cancer risk.[7]

Therefore, every cancer survivor who is advised to stop smoking and does so will reap some health benefit. A unique group is childhood cancer survivors, whose tendency to smoke is the same as their peers' but who are at risk of developing other malignancies. Depending on age at diagnosis and disease and treatment characteristics, survivors of childhood cancer may not know their cancer history, may be at risk of poorer school performance, and may be affected by lower self-esteem than their peers.[20] Risk-taking behaviors are similar. Therefore, this vulnerable group needs special attention during a long follow-up period.[20]

The promotion of smoking cessation has been most successful when multiple health providers use reinforcement to persuade smokers to maintain their "I quit" status.[21] Clinicians must be knowledgeable about both the process of change that influences a smoker to quit and the methods that are most effective in facilitating smoking cessation. The transtheoretic model (Fig. 24–2) proposed by Prochaska and DiClemente[22] is useful for examining the process that leads to behavioral change. According to this model, individuals move from precontemplation to contemplation, preparation, action, and maintenance. Health care providers can be instrumental in helping a smoker to at least contemplate quitting. If the person is ready to attempt to stop smoking, the provider can be helpful in the preparation and action phases, and then advise the former smoker about ways of maintaining his or her achievement.[21] More research is needed, but some evidence supports the effectiveness of using pharmaceutical nicotine replacement on a tapering-off basis in combination with behavioral approaches to address the psychological addiction.[21, 23] The Agency for Health Care Policy and Research guidelines offer information for clinicians, patients, and families regarding successful methods of smoking cessation.[23] Support and reinforcement

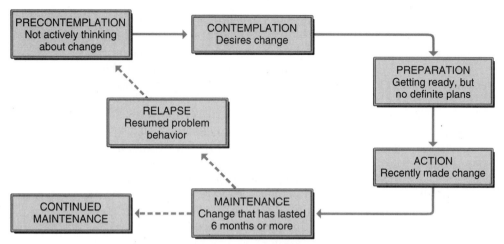

Figure 24-2. Transtheoretical framework for behavioral change. (Data from Prochaska J, DiClemente C: Stages and process of self-change and smoking: Toward an integrative model of change. J Consult Clin Psychol 1983;51:390.)

for the smoker are based on behavioral change principles; long-term follow-up and counseling to avoid relapse are essential to successful smoking cessation.

ACCIDENT PREVENTION AND INJURY CONTROL

Among the population at large, unintentional injuries are the fifth leading cause of death in the United States, and motor vehicle-related injuries alone are the eighth leading cause.[6] Unintentional injuries are the leading causes of death among children and young adults as well as an important source of disease and monetary expense.[6] In order of decreasing incidence, unintentional injuries are motor vehicle-related injuries, falls, poisoning, burns, drownings, suffocations, firearm-related injuries, and bicycling injuries. Cancer survivors share the general risks of unintentional injuries with the population at large, but factors related to disease and treatment may place them at higher risk. For example, the side effect of drowsiness from certain medications such as analgesics or antiemetics may increase the risk of motor vehicle accidents and falls; fatigue related to disease or treatment may contribute to inattentiveness to environmental dangers. Worry, preoccupation, and anxiety related to the diagnosis or outcome of cancer treatment could also result in inattention to hazards in the environment and thereby increase risk. Preventive actions related to unintentional injury have been scientifically documented and include use of automobile seat belts; avoidance of alcohol when driving, cycling, or operating machinery; use of safety helmets when motorcycling, bicycling, skateboarding, or skating; use of smoke detectors; and monitoring of the environment for risk factors, particularly for the elderly, who are at risk for falls. In general, the most effective interventions are those that do not require significant behavioral changes on the part of the potential victim,[6] such as installing a smoke alarm.

Counseling by health professionals about safety issues has been shown to be effective for parents of young children and somewhat effective for adults in other age groups. In general, counseling plus regulatory and community-based interventions (e.g., passive auto restraints, bicycle helmet regulations, infant car seat legislation, mandatory smoke detector installation in apartment complexes) are more effective for most age groups than counseling alone.[7] Cancer survivors need targeted advice about the increased risk of injury posed by treatment side effects, disease effects, and emotional factors. The health professional should include family members in this discussion because they are also at risk as a result of emotional stress and fatigue.

Use or abuse of certain substances is a major factor in the incidence of preventable deaths from injury.[4] It is estimated that more than half of fatally injured drivers have a blood alcohol level higher than 0.10 g/dL. Use of alcohol and other substances also increases the risk of other known potentiating behaviors, such as failure to use seat belts and motorcycle helmets. Additionally, alcohol is involved in 40% of all fatal fires and in an estimated 25% to 50% of deaths from drowning, shooting, and boating accidents. Persons who abuse alcohol and/or other substances need to be identified, counseled, monitored, and referred for treatment. Chronic alcohol use carries several health risks and also predisposes the user to poorer outcomes from trauma.[6]

Cancer survivors bring certain risky behaviors to their cancer experience. Some behaviors may be strongly associated with the particular cancer diagnosis (e.g., alcohol use with head and neck cancer).

IMMUNIZATIONS

Routine immunization for adults must be tailored to the individual circumstances of the cancer survivor. Immunocompromised persons are not harmed by killed or inactivated vaccines, and these should be administered as they are to healthy persons, although the cancer survivor's response may not be optimal.[24] Live vaccines, such as measles-mumps-rubella and polio vaccines, usually are contraindicated for persons who are immunosuppressed.[25] In addition, household members of immunosuppressed persons should not receive polio vaccine; however, measles-mumps-rubella vaccination is not contraindicated for those in close contact with the patient.[24]

Concerning young and midadult clients, if they are not immunocompromised (e.g., not taking high-dose or long-term steroids, have not been in active therapy for leukemia or lymphoma within the last 3 months, have not had a bone marrow transplant, do not have AIDS),[25] they should be immunized against measles and mumps. Similarly, rubella immunization should be offered to nonpregnant women of childbearing age and to women during the postpartum period. Tetanus and diphtheria boosters should be given to adults every 10 years throughout the lifespan, unless a serious injury warrants a booster in the interval. If an adult has not received the primary vaccination series, this should be completed at any age.[24] If cancer chemotherapy or immunosuppressive therapy is planned, vaccination is best done at least 2 weeks before therapy begins.[25] Vaccination for varicella is targeted to susceptible health care workers and family contacts of immunocompromised patients, as well as susceptible persons who live or work in areas in which transmission of the virus is likely.[6] Cancer survivors' immunity to varicella should be evaluated; this may necessitate serologic testing, and the decision regarding vaccination should be based on individual history, treatment variables, and family and environmental factors.

Hepatitis B vaccine should be provided to all young adults and others at high risk of infection (i.e., sexually active persons, substance abusers, those who frequently require blood transfusions or clotting factor concentrates, health care personnel, and travelers to areas where the disease is endemic).

Pneumococcal vaccination should be provided to all immunocompetent persons older than 65 years of age and to those at risk of the disease. Immunocompromised persons at high risk for development of pneumococcal disease should be vaccinated if they live or work in high-incidence areas[6]; such persons, including alcoholics, those with chronic renal failure, those with metastatic or hematologic malignancies, and those infected with the human immunodeficiency virus (HIV), may require higher doses or an increased number of doses.[25]

Finally, annual influenza vaccination is recommended for persons 65 years of age and older and for others in high-risk groups, such as chronically ill persons, health care workers, teachers, and young adults living in communities such as dormitories.[24] In cases of reduced immune response, prophylaxis with amantadine may be useful.[25] Family members of people in these high-risk groups should also be immunized annually against influenza.

SUBSTANCE ABUSE

Abuse of both illicit and legal drugs is an important medical problem in the United States. Approximately 6 million Americans are affected by drug use. A 1991 national survey found that almost 4% of the population met the criteria for a diagnosis of drug dependence.[6] The adverse effects of drug use range from cardiovascular and nasal damage in the cocaine user to AIDS in the intravenous drug user who shares needles.[6] Complications are greatest in heavy users. Indirectly, drug abuse also affects criminal activity and influences the rates of homicide, suicide, and motor vehicle injury. Trends indicate a rise in drug use among high school students.

Problem drinking also is increasingly recognized as an important health problem, affecting an estimated 1 in 3 Americans.[17] As many as three fourths of the alcoholics in the United States do not receive treatment for their alcoholism.[17] Alcohol abuse has been associated with increased mortality, hypertension, risk of cirrhosis, hemorrhagic stroke, and head and neck cancers.[6] An increased death rate from various causes has been associated with consumption of more than four drinks per day in men and more than two drinks per day in women.[6] Alcohol use is an increasing problem among adolescents and young adults.

Cancer patients, particularly adolescents and young adults, may comprise a vulnerable group with regard to substance use. Little research has been reported on the use of certain substances among cancer survivors specifically. Mulhern and colleagues[4] documented self-reported rate of alcohol use of 73% but no indication of problem drinking in a sample of 40 young adult survivors of cancer. Other studies of childhood cancer survivors indicate that their risk-taking behaviors are similar to those of their peers.[20] Research documentation of drug and alcohol use in adults surviving cancer is also scanty. Because of the cancer survivor's history and previous medical treatment, the potential for further damage to the immune, renal, and hepatic systems as a result of drug and alcohol use warrants particular concern on the part of health professionals caring for this population.

STRESS MANAGEMENT

Mental health problems, common in the United States population, are of particular concern to cancer patients. Anxiety, the frustrations that are part of an illness, and dysphoric mood related to social stresses are common symptoms.[17] Depression affects more than 6 million Americans. Among primary care patients, 3% to 8% are depressed, although up to one half of these depressed patients are not diagnosed as depressed.[7] Risk factors of depression include (1) previous diagnosis of depression, (2) positive family history, (3) previous suicide attempts, (4) other physical illness, (5) lack of social support, (6) stressful life events, and (7) current substance use.[26] Cancer survivors, in their routine monitoring, should be given information about stress management; how to deal with anger and develop outlets for one's emotions, including the use of relaxation techniques; and how to identify and avoid situations that may lead to depression.[27] Social support is critical while a client recovers from illness and later while he or she strives to maintain wellness.[4] Particularly for older adults, lack of social support is a risk factor of disease and a threat to functional independence.[7]

The *Guide to Clinical Preventive Services*[6] and the *Depression in Primary Care* guidelines of the Agency for Health Care Policy and Research[26] recommend the use of clinical interview and/or self-report questionnaires, such as the Short Beck Depression Inventory or the Center for Epidemiologic Studies Depression Scale. Clinicians working with cancer survivors should be alert to signs of depression and evaluate patients in whom they see indications of dysphoria.

An important stressor in today's society is violence—including family violence, child abuse, and spousal and elder abuse. In managing the follow-up care of cancer survivors, clinicians may need to discuss various factors that expose patients and families to violence: (1) history of violent injury to a child or other family members, (2) history of alcohol or other drug use, (3) guns or other weapons in the home, and (4) prevalence of violence in the community.[7] Counseling regarding avoidance of these risks or steps that the patient or family can take to modify risks should be based on the health care provider's assessment of the potential for violence in the patient's family or immediate surroundings.

OCCUPATIONAL SAFETY AND HEALTH

Now that growing numbers of cancer survivors are able to maintain extended disease-free periods, they will continue to work, their rights to employment protected by the Americans with Disabilities Act. Primary care providers are in an ideal position to help protect these persons from work-related illness and injury. Occupation-related cancers are estimated to account for only 2% to 8% of all cancers,[28] and they are almost entirely preventable. Although they cannot inspect the workplace for hazards, health care providers can discuss with the patient the work-related potential for stress and injury. Persons at risk of back injury should be counseled regarding preventive measures.[7] Another area of concern is exposure to environmental carcinogens. An excellent source of information on this topic is the International Agency for Research on Cancer, which has identified known and suspected carcinogens and compiled epidemiologic evidence related to industrial agents. Clinicians should assess the client's current and past workplace exposures to metals, dust, chemicals, fumes, radiation, loud noise, heat or cold, and biologic agents. The evaluation should include family members who may have been or are now being exposed to any of these substances or conditions, with as much specific information as possible. Clinicians should ask cancer survivors about the use of protective equipment and the quality of instruction in its use.[28] Finally, the client's own health habits, such as tobacco use and diet, should be correlated with any work-related exposure.

DENTAL HEALTH

Great numbers of Americans suffer from dental caries and periodontal disease. For cancer patients, dental health is a priority because decayed teeth and gums are a site of infection in the immunocompromised patient. Cancer survivors should be counseled to continue regular dental care after their treatment, use fluoridated toothpaste, floss and brush twice a day, and eat a healthy diet. They should receive routine oral screening during their regular visits to the dentist.

SEXUAL PRACTICES

Yearly, in the United States, an estimated 12 million people contract a sexually transmitted disease (STD), and 40,000 to 80,000 new cases of HIV infection are added annually to the estimated 1 million already affected.[6] As these figures show, precise numbers are not known. Nevertheless, it is known from surveys that risky sexual behaviors continue; significant numbers of men and women report having had two or more heterosexual partners without consistent use of condoms within the last year.[6] The "male risk factor," meaning the risk of cervical cancer for a woman in a monogamous relationship with a man who has multiple sexual partners, has become a focus of investigation.[29] Long-term effects of STDs include infertility, pelvic inflammatory disease, neurologic deficits (from syphilis), and death (from HIV infection and AIDS). High-risk groups include persons with multiple sexual partners, intravenous drug users, persons who exchange sex for money or drugs, and men who are homosexually or bisexually active.[7] Members of ethnic minorities, both heterosexual and homosexual, are at increased risk of STD, particularly HIV infection.[6] Immunocompromised persons are at high risk not only for STDs but for proinvasive disease of the vulva and cervix, with dysplasia. Cancer survivors are extremely vulnerable to infection with HIV and hepatitis B. Care providers for cancer survivors must include assessment of sexual function and activity as well as counseling in their surveillance of their patients' health needs during long term follow-up.

FAMILY PLANNING

An estimated two thirds of all American women are sexually active but do not intend to become pregnant. A survey of more than 8000 women aged 15 to 44 years indicated that 57% of all pregnancies in this group were unintended.[7] Teens are at special risk of unintended pregnancy: about 20% of sexually active teenaged girls become pregnant each year. At any age, lack of information about family planning and less than optimum prenatal care have ill effects on the health of clients and their families.

For the cancer survivor, all of these considerations are components of preventive counseling. In contrast, the problem of infertility, which is related to cancer site and treatment, is of great concern to young women and men who have survived cancer. Patients should be advised that mutational changes may be associated with some treatment modalities (i.e., irradiation and chemotherapy), but that the data are limited.[30] Counseling and referral regarding sexuality and fertility issues are an important aspect of preventive care and health promotion for cancer survivors and their families.

SCREENING RECOMMENDATIONS

When considering the use of screening tests, two critical questions must be answered: Does early detection benefit the condition to be screened? and Will early detection lead to intervention to prevent the condition or delay its progression? Treatment efficacy and the added benefit of early detection are then measured against waiting until symptoms arise and the patient seeks treatment.

The screening tests to be used must have an acceptable level of accuracy. Key issues are sensitivity (the ability of the test to give a correct, positive result when the person examined has the condition) and specificity (the ability of the test to give a correct, negative result when the person screened is free of the condition). In a test with low sensitivity, cases of disease will be missed, and the false-negative result may delay treatment and allow the disease to progress undetected. In a test with low specificity, false-positive results will cause those who are actually disease free to undergo further unnecessary testing.

Conditions that require periodic evaluation and screening include hypertension; hyperlipidemia; smoking behavior; colon, breast, and cervical cancer; and alcoholism.[6, 7] Cancer screening of obese patients is also recommended because of the relation of obesity to both cardiovascular disease and cancer. The recommendations of the U.S. Preventive Services Task Force,[6] the American Nurses Association,[7] and the American Cancer Society[31] are summarized in Tables 24–2 and 24–3. As noted in Table 24–4, selected groups deemed to be high risk should routinely be screened for a number of other conditions. Individual cancer survivors need to be evaluated regarding their specific risk of developing second cancers as well as other conditions.

Table 24–2. Conditions that Warrant Periodic Evaluation of Female Patients

CONDITION	SCREENING TESTS	POPULATION SUBGROUP	FREQUENCY
Hypertension	Blood pressure monitoring	>21 yr	Every 1–2 yr°
		Children/adolescents	At well-child visit
Hyperlipidemia	Blood cholesterol, fasting or nonfasting	45–65 yr	Annually
		>65 yr	Clinical discretion based on risk
Obesity	Height and weight measurement	All ages	At health check-up
Smoking	Assessment of smoking status, interest in cessation if smoker	All ages	At health check-up
		Smokers	At every visit
Cancer—breast	Mammography	>40°	Every 1–2 yr°
		>50	Annually
	Clinical breast examination	>40°	Every 1–2 yr°
		>50	Annually
	Breast self-examination	>20	Monthly°
Cancer—colon	Fecal occult blood Sigmoidoscopy	>50	Annually
Cancer—cervix	Papanicolaou smear	>18 or sexually active	Every 3 yr if within normal limits
		>65	May discharge if within normal limits
Alcoholism	History, questionnaires (CAGE or AUDIT)	All ages	At health check-up
		Pregnant women	At every visit

Data from U.S. Preventive Services Task Force[6] and American Nurses Association.[7]
°American Cancer Society recommendation; interval depends on identified risk factors.

Table 24–3. Conditions that Warrant Periodic Evaluation of Male Patients

CONDITION	SCREENING TEST	POPULATION GROUP	FREQUENCY
Hypertension	Blood pressure measurement	>21 yr	Every 1–2 yr
		Children, adolescents	At well-child visit
Hyperlipidemia	Blood cholesterol, fasting or nonfasting	>35–65 yr	Annually
Obesity	Height and weight	All ages	At health check-up
Smoking behavior	Assessment of smoking status, interest in cessation if smoker	All ages	At health check-up
		Father with children	Every visit
Cancer—colon	Fecal occult blood or sigmoidoscopy	>50 yr	Annually
Cancer—prostate°	Digital rectal examination, prostate-specific antigen	>50 yr	Annually
Alcoholism	History, questionnaires (CAGE or AUDIT)	All ages	At health check-up

Data from U.S. Preventive Services Task Force[6] and American Nurses Association.[7]
°American Cancer Society recommendation.

CANCER REHABILITATION

As the ranks of cancer survivors grow, health care providers will be increasingly concerned with issues related to survivorship. These include helping patients to live with effects of the disease and its treatment while also promoting a healthy lifestyle and, when necessary, teaching patients to manage other acute or chronic illnesses. In the broadest sense, cancer rehabilitation is concerned with promoting optimum wellness of the cancer survivor.[32]

One professional society has proposed that rehabilitation is a process by which individuals are helped to achieve optimal wellness within the limits imposed by cancer.[32] To accomplish this, those who monitor cancer survivors over the long term must provide access to rehabilitation services. These include physical, psychological, spiritual, social, vocational, and educational services that help the survivor to achieve his or her optimal functional status. These services are best provided by a team of health care professionals who are variously expert in these areas, coordinated by a team leader. Frequently, advanced practice clinicians have assumed the role of team leader. Providing liaison to other resources, such as other health professionals, community resources, and vocational services, is an important function of the leader of the rehabilitation team.

Further recommendations are that a range of services be provided to meet preventive, restorative, supportive, and/or palliative needs of the cancer survivor.[32] Beginning with the process of assessment, goal setting, and interventions, rehabilitation activities are planned to achieve measurable outcomes. All team members, the survivor, and family members collaborate in outcome planning. Health promotion and screening services are a vital component of the plan, as has been stressed in this chapter.

SUMMARY

More people are surviving cancer, but they are a vulnerable group because of their history and cancer-related treatment. Risks inherent in lifestyle, occupation,

Table 24–4. Conditions that Warrant Periodic Evaluation of Selected Persons at Risk

CONDITION	SCREENING TEST	POPULATION SUBGROUP
Human immunodeficiency virus (HIV)	Enzyme immunoassay; positives confirmed with western blot	Individuals seeking treatment for sexually transmitted disease (STD) Homosexuals or bisexuals Past or present intravenous drug users Persons who sell sex for money or drugs Infants born to HIV-positive mothers Sexual partners of HIV-infected intravenous drug users Transfusion history between 1978 and 1985
Tuberculosis	Mantoux test	HIV-positive individuals Close contacts of patients with tuberculosis (TB) Medical risk factors associated with TB Immigrants from countries with high TB incidence Medically underserved populations Alcoholics, intravenous drug users Residents of long-term care facilities
Chlamydia	Culture of endocervical specimen	Sexually active female adolescents and other women at high risk, including those with history of STD, new or multiple sex partners, <25 yr of age, inconsistent use of safe sex practices, unmarried, cervical ectopy
Hepatitis B	Hepatitis B surface antigen	Pregnant women
Diabetes	Fasting blood glucose Glucose challenge test	Members of high-risk groups at clinical discretion: obese men and women >40 yr; Native Americans, Hispanics, and African Americans; those with strong family history; pregnant women
Osteoporosis	Bone densitometry	High-risk postmenopausal women: Caucasians, those with premenopausal bilateral oophorectomy, slender build
Glaucoma	Tonometry, ophthalmoscopy	African Americans >40 yr; Caucasians >65 yr; those with family history, diabetics, patients with severe myopia
Hearing loss	Questioning about hearing and referral for further testing	Adults >65 yr Exposed to excessive occupational noise
Anemia		
Iron deficiency	Hemoglobin/hematocrit	Pregnant women, high-risk infants, African Americans, Mediterranean
Sickle cell	Two-tier hemoglobin electrophoresis	women who are pregnant or of childbearing age
Bacteriuria	Urine culture	Pregnant women
Cancer		
Thyroid	Palpation of thyroid	History of upper body (head and neck) radiation in childhood
Oral	Oral examination	Tobacco users Older frequent alcohol users All with suspicious oral lesions
Vaginal	Pelvic examination	Diethylstilbestrol exposure
Endometrial	Endometrial biopsy	>50 yr, obesity, abnormal bleeding
Testicular	Physical examination, testicular self-examination	History of cryptorchidism, atrophic testes
Depression	Beck Depression Inventory Center for Epidemiologic Studies Depression Scale	Adolescents, young adults Family or personal history of depression Persons with chronic illness Perceived or actual recent loss Sleep disorders, chronic pain

Data from U.S. Preventive Services Task Force[6] and American Nurses Association.[7]

or environment may lead to the development of second malignancies or other acute or chronic diseases. Clinicians who monitor cancer survivors during their long term of follow-up can influence health promotion by evaluation, counseling, and referral. By following the principles of cancer rehabilitation, the health care provider can guide the cancer survivor toward the goal of optimal functioning.

REFERENCES

1. American Cancer Society: Cancer Facts and Figures. Atlanta, American Cancer Society, 1996.
2. Anderson B: Surviving cancer. Cancer 1994;74:1484.
3. Kennedy BJ: Future manpower needs in caring for an older cancer-patient population. J Cancer Educ 1994;9:11.
4. Mulhern R, Tyc V, Phipps S, et al: Health related behaviors of survivors of childhood cancer. Med Pediatr Oncol 1995;25:159.
5. Public Health Service: Healthy People 2000. Washington, DC, U.S. Department of Health and Human Services, 1990.
6. U.S. Preventive Services Task Force: Guide to Clinical Preventive Services, 2nd ed. Baltimore, Williams & Wilkins, 1996.
7. American Nurses Association: Clinician's Handbook of Preventive Services: Put Prevention into Practice. Waldorf, MD, American Nurses Publishing, 1994.
8. Dryfoos J: Preventing high risk behavior. Am J Public Health 1991;81:157.
9. Rowan F: The high stakes of risk communication. Prev Med 1996;25:26.
10. Sutton S, Eisner E, Burklow J: Health communications to older Americans as a special population. Cancer 1994;74:2194.
11. Rankin S, Stallings K: Patient Education: Issues, Principles, Practices, 3rd ed. Philadelphia, Lippincott, 1996:147–169.
12. Bal D, Nixon D, Foerster S, et al: Cancer prevention. In Murphy G, Lawrence W, Lenhard R (eds): Clinical Oncology. Atlanta, American Cancer Society, 1995.
13. Frank-Stromberg M, Olsen S: Cancer prevention in minority populations: Cultural implications for health professionals. St. Louis, Mosby, 1993.
14. Castro FG, Elder J, Coe K, et al: Mobilizing churches for health promotion in Latino communities: Compãneros en la salud. J Natl Cancer Inst Monogr 1995;18:127.
15. NIH Consensus Development Panel: Physical activity and cardiovascular health. JAMA 1996;276:241.
16. Cohen L: Physical activity and cancer. Cancer Prevention 1991;1–10.
17. Barker LR, Burton J, Zieve P: Principles of Ambulatory Medicine, 4th ed. Baltimore, Williams & Wilkins, 1995.
18. Spitz M, Fueger J, Eriksen M, et al: Cigarette smoking patterns of cancer patients. In: Engstrom P, Rimer B, Mortenson L (eds): Advances in Cancer Control: Screening and Prevention Research. New York, Wiley-Liss, 1990:49.
19. Hecht J, Emmons K, Brown R, et al: Smoking interventions for patients with cancer: Guidelines for nursing practice. Oncol Nurs Forum 1994;21:1657.
20. Bolinger C: Smoking prevention in childhood cancer survivors. J Pediatr Oncol Nurs 1994;11:167.
21. Shelton G: Smoking cessation modalities: A comparison for health professionals. Cancer Practice 1993;1:49.
22. Prochaska J, DiClemente C: Stages and process of self-change of smoking: Toward an integrative model of change. J Consult Clin Psychol 1983;51:390.
23. Fiore MC, Bailey WC, Cohen SJ, et al: Smoking cessation: Information for specialists. Clinical Practice Guidelines, No. 18. AHCPR Pub. No. 96-0694. Rockville, MD, U.S. Department of Health and Human Services, Public Health Service, Agency for Health Care Policy and Research and Centers for Disease Control and Prevention, April, 1996.
24. Osguthorpe N, Morgan E: An immunization update for primary health care providers. Nurse Pract 95;20:52.
25. Advisory Committee on Immunization Practices (ACIP): Use of vaccines and immune globulins for person with altered immunocompetence. MMWR Morb Mortal Wkly Rep 1993;42(RR-4):1.
26. Depression Guideline Panel: Depression in Primary Care. Vol 1: Detection and Diagnosis. Clinical Practice Guidelines, No. 5. AHCPR Pub. 93-0551. Rockville, MD, U.S. Department of Health and Human Services, Public Health Service, Agency for Health Care Policy and Research and Centers for Disease Control and Prevention, April, 1993.
27. Pender N: Health promotion in Nursing Practice, 2nd ed. Norwalk, CT, Appleton & Lange, 1995.
28. Stellman J, Stellman S: Cancer and the workplace. CA Can J Clin 1996;46:70.
29. Lovejoy N: Precancerous and cancerous cervical lesions: The multicultural "male" risk factor. Oncol Nurs Forum 1994;21:497.
30. Mulvihill J, Byrne J: Genetic counseling for the cancer survivor: Possible germ cell effects of

cancer therapy. In Green D, D'Angio G (eds). Late effects of treatment for childhood cancer. New York, Wiley-Liss, 1992:113.

31. Fink D, Mettlin C: Cancer detection: The cancer-related checkup guidelines. In Murphy G, Lawrence W, Lenhard E (eds): Clinical Oncology. Atlanta, American Cancer Society, 1995:178.

32. Mayer D, O'Connor L: Rehabilitation of persons with cancer: An ONS position statement. Oncol Nurs Forum 1989;16:433.

Index

Note: Page numbers in *italics* refer to illustrations; page numbers followed by t refer to tables.

ISBN 0-7216-7316-3